WIT

60 HIKES
WITHIN 60 MILES

4TH Edition

SAN FRANCISCO

Including North Bay, East Bay, Peninsula, and South Bay

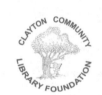
Jane Huber

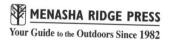
MENASHA RIDGE PRESS
Your Guide to the Outdoors Since 1982

Dedication

For my mom, who taught me about lady's slippers and wrens

60 HIKES WITHIN 60 MILES: San Francisco

Editor: Kate Johnson
Cover design: Jonathan Norberg and Scott McGrew
Cartography: Steve Jones
Interior design: Jonathan Norberg
Interior photos: Jane Huber except where noted on page
Proofreader: Emily Beaumont
Indexer: Rich Carlson

Library of Congress Cataloging-in-Publication Data

Names: Huber, Jane, 1965– author.
Title: 60 hikes within 60 miles : San Francisco.
Other titles: San Francisco
Description: Fourth edition. | Birmingham, AL : Menasha Ridge Press, [2019] | Includes index.
   Summary: "Huber finds the 60 best hiking spots within roughly an hour's drive from central San Francisco. By keeping its focus on the immediately local area, this new edition highlights even more of the lesser known hiking parks and open-space preserves—especially those surrounding the Bay Area's most densely packed cities of San Jose, San Francisco, and Oakland—while still including major tourism draws, making it perfect for city natives and visitors alike." — Provided by publisher
Identifiers: LCCN 2019018569 | ISBN 9781634041263 (pbk.) | ISBN 9781634041270 (ebook)
Subjects: LCSH: Hiking—California—San Francisco Bay Area—Guidebooks. | Trails—California—San Francisco Bay Area—Guidebooks. | San Francisco Bay Area (Calif.)—Guidebooks.
Classification: LCC GV199.42.C22 S269443 2019 | DDC 796.5109794/61—dc23
LC record available at https://lccn.loc.gov/2019018569

 MENASHA RIDGE PRESS
An imprint of AdventureKEEN
2204 First Ave. S., Ste. 102
Birmingham, AL 35233

Visit menasharidge.com for a complete listing of our books and for ordering information. Contact us at our website, at facebook.com/menasharidge, or at twitter.com/menasharidge with questions or comments. To find out more about who we are and what we're doing, visit blog.menasharidge.com.

Cover photo: Panoramic view on a sunny day in winter from the Mary Bowerman Trail in Mount Diablo State Park (Hike 29, page 146). © Dreamframer/Shutterstock
Back cover photos: (left to right) Hike 60, The Presidio: Batteries to Bluffs Trail (page 284); Hike 19, Black Diamond Mines Regional Preserve (page 103); Hike 56, Golden Gate Park: Stow Lake (page 268)

DISCLAIMER This book is meant only as a guide to select trails in the San Francisco area and does not guarantee hiker safety—you hike at your own risk. Neither Menasha Ridge Press nor Jane Huber is liable for property loss or damage, personal injury, or death that may result from accessing or hiking the trails described in this guide. Be especially cautious when walking in potentially hazardous terrains with, for example, steep inclines or drop-offs. Do not attempt to explore terrain that may be beyond your abilities. Please read carefully the introduction to this book, as well as safety information from other sources. Familiarize yourself with current weather reports and maps of the area you plan to visit (in addition to the maps provided in this guidebook). Be cognizant of park regulations, and always follow them. While every effort has been made to ensure the accuracy of the information in this guidebook, land and road conditions, phone numbers and websites, and other information can change from year to year.

TABLE OF CONTENTS

60 Hikes Within 60 Miles: San Francisco

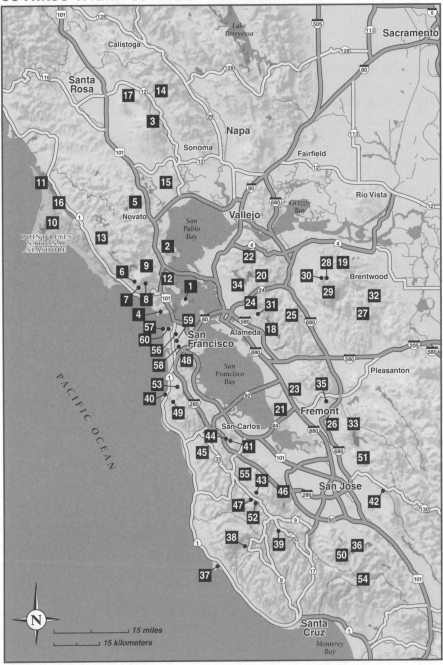

↔ ➡ Directional arrows	▬▬▬▬▬ Featured trail	∙∙∙∙∙∙∙∙∙∙∙∙ Alternate trail
▬▬▬▬▬ Freeway	▬▬▬═▬▬▬ Highway with bridge	▬▬▬▬▬ Minor road
▭▭▭▭▭▭ Boardwalk	▬▬▬▬▬▬ Unpaved road	┼┼┼┼┼┼┼┼ Railroad
•─•─•─• Power line	▬·─·─·─· Boundary line	
Park/forest	Water body	River/creek/ intermittent stream

✈	Airport	H	Hospital	⌐ᶠ	Radio tower
🕺	Baseball field	?	Information	⚦	Restroom
⛹	Basketball court	🗼	Lighthouse	∴	Ruins
⛱	Beach access	🗼	Monument	📷	Scenic view
⌐	Bench	◀	One-way (road)	⚽	Soccer field
🚢	Boat launch	▲	Overlook	🏇	Stable
⛺	Campground	P	Parking	🛒	Store
⸸	Cemetery	⌂	Park office	🏊	Swimming
⛪	Church	▲▲	Peak/summit	🎾	Tennis court
⚒	Dam	🍽	Picnic area	🥾	Trailhead
⋈	Footbridge	🏠	Picnic shelter	🔭	Viewing platform
✳	Garden	🛝	Playground	//	Waterfall
🏌	Golf course	●	Point of interest		

ACKNOWLEDGMENTS

Thanks once again to all the Bay Area Hikers who generously shared trail conditions and observations. Special kudos to my Patreon patrons for their support.

Cheers to everyone at Menasha Ridge Press for their help, and a tip of the map to Scott McGrew for his fine cartography. Kate Johnson edited the project, and her suggestions made a better book.

I'm so lucky to have two cartographer friends who are incredible mapmakers with deep knowledge of Bay Area trails: Ben Pease and Dave Baselt—thanks.

My husband, Hans Huber, has always been my biggest supporter and continues to help me whenever and however I need him. Our son, Jack, is a determined and tough hiker who warms my heart with his love of nature. Dorothy Greco continues to be an excellent sounding board and all-around great sister.

—*Jane Huber*

Buckeye butterfly resting on coyote brush

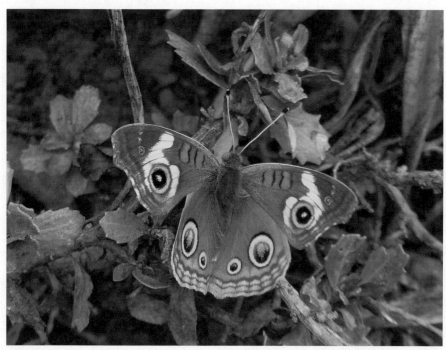

Welcome to Menasha Ridge Press's 60 Hikes Within 60 Miles, a series designed to provide hikers with the information they need to find and hike the very best trails surrounding metropolitan areas.

Our strategy is simple: First, find a hiker who knows the area and loves to hike. Second, ask that person to spend a year researching the most popular and very best trails around. And third, have that person describe each trail in terms of difficulty, scenery, condition, elevation change, and other categories of information that are important to hikers. "Pretend you've just completed a hike and met up with other hikers at the trailhead," we tell each author. "Imagine their questions, and be clear in your answers."

An experienced hiker and writer, Jane Huber has selected 60 of the best hikes in and around the San Francisco metropolitan area. From greenways and urban trails that make use of parklands to flora- and fauna-rich treks along the cliffs and hills in the hinterlands, Jane provides hikers (and walkers) with a great variety of options—all within roughly 60 miles of San Francisco.

You'll get the most from this book if you take a moment to read the Introduction, which explains how to read the trail listings. The "Topographic Maps" section (page 4) will help you understand how useful topos are on a hike and will also tell you where to get them. And though this is a where-to rather than a how-to guide, readers who haven't hiked extensively will find the Introduction of particular value.

As much to free the spirit as to free the body, let these hikes elevate you above the urban fray.

All the best,
The Editors at Menasha Ridge Press

PREFACE

I remember my first Bay Area hike well. On my premier trip to San Francisco, I accompanied two friends on what they promoted as a "walk on the beach." When I showed up with sandals on, they laughed and sent me back for sneakers—this was to be a walk *to* the beach. We drove across the Golden Gate Bridge, then wound uphill through woods on a tiny, curvy road. We finally stopped at a parking lot (Mount Tamalpais, Pantoll) and began hiking on Steep Ravine Trail.

I grew up near High Point, the tallest elevation in New Jersey (all of 1,803 feet), and I spent my youth walking along country roads and romping through rural woods. Even when I left New Jersey for six years of city living in Boston and New York, I always walked whenever possible, usually several miles daily. None of this walking had prepared me for Steep Ravine, a footpath plummeting through a wooded canyon, where I had to stop and rest (going downhill) because my quads were quivering. I marveled at the foreign scenery—unknown tall trees and lush shrubs—and was suitably impressed by the throngs of happy people on the trail, but in no way did the experience pique my interest in hiking.

I eventually got the nerve to pull up stakes and move to San Francisco, and a few years later a stray impulse triggered an interest in hiking. Once I started, I found I couldn't stop: my passion raged like a fever. I sought out maps and devoured them, studying the contour lines and squiggling trails, awed at the possibilities. I acquired hiking boots, wildflower guides, and sunscreen. I ignored the

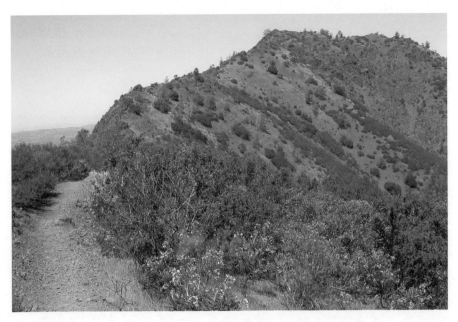

Eagle Peak Trail: an unforgettable adventure at Mount Diablo (see Hike 30, page 150)

worried pleas of friends and family who were sure I'd be stalked by psychopaths roaming the trails as I hiked alone. I began learning about the different vegetation and landscapes of the Bay Area: the rolling grassy ridges, steep-sided redwood canyons, and sunbaked hillsides covered with a curious mix of shrubs I would later learn was called chaparral. I'm still exploring today, chasing fragments of second-hand information about obscure trails, identifying new wildflowers, and learning to tell the difference between painted lady and American lady butterflies.

Consider yourself warned: Hiking in the Bay Area can be intense and addictive. Sure, other areas of California are home to more-esteemed landforms and parks—Yosemite is one of many world-class parks within a day's drive, and backpackers traverse the state on the Pacific Crest Trail. Throughout the Bay Area are many "destination parks," where people from all over the world flock to walk among giant redwoods or whale-watch from a wildflower-dotted coastal bluff. But there are also hundreds of smaller parks unknown to most tourists and even lifelong residents, and short drives (or in some cases bus trips, walks, or bike rides) lead to numerous parks and preserves with stunning views, bountiful wildlife, and quiet trails. These "backyard" preserves are especially beneficial to the residents of the Bay Area's most densely packed cities: San Jose, San Francisco, and Oakland. Local parks provide close-to-home outlets for daily exercise and nature exploration—thousands of people living in the foothills of Mount Tamalpais can literally walk from their front door all the way to the top of the mountain if they like. Every day, locals hike parks and open-space preserves bordering the towns of Berkeley, Mill Valley, and Woodside, and they take an active role in maintaining the trails. Getting to know your backyard means getting to love your backyard—and we fight for what we love.

This dedication to open space has led many ordinary citizens to work to save some of our most cherished Bay Area spots. The campaign to preserve open space began in the era of John Muir, and the list of protected parklands is long and impressive. Battles continue, and development still threatens many special areas. As you make your way over trails throughout the Bay Area, think of what we could have lost and what we've already preserved: old-growth redwoods in Muir Woods saved from logging; Point Reyes National Seashore and the Marin Headlands saved from huge housing complexes; various small parks, including Edgewood, saved from development as golf courses; and many other "common" plots of land preserved to make life a little better for the surrounding community.

What difference does open space make to the Bay Area? It permits residents to depart from the edge of a suburban development onto a path climbing a hillside peppered with wildflowers, where butterflies and damselflies flutter. It beckons hikers off bustling city streets to a park where bobcat prints mark the trail, hawks perch in hundred-year-old oaks, and salmon spawn in clear, cold creeks. It draws nature lovers from all over the world to redwood canyons so majestic that some find themselves overwhelmed with emotion. These preserved lands will stand long after we're gone, and although the tallest trees will eventually fall, a new generation of saplings will find a protected home in these parks, where manzanitas will put forth sweet-smelling blossoms yearly, mountain lions will roam with stealth and grace, and carpets of wildflowers will bloom whether anyone sees them or not.

Take care of these parks and preserves, and treat nature with reverence—you will be handsomely rewarded with memories that will last a lifetime. I think of all I've experienced in less than 20 years of hiking Bay Area trails: whales lumbering through the waters off Point Reyes' Chimney Rock; the soft sound of raindrops pattering through woods at Castle Rock; a bobcat close enough to pet, transfixed at the edge of a lake at Skyline Ridge; a coyote stepping out of the woods then vanishing back into the trees on the high slopes of Mount Tam; fresh drifts of snow covering soaring Douglas-firs after an unusual Bay Area winter storm along Skyline Boulevard; dazzling flowers everywhere—so many incredible springtime displays that I often felt giddy from the splendor.

We never made it all the way to the beach that fateful day, but I've been back to Steep Ravine since. I now know the plants that line the trail and the creatures that roam the woods, and I sometimes utter their names under my breath in passing, as if greeting old friends. My fingers lightly linger on blossoms of trillium, hound's tongue, and violet; trail over the shaggy bark on redwoods and Douglas-firs; and caress the smooth trunks of aromatic bay. I watch the silent flutter of a buckeye butterfly and the slow, languid crawl of a banana slug. Unseen mammals who creep about at night have left their calling cards, and I look for coyote scat at the trail junctions and raccoon footprints in mud along the creek.

The hike through Steep Ravine to Stinson Beach, combined with a return ascent through Douglas-fir woods and the high, grassy ridges of Mount Tam, is one of the hikes I've included in this book (Hike 7, page 45). It's an incredible trek that highlights the best of Bay Area hiking—easy access from San Francisco, a variety of vegetation, and a sense of peacefulness weaving through a wild landscape.

San Francisco Bay Area trails are incredibly diverse and beautiful. Whether you hike for exercise, for nature study, or in companionship with others, I hope you'll delight in discovering these parks and preserves.

Sticky monkeyflower and coyote mint are just a few of the wildflowers that add fragrance and color to Bay Area trails.

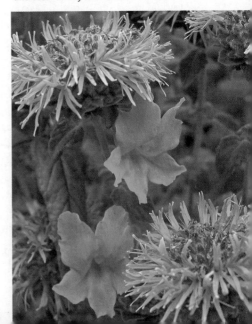

60 HIKES BY CATEGORY

Hike Number/Hike Name	Page	Mileage	Difficulty*	Kid-Friendly	Dogs Allowed	Wheelchair Access**	Public Transit
NORTH BAY							
1 Angel Island State Park	16	5.1	E	✔			✔
2 China Camp State Park	21	6.5	M			✔	
3 Jack London State Historic Park	26	8.9	M			✔	
4 Marin Headlands	30	5.9	M	✔		✔	✔
5 Mt. Burdell Open Space Preserve	35	5.1	M		✔		
6 Mt. Tamalpais: Cataract Falls–Potrero Meadows Loop	40	6.3	M–S		✔		
7 Mt. Tamalpais: Matt Davis–Steep Ravine Loop	45	6.5	M				✔
8 Mt. Tamalpais: Mountain Home–Muir Woods Loop	50	4.5	M	✔			✔
9 Mt. Tamalpais: Phoenix Lake	55	4.8	E	✔	✔		
10 Point Reyes National Seashore: Muddy Hollow	60	7.4	M	✔			
11 Point Reyes National Seashore: Tomales Point	64	7.6	M	✔			
12 Ring Mountain Open Space Preserve	68	1.9	E	✔	✔		
13 Samuel P. Taylor State Park	72	6.2	M	✔		✔	
14 Sugarloaf Ridge State Park	77	6.4	M	✔			
15 Tolay Lake Regional Park	83	3.0	E	✔	✔		
16 Tomales Bay State Park	87	2.6	E	✔			
17 Trione-Annadel State Park	91	6.2	M				
EAST BAY							
18 Anthony Chabot Regional Park	98	6.3	M	✔	✔		
19 Black Diamond Mines Regional Preserve	103	3.7	E–M	✔	✔	✔	
20 Briones Regional Park	108	4.3	E	✔	✔	✔	
21 Coyote Hills Regional Park	112	5.0	E	✔		✔	
22 Fernandez Ranch	117	3.7	E	✔	✔	✔	
23 Garin Regional Park	121	3.3	E	✔	✔	✔	
24 Huckleberry Botanic Regional Preserve	125	1.8	E	✔			
25 Las Trampas Wilderness Regional Preserve	129	4.7	M		✔		
26 Mission Peak Regional Preserve	133	6.1	S		✔		
27 Morgan Territory Regional Preserve	137	5.1	E		✔		
28 Mt. Diablo State Park: Donner Canyon Waterfall Loop	141	7.4	S				
29 Mt. Diablo State Park: Mary Bowerman Trail	146	0.7	E	✔		✔	
30 Mt. Diablo State Park: Mitchell Canyon–Eagle Peak Loop	150	7.7	S				

* E = Easy; M = Moderate; S = Strenuous ** A check mark indicates that the trail is at least partially accessible. Refer to the hike's Key Information for details.

Hike Number/ Hike Name	Page	Mileage	Difficulty*	Kid-Friendly	Dogs Allowed	Wheelchair Access**	Public Transit
31 Redwood Regional Park	155	4.1	E	✔	✔	✔	
32 Round Valley Regional Preserve	160	4.4	M	✔			
33 Sunol Regional Wilderness	164	2.7	E	✔	✔	✔	
34 Tilden Regional Park	168	3.9	E	✔	✔	✔	
35 Vargas Plateau Regional Park	172	3.8	E	✔	✔		
PENINSULA AND SOUTH BAY							
36 Almaden Quicksilver County Park	178	8.9	M		✔		
37 Año Nuevo State Park	183	3.6	E	✔		✔	
38 Big Basin Redwoods State Park: Waterfall Loop	187	9.6	S			✔	
39 Castle Rock State Park	192	5.3	M	✔			
40 Devil's Slide Trail	197	2.0	E	✔	✔	✔	
41 Edgewood County Park and Natural Preserve	200	3.5	E	✔			
42 Joseph D. Grant County Park	204	7.6	M				
43 Monte Bello Open Space Preserve	209	6.9	M	✔		✔	
44 Pulgas Ridge Open Space Preserve	214	2.6	E	✔	✔	✔	
45 Purisima Creek Redwoods Open Space Preserve	218	6.9	M			✔	
46 Rancho San Antonio Open Space Preserve	222	6.3	M	✔		✔	
47 Russian Ridge Open Space Preserve	227	3.7	E	✔		✔	
48 San Bruno Mountain State & County Park	231	3.6	E	✔		✔	
49 San Pedro Valley County Park	235	4.7	M	✔		✔	
50 Sierra Azul Open Space Preserve	239	7.8	M	✔		✔	
51 Sierra Vista Open Space Preserve	243	1.1	E	✔			
52 Skyline Ridge Open Space Preserve	247	4.4	M	✔		✔	
53 Sweeney Ridge	252	3.0	E	✔			
54 Uvas Canyon County Park	258	4.4	M	✔	✔		
55 Windy Hill Open Space Preserve	261	7.1	M		✔	✔	
CITY OF SAN FRANCISCO							
56 Golden Gate Park: Stow Lake	268	2.1	E	✔	✔	✔	✔
57 Lands End: Coastal Trail	272	2.8	E	✔	✔	✔	✔
58 Mt. Davidson	276	0.9	E	✔	✔		✔
59 Mount Sutro Open Space Reserve	280	2.1	E	✔	✔		✔
60 The Presidio: Batteries to Bluffs Trail	284	1.6	E	✔		✔	✔

More Recommended Hikes Categories

Hike Number/ Hike Name	Page	Wildlife	Wild-flowers	Red-woods	Good for Runners	Scenic Views	Waterfalls
NORTH BAY							
1 Angel Island State Park	16		✔			✔	
2 China Camp State Park	21	✔	✔		✔	✔	
3 Jack London State Historic Park	26		✔	✔			
4 Marin Headlands	30				✔	✔	
5 Mt. Burdell Open Space Preserve	35		✔				
6 Mt. Tamalpais: Cataract Falls–Potrero Meadows Loop	40		✔	✔			✔
7 Mt. Tamalpais: Matt Davis–Steep Ravine Loop	45		✔	✔		✔	✔
8 Mt. Tamalpais: Mountain Home–Muir Woods Loop	50			✔			✔
9 Mt. Tamalpais: Phoenix Lake	55		✔		✔		
10 Point Reyes National Seashore: Muddy Hollow	60	✔	✔			✔	
11 Point Reyes National Seashore: Tomales Point	64	✔	✔			✔	
12 Ring Mountain Open Space Preserve	68		✔			✔	
13 Samuel P. Taylor State Park	72		✔	✔		✔	✔
14 Sugarloaf Ridge State Park	77		✔			✔	
15 Tolay Lake Regional Park	83		✔			✔	
16 Tomales Bay State Park	87					✔	
17 Trione-Annadel State Park	91	✔	✔				
EAST BAY							
18 Anthony Chabot Regional Park	98		✔				
19 Black Diamond Mines Regional Preserve	103		✔				
20 Briones Regional Park	108		✔		✔		
21 Coyote Hills Regional Park	112				✔	✔	
22 Fernandez Ranch	117	✔	✔			✔	
23 Garin Regional Park	121		✔			✔	
24 Huckleberry Botanic Regional Preserve	125		✔				
25 Las Trampas Wilderness Regional Preserve	129		✔		✔	✔	
26 Mission Peak Regional Preserve	133	✔				✔	
27 Morgan Territory Regional Preserve	137		✔				
28 Mt. Diablo State Park: Donner Canyon Waterfall Loop	141		✔			✔	✔
29 Mt. Diablo State Park: Mary Bowerman Trail	146					✔	

Hike Number/ Hike Name	Page	Wildlife	Wild-flowers	Red-woods	Good for Runners	Scenic Views	Waterfalls
EAST BAY *(continued)*							
30 Mt. Diablo State Park: Mitchell Canyon–Eagle Peak Loop	150		✔			✔	
31 Redwood Regional Park	155			✔			
32 Round Valley Regional Preserve	160	✔					
33 Sunol Regional Wilderness	164		✔			✔	
34 Tilden Regional Park	168				✔	✔	
35 Vargas Plateau Regional Park	172		✔			✔	
PENINSULA AND SOUTH BAY							
36 Almaden Quicksilver County Park	178		✔				
37 Año Nuevo State Park	183	✔					
38 Big Basin Redwoods State Park: Waterfall Loop	187			✔			✔
39 Castle Rock State Park	192		✔			✔	✔
40 Devil's Slide	197	✔				✔	
41 Edgewood County Park and Natural Preserve	200		✔		✔		
42 Joseph D. Grant County Park	204		✔			✔	
43 Monte Bello Open Space Preserve	209		✔			✔	
44 Pulgas Ridge Open Space Preserve	214		✔		✔		
45 Purisima Creek Redwoods Open Space Preserve	218			✔			
46 Rancho San Antonio Open Space Preserve	222	✔	✔		✔		
47 Russian Ridge Open Space Preserve	227		✔		✔	✔	
48 San Bruno Mountain State & County Park	231		✔			✔	
49 San Pedro Valley County Park	235		✔			✔	
50 Sierra Azul Open Space Preserve	239		✔		✔	✔	
51 Sierra Vista Open Space Preserve	243		✔		✔	✔	
52 Skyline Ridge Open Space Preserve	247		✔		✔	✔	
53 Sweeney Ridge	252		✔			✔	
54 Uvas Canyon County Park	258			✔			✔
55 Windy Hill Open Space Preserve	261		✔			✔	
CITY OF SAN FRANCISCO							
56 Golden Gate Park: Stow Lake	268				✔		
57 Lands End: Coastal Trail	272				✔	✔	
58 Mt. Davidson	276					✔	
59 Mount Sutro Open Space Reserve	280				✔		
60 The Presidio: Batteries to Bluffs Trail	284		✔		✔	✔	

Welcome to *60 Hikes Within 60 Miles: San Francisco.* If you're new to hiking or even if you're a seasoned trailsmith, take a few minutes to read the following pages. They explain how this book is organized and how to use it.

How to Use This Guidebook
OVERVIEW MAP AND MAP LEGEND

The overview map on page vi shows the primary trailheads for all 60 hikes. Each hike's number appears on the overview map and in the table of contents. As you flip through the book, a hike's full profile is easy to locate by watching for the hike number at the top of each left-hand page. The book is organized by region, as indicated in the table of contents. A legend explaining the map symbols used throughout the book appears on page vii.

REGIONAL MAPS

The book is divided into regions, and prefacing each regional section is an overview map. The regional maps provide more detail than the overview map, bringing you closer to the hikes.

TRAIL MAPS

A detailed map of each hike's route appears with its profile. On each of these maps, symbols indicate the trailhead, the complete route, significant features, facilities, and topographic landmarks such as creeks, overlooks, and peaks.

To produce the highly accurate maps in this book, I created maps on CalTopo, then sent that data to Menasha Ridge Press's expert cartographers. Be aware, if you navigate with a mapping app on your phone or a GPS, that neither is a substitute for sound, sensible navigation that takes into account the conditions that you observe while hiking.

Further, despite the high quality of the maps in this guidebook, I strongly recommend that you always carry an additional map, such as the ones noted in "Maps" in each hike's Key Information.

ELEVATION PROFILES

Each hike contains a detailed elevation profile that corresponds directly to the trail map. This graphical element provides a quick look at the trail from the side, enabling you to visualize how the trail rises and falls. On the diagram's vertical axis, or height scale, the number of feet indicated between each tick mark lets you visualize the climb. To avoid making flat hikes look steep and steep hikes appear flat, varying height scales provide an accurate image of each hike's climbing challenge. Elevation profiles for loop hikes show total distance; those for out-and-back hikes show only one-way distance.

The Hike Profile

Each hike contains a brief overview of the trail; a description of the route from start to finish; key information—from the trail's distance and configuration to contacts for local information; GPS trailhead coordinates; and directions for driving to the trailhead area. Each profile also includes a map (see "Trail Maps," page 1) and elevation profile. Some hike profiles also include notes on nearby activities.

IN BRIEF

Think of this section as a taste of the trail, a snapshot focused on the historical landmarks, beautiful vistas, and other sights you may encounter on the hike.

KEY INFORMATION

The information in this box gives you a quick idea of the specifics of each hike.

DISTANCE & CONFIGURATION *Distance* notes the length of the hike round-trip, from start to finish. If the hike description includes options to shorten or extend the hike, those round-trip distances will also be factored here. *Configuration* defines the trail as a loop, an out-and-back (taking you in and out via the same route), a figure eight, or a balloon.

DIFFICULTY The degree of effort an average hiker should expect on a given hike. For simplicity, the trails are rated as *easy, moderate,* or *strenuous.*

SCENERY A short summary of the attractions offered by the hike and what to expect in terms of plant life, wildlife, natural wonders, and historical features.

EXPOSURE A quick check of how much sun you can expect on your shoulders during the hike.

TRAIL TRAFFIC Indicates how busy the trail might be on an average day. Trail traffic, of course, varies from day to day and season to season.

TRAIL SURFACE Indicates whether the path is paved, rocky, gravel, dirt, boardwalk, or a mixture of elements.

HIKING TIME How long it took me to hike the trail. I like to dawdle, and I can easily fritter away time watching butterflies or admiring wildflowers. On average, I cover 2 miles an hour (more mileage hiking downhill, less on steady ascents, particularly during hot weather). If you're an experienced hiker in great shape, you'll finish the hikes with time to spare, but if you're a beginner or you like to stop and smell the manzanitas, allow for a little extra.

DRIVING DISTANCE Listed in miles from a major intersection or landmark—for example, the Golden Gate Bridge toll plaza.

ACCESS A listing of any required fees or permits.

WHEELCHAIR ACCESS In a select few cases, I've noted sections of trail that are wheelchair accessible. While some other hikes in this book are technically accessible, meaning they contain no impediments such as stairs, they involve considerable changes in elevation that would likely challenge even those with exceptional maneuvering abilities.

MAPS Which supplementary map is the best or easiest to use (in my opinion) for a particular hike, and where to get it.

FACILITIES Restrooms, phones, water, and other niceties available at the trailhead or nearby.

CONTACT Phone numbers and/or websites for checking trail conditions and gleaning other basic information.

LOCATION The city or nearby community in which the trail is located. Street addresses are provided when applicable.

COMMENTS Provides you with those little extra details that don't fit into any of the above categories. These may include insider information or special considerations about the trail, warnings, or ideas for enhancing your hiking experience.

DESCRIPTION

This is the heart of the hike, summarizing the trail's essence and highlighting any special traits the hike has to offer. The route is clearly outlined, including landmarks, side trips, and possible alternate routes along the way. Ultimately, the Description will help you choose which hikes are best for you.

NEARBY ACTIVITIES

Not every hike has this listing, but for hikes that do, look here for information about appealing attractions in the vicinity of the trail.

DIRECTIONS

Used in conjunction with the GPS trailhead coordinates, these will help you locate each trailhead. California numbers its freeway exits; when pertinent, exit numbers are included.

GPS TRAILHEAD COORDINATES

As noted in "Trail Maps," page 1, the author used CalTopo to obtain geographic data and sent the information to the publisher's cartographers. The trailhead coordinates—the intersection of latitude (north) and longitude (west)—will orient you from the trailhead. In some cases, you can park within viewing distance of a trailhead. Other hiking routes require a short walk to the trailhead from a parking area. As a complementary aid to navigation, I've also provided street addresses where appropriate.

You will also note that this guidebook uses the degree–decimal minute format for presenting the latitude and longitude GPS coordinates.

N37° 52.110' W122° 26.083'

The latitude–longitude grid system is likely quite familiar to you, but here's a refresher, pertinent to visualizing the coordinates:

Imaginary lines of latitude—called parallels and approximately 69 miles apart from each other—run horizontally around the globe. The equator is established to be 0°, and each parallel is indicated by degrees from the equator: up to 90°N at the North Pole, and down to 90°S at the South Pole.

Imaginary lines of longitude—called meridians—run perpendicular to lines of latitude and are likewise indicated by degrees. Starting from 0° at the Prime Meridian in Greenwich, England, they continue to the east and west until they meet 180° later at the International Date Line in the Pacific Ocean. At the equator, longitude lines also are approximately 69 miles apart, but that distance narrows as the meridians converge toward the North and South Poles.

To convert GPS coordinates given in degrees, minutes, and seconds to degrees and decimal minutes, divide the seconds by 60. For more on GPS technology, visit usgs.gov.

Topographic Maps

The maps in this book have been produced with great care and, used with the hike text, will direct you to the trail and help you stay on course. However, you'll find superior detail and valuable information in the U.S. Geological Survey's 7.5-minute-series topographic maps. At mytopo.com, for example, you can view and print free USGS topos of the entire United States. Online services such as Trails.com charge annual fees for additional features such as shaded relief, which makes the topography stand out more. If you expect to print out many topo maps each year, it might be worth paying for such extras. The downside to USGS maps is that most are outdated, having been created 20–30 years ago; nevertheless, they provide excellent topographic detail. Of course, Google Earth (earth.google.com) does away with topo maps and their inaccuracies . . . replacing them with satellite imagery and its inaccuracies. Regardless, what one lacks, the other augments. Google Earth is an excellent tool whether you have difficulty with topos or not.

If you're new to hiking, you might be wondering, "What's a topo map?" In short, it indicates not only linear distance but elevation as well, using contour lines. These lines spread across the map like dozens of intricate spiderwebs. Each line represents a particular elevation, and at the base of each topo a contour's interval designation is given. If, for example, the contour interval is 20 feet, then the distance between each contour line is 20 feet. Follow five contour lines up on the same map, and the elevation has increased by 100 feet. In addition to the sources listed previously and in Appendix B, you'll find topos at major universities, outdoors shops, and some public libraries, as well as online at nationalmap.gov and store.usgs.gov.

Weather

Bay Area weather is mild, with a Mediterranean-like climate that generally ranges from the 40s to the 80s, inviting year-round hikes. Microclimates throughout the Bay Area span a wide range of temperatures and conditions, particularly in summer and winter (see table on next page). On a typical summer day, the weather may be clear and warm along the Sonoma coast, scorchingly hot and dry inland around Mount Diablo, and completely fogbound in San Francisco. During the rainy season, generally November–March, coastal mountains are inundated with rainfall, and the Bay Area's highest peaks are occasionally dusted with snow. City residents may go for a week without even switching on the heater. Locals learn to avoid getting caught out in weather shifts by carrying layers wherever they go, and this is a practical solution for hikers as well. Stuff a lightweight fleece jacket, one of those anoraks that compress down to nearly nothing, and a hat into your backpack, and you're generally prepared for light rain and cool snaps. Beware of fog, which commonly collects on high ridges near the coast, mostly in summer; it often blows in very quickly and can make for a nasty hike, as it completely obscures landmarks and trail junctions. A safe policy is to descend as soon as you see the fog headed your way.

Because heavy storms almost always damage trails, particularly in forested canyon parks, you should check weather conditions before you head out in winter and early spring. Trails get substantially less use in winter, but I adore hiking through forests in light rain (Castle Rock State Park in the fog is particularly enchanting). In summer, unless you prefer hot, dry heat, avoid exposed destinations in Alameda, Contra Costa, Napa, Santa Clara, and Sonoma Counties, where temperatures can soar to nearly 100° F. Summer is a good time to visit forested parks, particularly near the coast. Spring and autumn are the most easygoing seasons, although some parks close during times of high fire danger (red-flag days), until the rains begin in late fall.

AVERAGE DAILY TEMPERATURE						
MONTH	JAN	FEB	MAR	APR	MAY	JUN
HIGH	57° F	60° F	62° F	63° F	64° F	66° F
LOW	46° F	47° F	49° F	49° F	51°F	53° F
MONTH	JUL	AUG	SEP	OCT	NOV	DEC
HIGH	67° F	68° F	70° F	69° F	63° F	57° F
LOW	54° F	55° F	55° F	54° F	50° F	46° F
AVERAGE PRECIPITATION						
MONTH	JAN	FEB	MAR	APR	MAY	JUN
	4.5"	4.4"	3.3"	1.5"	0.7"	0.2"
MONTH	JUL	AUG	SEP	OCT	NOV	DEC
	0.0"	0.1"	0.2"	1.1"	3.2"	4.6"

Source: usclimatedata.com

Water

How much is enough? Well, one simple physiological fact should convince you to err on the side of excess when deciding how much water to pack: a hiker walking steadily in 90° F heat needs about 10 quarts of fluid per day—that's 2.5 gallons. A good rule of thumb is to hydrate before your hike, carry (and drink) 6 ounces of water for every mile you plan to hike, and hydrate again after the hike. For most people, the pleasures of hiking make carrying water a relatively minor price to pay to remain safe and healthy, so pack more water than you anticipate needing, even for short hikes.

If you find yourself tempted to drink "found water," proceed with extreme caution. Many ponds and lakes you'll encounter are fairly stagnant, and the water tastes terrible. Drinking such water also presents inherent risks for thirsty trekkers. Giardia parasites contaminate many water sources and cause the intestinal ailment giardiasis, which can last for weeks after onset. For more information, visit the Centers for Disease Control and Prevention website: cdc.gov/parasites/giardia.

Effective treatment is essential before you use any water source you've found along the trail. Boiling water for 2–3 minutes is always a safe measure for camping, but day hikers can consider iodine tablets, approved chemical mixes, filtration units rated for giardia, and ultraviolet filtration. Some of these methods (for example, filtration with an added carbon filter) remove bad tastes typical in stagnant water, while others add their own taste. Even if you've brought your own water, consider bringing along a means of water purification in case you've underestimated your consumption needs.

CLOTHING

Weather, unexpected trail conditions, fatigue, extended hiking duration, and wrong turns can individually or collectively turn a great outing into a very uncomfortable one at best. Following are some helpful guidelines.

➤ **Choose silk, wool, or moisture-wicking synthetics** for maximum comfort in all of your hiking attire—from hats to socks. Cotton is fine if the weather remains dry and stable, but you won't be happy if that fabric gets wet.

➤ **Always wear a hat,** or at least tuck one into your day pack or hitch it to your belt. Hats offer all-weather sun and wind protection as well as warmth if it turns cold.

➤ **Be ready to layer up** or down as the day progresses and the mercury rises or falls. Today's outdoor wear makes layering easy, with such designs as jackets that convert to vests and zip-off or button-up legs.

➤ **Mosquitoes, poison oak,** and thorny bushes found along many trails can generate short-term discomfort and long-term agony. A lightweight pair of pants and a long-sleeved shirt can go a long way toward protecting you from these pests.

➤ **Wear hiking boots** or sturdy hiking sandals with toe protection. Flip-flopping along a paved urban greenway is one thing, but you should never hike a trail in open sandals or casual sneakers. Your bones and arches need support, and your skin needs protection.

➤ **Pair that footwear with good socks.** If you prefer not to sheathe your feet when wearing hiking sandals, tuck the socks into your day pack—you may need them if temperatures plummet or if you hit rocky turf and pebbles begin to irritate your feet.

➤ **Don't leave rainwear behind,** even if the day dawns clear and sunny. Tuck into your day pack, or tie around your waist, a jacket that's breathable and either water-resistant or waterproof. Investigate different choices at your local outdoors retailer. If you're a frequent hiker, ideally you'll have more than one rainwear weight, material, and style in your closet to protect you in all seasons in your regional climate and hiking microclimates.

ESSENTIAL GEAR

Today you can buy outdoor vests that have up to 20 pockets shaped and sized to carry everything from toothpicks to binoculars. Or, if you don't aspire to feel like a burro, you can neatly stow all of these items in your day pack or backpack. The following list showcases never-hike-without-them items, in alphabetical order, as all are important.

➤ **Extra clothes** Rain gear, warm hat, gloves, and change of socks and shirt

➤ **Extra food** Trail mix, granola bars, or other high-energy foods

➤ **Flashlight or headlamp** with extra bulb and batteries

➤ **Insect repellent** For some areas and seasons, this is extremely vital.

➤ **Maps and a high-quality compass** Even if you know the terrain from previous hikes, don't leave home without these tools. And, as previously noted, bring maps in addition to those in this guidebook, and consult your maps prior to the hike. If you are versed in GPS usage, bring that device too, but don't rely on it as your sole navigational tool, as battery life can dwindle or run out, and be sure to compare its guidance with that of your maps.

➤ **Pocketknife and/or multitool**

➤ **Sunscreen** Note the expiration date on the tube or bottle; it's usually embossed on the top.

➤ **Water** As emphasized more than once in this book, bring more than you think you will drink. Depending on your destination, you may want to bring a container and iodine or a filter for purifying water in case you run out.

➤ **Whistle** This little gadget will be your best friend in an emergency.

➤ **Windproof matches** and/or a lighter, as well as a fire starter

First Aid Kit

In addition to the preceding items, the ones that follow may seem daunting to carry along for a day hike. But any paramedic will tell you that the products listed here are just the basics. The reality of hiking is that you can be out for a week of backpacking and acquire only a mosquito bite . . . or you can hike for an hour, slip, and suffer a cut or broken bone. Fortunately, the items listed pack into a very small space. Convenient prepackaged kits are available at your pharmacy or online.

➤ **Ace bandages** or Spenco joint wraps

➤ **Adhesive bandages**

➤ **Antibiotic ointment** (such as Neosporin)

➤ **Aspirin, acetaminophen (Tylenol), or ibuprofen (Advil)**

➤ **Athletic tape**

➤ **Blister kit** (such as Moleskin or Spenco 2nd Skin)

➤ **Butterfly-closure bandages**

➤ **Diphenhydramine (Benadryl),** in case of allergic reactions

➤ **Epinephrine in a prefilled syringe (EpiPen),** typically available by prescription only, for people known to have severe allergic reactions to hiking mishaps such as bee stings

➤ **Gauze** (one roll and a half-dozen 4-by-4-inch pads)

➤ **Hydrogen peroxide** or iodine

Hiking with Children

No one is too young for a hike in the outdoors. Be mindful, though. Flat, short, and shaded trails are best with an infant. Toddlers who haven't quite mastered walking can still tag along, riding on an adult's back in a child carrier. Use common sense to judge a youngster's capacity to hike a particular trail, and be ready for the child to tire quickly and need to be carried.

When packing for the hike, remember the child's needs as well as your own. Make sure children are adequately clothed for the weather, have proper shoes, and are protected from the sun with sunscreen. Kids dehydrate quickly, so make sure you have plenty of fluids for everyone. Hikes suitable for children are noted in the 60 Hikes by Category table on pages xiii–xvi.

Finally, when hiking with kids, remember that the trip will be a compromise. A child will alternate between bursts of speed and long stops to examine snails, sticks, dirt, and other attractions.

General Safety

While many hikers hit the trail full of enthusiasm and energy, others may find themselves feeling apprehensive about possible outdoor hazards. Although potentially dangerous situations can occur anywhere, your hike can be as safe and enjoyable as you had hoped, as long as you use sound judgment and prepare yourself before hitting the trail. Here are a few tips to make your trip safer and easier.

➤ **Hike with a buddy.** Not only is there safety in numbers, but a hiking companion can help you if you twist an ankle on the trail or if you get lost, can assist in carrying food and water, and can be a partner in discovery. A buddy is good to bring along not only to infrequently traveled or remote areas but also to urban areas.

➤ **If you're hiking alone,** leave your hiking itinerary with someone you trust, and let that person know when you return.

➤ **Don't count on a mobile phone for your safety.** Reception may be spotty or nonexistent on the trail, even on an urban walk—especially one embraced by towering trees.

➤ **Always carry food and water, even on short hikes.** Food will give you energy and sustain you in an emergency until help arrives. Bring more water than you think you'll need—we can't emphasize this enough. Hydrate throughout your hike and at regular intervals; don't wait until you feel thirsty. Treat water from a stream or other source before drinking it.

➤ **Ask questions.** Public-land employees are on hand to help. It's a lot easier to solicit advice before a problem occurs, and it will help you avoid a mishap away from civilization when it's too late to amend an error.

➤ **Stay on designated trails.** Most hikers get lost when they leave the path. Even on the most clearly marked trails, you usually reach a point where you have to stop and consider which direction to head. If you become disoriented, don't panic. As soon as you think you may be off-track, stop, assess your current direction, and then retrace your steps back to the point where you went awry. Using a map, a compass, and this book—and keeping in mind what you've passed thus far—reorient yourself and trust your judgment about which way to continue. If you become absolutely unsure of how to continue, return to your vehicle the way you came in. Should you become completely lost and have no idea how to return to the trailhead, remaining in place along the trail and waiting for help is most often the best option for adults and always the best option for children.

➤ **Always carry a whistle.** It may become a lifesaver if you get lost or hurt.

➤ **Be especially careful when crossing streams.** Whether you're fording the stream or crossing on a log, make every step count. If you have any doubt about maintaining your balance on a foot log, go ahead and ford the stream instead. When fording a stream, use a trekking pole or stout stick for balance and face upstream as you cross. If a stream seems too deep to ford, turn back. Whatever is on the other side isn't worth risking your life for.

➤ **Be careful at overlooks.** While these areas may provide spectacular views, they are potentially hazardous. Stay back from the edge of outcrops, and be absolutely sure of your footing.

➤ **Standing dead trees and storm-damaged living trees pose a hazard to hikers and tent campers.** These trees may have loose or broken limbs that could fall at any time. When choosing a spot to rest, camp, or snack, look up.

➤ **Know the symptoms of heat exhaustion, or hyperthermia.** Light-headedness and loss of energy are the first two indicators. If you feel these symptoms coming on, find some shade, drink your water, remove as many layers of clothing as practical, and stay put until you cool down. Marching through heat exhaustion leads to heatstroke—which can be deadly. If you should be sweating and you're not, that's the signature warning sign. If you or a companion reaches this point, your hike is over: do whatever you can to cool down, and seek medical help immediately.

➤ **Likewise, know the symptoms of subnormal body temperature, or hypothermia.** Shivering and forgetfulness are the two most common indicators of this stealthy killer. Hypothermia can occur at any elevation, even in the summer—especially if you're wearing lightweight cotton clothing. If symptoms develop, get to shelter, hot liquids, and dry clothes as soon as possible.

➤ **Most important, take along your brain.** A cool, calculating mind is the single most important asset on the trail. Think before you act. Watch your step. Plan ahead. Avoiding accidents before they happen is the best way to ensure a rewarding and relaxing hike.

Watchwords for Flora and Fauna

Hikers should be aware of the concerns on the following pages regarding plant life and wildlife, described in alphabetical order.

POISON OAK This deciduous plant (right) grows as a sparse ground cover, vine, or shrub; regardless of its form, poison oak always has three leaflets. It's easiest to spot in summer and early autumn, when the leaves flush bright red. Beware of unknown bare-branched shrubs and vines in winter—the entire plant can cause a rash, no matter what the season.

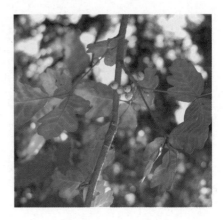

Urushiol, the oil in the sap of the plant, is responsible for the rash. Reactions may start almost immediately or not appear until a week after exposure. Raised lines and/or blisters will appear, accompanied by a terrible itch. Try to refrain from scratching, though, because bacteria under your fingernails can cause an infection. Wash and dry the affected area thoroughly, applying calamine lotion to help dry out the rash. If the itching or blistering is severe, seek medical attention.

Most people come into contact with poison oak while bushwhacking or traveling off-trail, so stay on established trails whenever possible. If you do knowingly touch the plant, you must remove the oil within 15–20 minutes to avoid a reaction. Rinsing off the oil with cool water (hot water spreads it) is impractical on the trail, but some commercial products such as Tecnu are effective in removing urushiol from your skin. To keep from spreading the misery to someone else, wash not only any exposed parts of your body but also any oil-contaminated clothes, hiking gear, and pets.

SNAKES The most common snakes you'll encounter along Bay Area trails are nonvenomous gopher and garter snakes. The only venomous snakes in the Bay Area are rattlesnakes, but sightings of these pit vipers are generally infrequent, occurring most commonly in dry, rocky, or exposed zones during the warmest months of the year. Following is the standard advice for hiking in rattlesnake territory.

- ➤ Don't put your hands or feet where you can't see them—at the top of a rock outcrop, for example, or in tall grass or a log pile.
- ➤ Be extra cautious in hot weather, when snakes are more active.
- ➤ Scan the trail continuously as you hike.
- ➤ Keep kids from running ahead on the trail. Bites to children are more severe than those to adults.

Should you encounter a rattlesnake, its body language will reveal its mood. A coiled rattler is primed for a strike, while a relaxed rattler is more sanguine (although snakes have been reported to lunge). If the snake is within striking distance, stand motionless and wait for it to calm down and move on. Taking small, slow steps backward is another

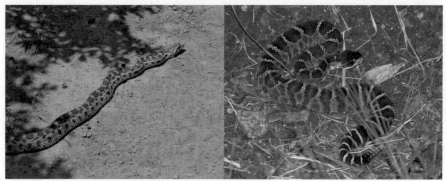

Gopher snake   Rattlesnake

smart strategy. If you're out of immediate range, you can either skirt the snake or wait for it to move. Some people believe tapping the ground with a stick (from a safe distance, rather than in the snake's face) will encourage the snake to move on.

Gopher snakes resemble rattlesnakes; both species have a cream, tan, and brown pattern. The easiest way to tell them apart—again, of course, from a safe distance—is by head shape: a gopher snake (above left) has no distinction from its "neck" to its head, while a rattler (above right) has a diamond-shaped head. Both, by the way, make noises to warn off predators, rattlesnakes by shaking their rattles and gopher snakes by vibrating their tails against the ground.

TICKS These arachnids like to hang out in the brush that grows along trails. July is the peak month for ticks in the Bay Area, but you should be tick-aware throughout the spring, summer, and fall. The ticks that alight onto you while hiking will be very small, sometimes so tiny that you won't be able to spot them. All ticks need to attach for several hours before they can transmit disease.

A few precautions: Use insect repellent that contains DEET. Wear light-colored clothing, which will make it easy for you to spot ticks before they migrate to your skin. When your hike is done, inspect your hair, the back of your neck, your armpits, and your socks. During your posthike shower, take a moment to do a more complete body check. To remove a tick that is already embedded, use fine-tipped tweezers to grasp the tick as close to the skin's surface as possible, and pull upward with steady, even pressure. Treat the bite with disinfectant solution.

Trail Etiquette

Whether you're hiking in a city, county, state, or national park, always remember that great care and resources (from nature as well as your tax dollars) have gone into creating these spaces. Treat the trail, wildlife, and fellow hikers with respect. Here are a few general principles to keep in mind while you're on the trail.

➤ **Hike on open trails only.** Respect trail and road closures (ask if you're not sure), avoid trespassing on private land, and obtain all permits and authorization as required. Leave gates as you found them or as marked.

➤ **Be sensitive to the ground beneath you.** This also means staying on the existing trail and not blazing any new trails. Pack out what you pack in. Leave No Trace ethics make hiking and camping more fun for others (visit lnt.org for details).

➤ **Never spook animals.** An unannounced approach, a sudden movement, or a loud noise can startle them. A surprised cow, snake, or skunk can be dangerous to you, others, and itself. Give animals extra room and time to adjust to your presence.

➤ **Plan ahead.** Know your equipment, your ability, and the area in which you are hiking—and prepare accordingly. Be self-sufficient at all times; carry necessary supplies for changes in weather or other conditions. A well-executed trip is a satisfaction to you and to others.

➤ **Be courteous to others you encounter on the trails.** Hikers and bikers should yield to equestrians; bikers should yield to hikers; and, whenever safe, everyone should yield to uphill hikers, bikers, or equestrians.

A tight switchback with a view at Round Valley Preserve (Hike 32, page 160)

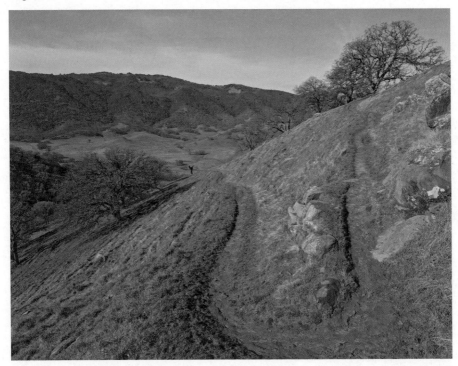

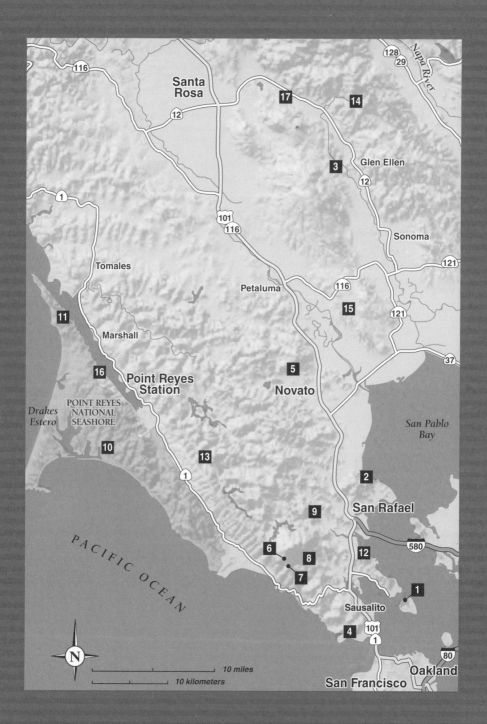

NORTH BAY

(Including Marin, Napa, and Sonoma Counties)

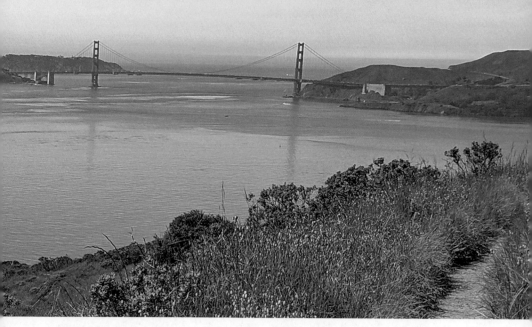

Angel Island's Sunset Trail affords 360-degree views of Bay Area landmarks, including the Golden Gate Bridge.

ANGEL ISLAND IS a perfect day trip, where the journey to the trailhead rivals the hike for sheer relaxation and beauty. Because you can reach Angel Island only by boat, sit back and enjoy the ferry ride, then climb to the top of the island and back, with incredible views nearly the entire trip. Just keep an eye on the clock to make sure you catch that last ferry.

DESCRIPTION

San Francisco Bay's largest island, rising out of the water between Marin and San Francisco, has served as a cattle ranch, a military base, a quarantine station, an immigration facility, a prisoner-of-war detention center, and a Nike missile site. When the federal government abandoned the island in the late 1940s, it became part of the state-park system, though missile sites operated until 1962. Years of restoration, the elimination of planted non-native vegetation, and the passage of time have allowed coast live oak woods and grassland to make a comeback. Park staff returned the island's highest peak, Mount Livermore, to its original state by restoring acres of dirt pushed off the summit by the military.

Angel Island offers two main hikes: a nearly level 5-mile circuit around the island on a fire road, and this loop, a combination of the North Ridge and Sunset Trails, with

DISTANCE & CONFIGURATION: 5.1-mile loop with 1 out-and-back segment

DIFFICULTY: Easy

SCENERY: Coast live oak and California bay woods, grassland and chaparral, and 360-degree views of the Bay Area from the top of Mount Livermore

EXPOSURE: Mix of sun and shade, with full sun at top

TRAIL TRAFFIC: Moderate–heavy in summer; lighter in the off-season

TRAIL SURFACE: Dirt

HIKING TIME: 3 hours

DRIVING DISTANCE: About 3.75 miles from the Golden Gate Bridge toll plaza to parking at Fisherman's Wharf (trail accessible only by boat)

ACCESS: Daily, 8 a.m.–sunset, but ferry service is limited during the off-season, generally September–May. Good year-round. Blue and Gold Fleet's $19.50 round-trip ferry ticket ($11 for seniors and children ages 5–11) includes park admission.

WHEELCHAIR ACCESS: Some of the trails at Angel Island are wheelchair accessible, but for the hike described here, wheelchairs are not recommended.

MAPS: Available at park visitor center, ferry landing, and parks.ca.gov

FACILITIES: Restrooms and drinking water at trailhead; picnic tables

CONTACT: 415-435-5390, parks.ca.gov. Contact Blue and Gold Fleet, 415-705-8200 or blueandgoldfleet.com, for a ferry schedule.

LOCATION: Angel Island

COMMENTS: No dogs allowed on the island except service animals

a short out-and-back spur to the summit. The park is busy during tourist season, but once when I visited with a friend in early summer, we disembarked from a nearly full ferry, then watched as the crowds made a beeline for the visitor center; on the trails, we crossed paths with only a dozen other hikers. Trails are even quieter in winter, when clear days promise long views, and early spring, when the wildflower displays are legendary.

Begin from the ferry landing on North Ridge Trail, which sets off to the left (north) of the restrooms. As it leaves the shoreline area, this path climbs through pine, toyon, and coast live oak, ascends some long, steep stairs past a few picnic tables and then reaches a cluster of eucalyptus and the paved Perimeter Road at 0.1 mile. Turn right and walk about 20 feet on the pavement, then turn left to continue on North Ridge Trail. The narrow path winds uphill through shaded woods of California bay and hazelnut, where clarkia and Indian pink bloom in early summer. When North Ridge Trail emerges from the woods on the northernmost flank of the island, enjoy views north across Raccoon Strait to the Tiburon Peninsula. Wind through some chaparral with lots of manzanita and chamise, then continue through woods to a junction at 0.9 mile where you turn left onto a fire road. After a few feet, veer right, continuing on North Ridge Trail.

After one last foray through chaparral, the path, still ascending easily, takes a long tour through quiet woods of coast live oak, where you might also see madrone, gooseberry, huge thickets of hazelnut, and poison oak. North Ridge Trail levels out as it reaches a grassy plateau dotted with coyote brush; here, iris and paintbrush bloom in spring, and coyote mint, venus thistle, and buckwheat flower in summer.

Angel Island State Park

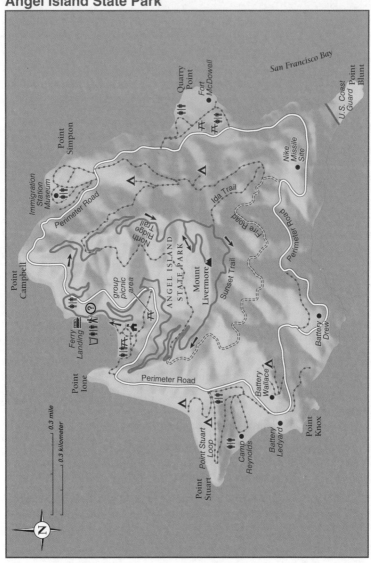

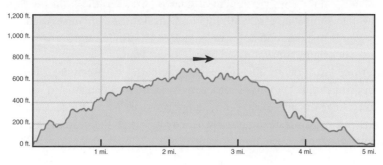

There are good views too—west to Mount Tamalpais and uphill to Mount Livermore's summit. Under a few pines at 1.8 miles, North Ridge Trail ends at a T-junction. Turn right, following the sign to Mount Livermore.

At an easygoing rate, the trail climbs past coast live oaks into grassland. You'll likely see butterflies, including California sister and a variety of swallowtails, fluttering about in summer, along with fast-moving swifts and more-languid vultures and hawks riding the thermal currents. After two bends in the trail, the path makes a final push to the summit, climbing through grassy slopes dotted with coyote brush. At 2.1 miles, you'll reach the top of Mount Livermore, where views are simply incredible and, even in summer's haze, include Alcatraz Island, Mount Tamalpais, the downtown San Francisco skyline, Mount Diablo, Treasure Island, the Bay Bridge, and the Golden Gate Bridge stretching from San Francisco's Presidio to Marin's rolling Headlands. Descend back to the previous junction, then continue right on Sunset Trail.

As you drop down onto the island's south slope, unobstructed views extend downhill to Point Blunt, an active Coast Guard station. Sunset Trail crosses an old, closed road and begins to angle across a hillside, heading west. Bushes of sticky monkeyflower, coyote brush, poison oak, and sagebrush frame awesome views of the world's most famous span, its signature "international orange" paint scheme so pretty against a clear blue sky. The trail descends a ridge, offering splendid views of Sausalito, Belvedere Island, the Marin Headlands, and Mount Tam, then veers right into coast live oak woods.

At one last little sunny viewpoint, a bench invites a lingering break before the trail begins a campaign of switchbacks. Some shortcuts are worn into the hillside, but please stay on the trail, which is well-graded. Poison oak and Italian thistle will crowd the trail in places in summer. At 3.4 miles, veer right on a fire road a few feet, and then turn left, back onto Sunset Trail. Switchbacks continue, mostly through California bay and coast live oak woods. Just past a water tank and a cluster of picnic tables, Sunset Trail bends left, runs along the road, then ends at 4.5 miles. Cross the road near a paved route descending to group picnic areas, then veer right, toward the dock area.

As you descend toward the visitor center, you might notice several non-native plants, including pride of Madeira, a shrub with big purple flower spikes, and broom, a wispy bush that bears yellow, sweet-smelling, pealike blossoms. The route turns sharply left and then ends at the side of the visitor center, where a grassy picnic area fronts the shoreline at Ayala Cove. Turn right and walk on a paved road the remaining distance back to the ferry landing.

• •

GPS TRAILHEAD COORDINATES N37° 52.110' W122° 26.083'

DIRECTIONS Angel Island is accessible by boat only. If you start a journey to Angel Island from a location served by BART or Muni trains, it makes perfect sense to take public transportation to the ferry landing at San Francisco's Pier 41. Take BART or Muni to the Embarcadero station, come aboveground and transfer to the F Line (on The Embarcadero across from the Ferry Building), and proceed west to the Fisherman's Wharf stop. Ferries to Angel Island also depart from Tiburon. To drive to the ferry from the East Bay via the Bay Bridge, take Exit 2C, Fremont Street. Use the middle lane and turn left onto Fremont Street, then turn right onto Howard Street. At the end of Howard, turn left onto The Embarcadero. Continue about 1.5 miles to Pier 41 and the parking garages at Fisherman's Wharf. From the Golden Gate Bridge, take Lombard Street to Van Ness Avenue. Turn left and go 4 blocks to North Point Street. Turn right on North Point, go about 5 blocks, and park in one of the parking garages at Fisherman's Wharf.

Blooming ceanothus frames a view from Angel Island to Mount Tamalpais.

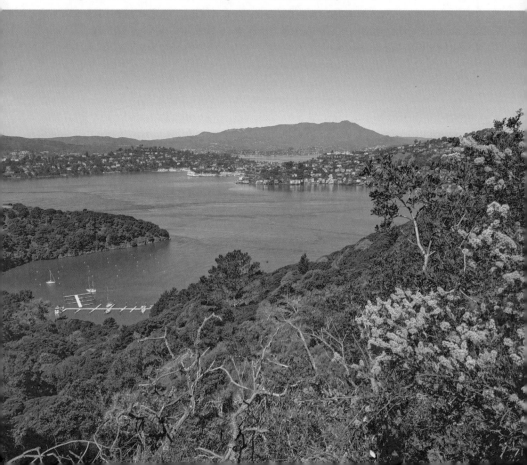

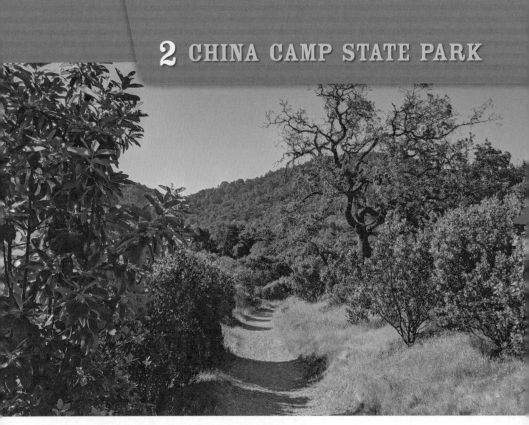

This flat stretch of Shoreline Trail makes for easy walking.

CHINA CAMP'S ROLLING, forested hills front San Pablo Bay just minutes from the hustle and bustle of San Rafael. Unlike some other destinations where the trip to the start of your hike seems to take forever, the coffee nestled in your cup holder may still be warm when you pull into this trailhead.

DESCRIPTION

China Camp can feel rather sleepy in autumn and winter, but summer draws loads of visitors for hiking, biking, picnicking, and camping. Miwok Meadows Picnic Area is a popular day-use site for family gatherings and parties (reservations required). Back Ranch Meadows Campground has 35 walk-in sites strewn throughout pretty woods. It is an extremely popular destination in summer, but you can often snag a site at the last minute on an autumn or early-spring weekday; in winter the place is mostly deserted.

Before you start your hike here, take a minute to discuss trail-sharing etiquette with your hiking partners. China Camp is an unusual Bay Area state park, with all but one trail open to hikers, equestrians, and cyclists (most state parks prohibit bikes from narrow trails). You probably won't see many horses, but cycling is popular here, and you'll likely cross paths with lots of bikes. The protocol for multiuse trails is that bikers yield to hikers and everyone steps aside for horses. However, on China

21

DISTANCE & CONFIGURATION: 6.5-mile loop

DIFFICULTY: Moderate

SCENERY: Mixed woods and views

EXPOSURE: Mostly shaded; some full sun

TRAIL TRAFFIC: Moderate

TRAIL SURFACE: Dirt fire roads and trails

HIKING TIME: 3 hours

DRIVING DISTANCE: 18 miles from the Golden Gate Bridge toll plaza

ACCESS: Daily, 8 a.m.–sunset. Good year-round. Pay the $5 day-use fee at the entrance kiosk. There is designated handicapped parking.

WHEELCHAIR ACCESS: There are designated handicapped parking spots. Wheelchair users should be able to navigate the first 1.3 miles of this hike (note that trails are muddy in winter and spring).

MAPS: At entrance kiosk and parks.ca.gov

FACILITIES: Restrooms and drinking water at the campground

CONTACT: 415-456-0766, parks.ca.gov

LOCATION: 739 North San Pedro Road, San Rafael, CA 94901

COMMENTS: Dogs are not allowed on the trails. The park's name dates back to the Chinese shrimp-fishing village that existed here in the 1880s. If you want to learn more about the history of China Camp, visit the Village Area: continue east on North San Pablo Road, past the campground trailhead and ranger station, to the signed China Camp Village Area on the left.

Camp's narrow trails, I find it simpler to step aside for the bikes, particularly when riders are slogging uphill, where momentum is important. In a group, the first hiker who spots a cyclist is advised to call out, "Bike!" to the rest of the party, who should then veer onto the right edge of the trail. When hiking with several people, try to remain single-file rather than stretching across the trail. Use special caution near blind corners on the upper trails—down in the flats cyclists expect heavy hiker use, but farther afield they don't seem as prepared for encounters.

Begin from the day-use lot and walk on the paved park road toward the campground. (You can skirt the campground completely via Shoreline Trail, but that option is longer and does not access some of the nicest park restrooms in the Bay Area, at the campground.) When we hiked here one summer, the smell of morning-campfire smoke drifted our way as a wild turkey trotted across the road. When you reach the campground parking lot, look for a signed path (pointing toward Shoreline Trail) departing from the east edge of the lot. After a few steps, Shoreline Trail feeds in from the right. The nearly level path runs above a damp area on the left, through grassland dotted with young buckeyes and coyote brush. Deer are common throughout the park, and we saw the first of several here on a summer morning. Without tall trees blocking views, uninterrupted vistas stretch north to the shores of San Pablo Bay and south to the park's tallest hills.

At 0.3 mile continue straight on Shoreline Trail, from a junction where a path heads left toward Turtle Back Nature Trail. Shoreline Trail runs near North San Pedro Road briefly, then veers right as it skirts a marshy meadow. Look for a pretty buckeye standing alone off to the left, conspicuous in early summer when ablaze with clusters of white flowers. At 0.7 mile stay right as a trail doubles back toward Bullet Hill. Shoreline Trail passes through pockets of California bays and oaks, crosses a

China Camp State Park

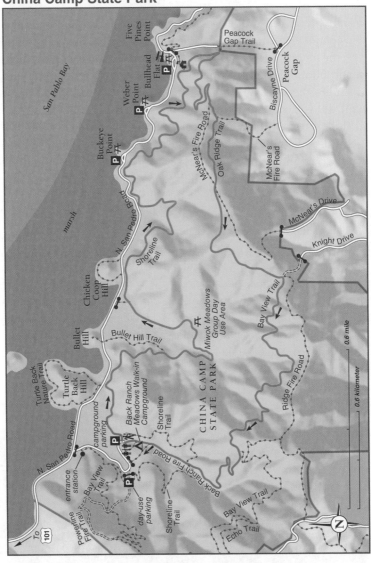

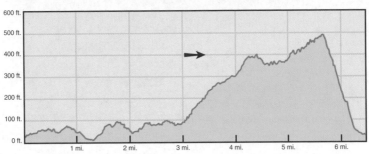

creek, then reaches the edge of Miwok Meadows Picnic Area. Pass through the parking lot and continue on Shoreline Trail, here a wide dirt road (watch for cars). At a level grade, the trail runs along the edge of sloping woods on the right, where orange sticky monkeyflower blooms in spring and summer.

At 1.3 miles the service road veers left (years ago Miwok Trail used to head uphill here), but you continue to the right, following the TO RANGER STATION signs. The trail shrinks back to footpath size and once again parallels North San Pedro Road briefly. In early summer, look for yellow mariposa lilies. Shoreline Trail pulls away from the road and heads into woods again, giving hikers an opportunity to see or hear some of the songbirds that call China Camp home. Chickadees are common—listen for their *chick-a-dee-dee-dee* call as they flit through the trees. I've also seen a black phoebe and spotted towhee in this area. With dark-gray heads and backs and white bellies, black phoebes are flycatchers, so look for them perched on tree or shrub branches, while spotted towhees shuffle through the leaf litter on the ground. Spotted towhees are about robin-size and have rusty bellies. Their black wings are speckled with white, which is most obvious when they are in flight. Shoreline Trail winds through patches of grassland and a forest of natives, including madrone, coast live and black oak, and California bay. At 2.9 miles you'll reach a junction with Peacock Gap Trail. Bear right and ascend to a second junction at 3.1 miles, where Peacock Gap Trail continues straight to the park boundary. Bear right, now on Oak Ridge Trail.

A small pond at China Camp State Park

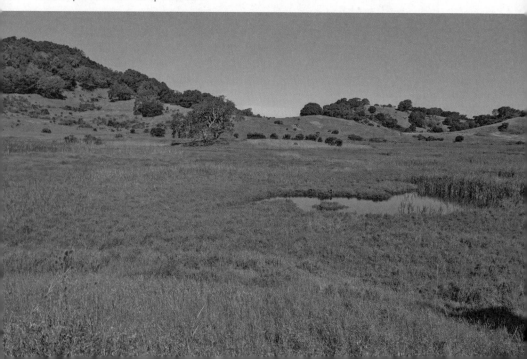

The narrow trail weaves uphill through woods dominated by California bays. Switchbacks ease the climb, and soon you'll emerge from the woods at a junction at 3.6 miles. McNear's Fire Road heads left and right—continue straight on Oak Ridge Trail. Slightly off the ridgeline, Oak Ridge Trail sweeps across a sloping hillside dotted with oaks and a few manzanita shrubs. Early wildflowers here include milkmaids and shooting stars. Where breaks in the vegetation permit, look off to the left for great views of San Rafael Bay and the Richmond–San Rafael Bridge. Oak Ridge Trail meets McNear's Fire Road again at 4 miles. The fire road climbs steeply to the left, up a ridge once dominated by non-native eucalyptus. In 2001 the park removed the trees; for a few years the ridgeline was bare, but now coast live oaks are beginning to dominate. Continue straight, still on Oak Ridge Trail. Back in the pretty mixed woods, the trail keeps to a nearly level grade. The shade is welcome on a warm summer day, but in the winter expect mud in this section. Oak Ridge Trail ends at 4.6 miles. Turn right onto Bay View Trail.

Another singletrack trail, Bay View is one of the park's quietest. Far uphill from the developed area, the trail provides easy and peaceful strolling under cover of oaks, madrone, and California bay woods. In spring blue-eyed grass blooms along the trail, and in summer look for California milkwort, a native wildflower with rose-pink petals. Bay View Trail meets Back Ranch Fire Road at 5.7 miles. Bear right.

This steep fire road descends rapidly, switchbacking under power lines. The black oaks mixed in with madrone and California bays along the trail shed gorgeous orange leaves here in autumn. After one last steep and slippery patch, Back Ranch Fire Road ends at a junction with Shoreline Trail at 6.2 miles (the leg left skirts the campground and is an optional route back to the parking lot). Continue straight, and the trail drops into the campground (if you camped here you'd be home now). A spur heads left near the restrooms, but keep going straight to the bridge at 6.4 miles, then turn left and retrace your steps back to the trailhead.

• •

GPS TRAILHEAD COORDINATES N38° 00.388' W122° 29.671'

DIRECTIONS From the Golden Gate Bridge toll plaza, drive north on US 101 about 14 miles, then take Exit 454, North San Pedro Road. Continue east on North San Pedro Road 3 miles, turn right into the park at the BACK RANCH MEADOWS sign, and then drive a short distance on the park road to trailhead parking on the right.

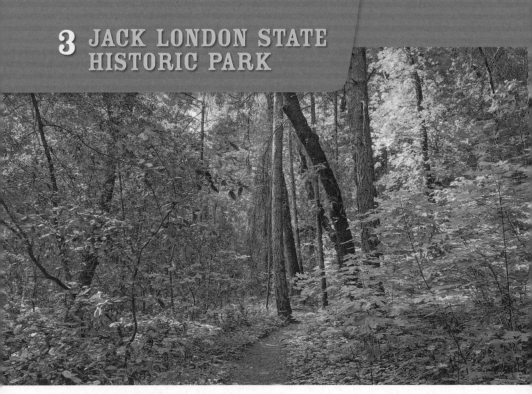

Walk in Jack London's footsteps on Lake Trail.

THIS BAY AREA RIDGE TRAIL segment begins on old ranch roads then ascends on a narrow path through an unspoiled forest of madrone, black oak, bigleaf maple, buckeye, redwood, and California bay. After 4.5 miles you'll reach the end of the trail, and the return segment is downhill almost all the way.

DESCRIPTION

Just minutes from the charming wine country village of Glen Ellen, hikers can walk up the forested slopes of Sonoma Mountain, literally following in the footsteps of Jack London, author of *The Call of the Wild*. The property, containing London's home and ranch buildings, as well as many surrounding wooded acres, became a state park after London's wife, Charmian, died in 1955. Visitors can tour the House of Happy Walls Museum; London's grave site; and the remains of Wolf House, London's dream home, which was destroyed by fire before it was ever occupied. For many, that's an adequate day trip, but hikers should press on, up the hillsides of Sonoma Mountain and into a gorgeous forest.

This hike adds up to nearly 9 miles, but the trails are so well graded that it's a moderate excursion. The park is a popular stop for summer visitors, but once you get away from the developed areas, you might see more squirrels than people. Spring hikes are tempting, and the gentle temperatures and colorful foliage of Indian summer make autumn hikes very enjoyable.

DISTANCE & CONFIGURATION: 8.9-mile out-and-back with 2 short loops

DIFFICULTY: Moderate, despite the length

SCENERY: Woods with some grassland

EXPOSURE: Almost completely shaded

TRAIL TRAFFIC: Moderate around ranch; light on upper trails

TRAIL SURFACE: Dirt fire roads and trails

HIKING TIME: 6 hours

DRIVING DISTANCE: 46 miles from the Golden Gate Bridge toll plaza

ACCESS: Daily, 9 a.m.–5 p.m.; closed December 25. Anytime is good, but autumn is perfect. Pay $10 fee at entrance kiosk.

WHEELCHAIR ACCESS: Wheelchair users should be able to navigate the trails in the developed part of the park. There is no designated handicapped parking at this trailhead.

MAPS: At the entrance kiosk, the park museum, and jacklondonpark.com/park-trails-hikes

FACILITIES: Pit toilets and water near trailhead

CONTACT: 707-938-5216, jacklondonpark.com

LOCATION: 2400 London Ranch Road, Glen Ellen, CA 95442

COMMENTS: Dogs are permitted on some park trails, but not on every trail in this hike.

Begin from the parking lot, following the Bay Area Ridge Trail (BART) symbol. When the path ends at a T-junction with a wide gravel road, turn right. London's cottage and the winery ruins are on your left. (If you care to explore them, return to the ranch road when you're done and keep following the signs for BART and the lake.) As you skirt a vineyard on the left, a few more paths on the right depart to the Pig Palace and other old farm buildings. All of these are optional side hikes.

After the trail makes a sharp turn with the vineyard still on the left, a gate stretches across the fire road, also known as Lake Service Road, and you'll reach a signed junction with Lake Trail. At this point you'll have traveled about 0.5 mile from the parking lot. Turn right, still on Lake Trail.

The narrow path begins an easy climb through the woods. On sunny days, light filters down to highlight a few stately redwoods nestled in a forest of madrone, big-leaf maple, black oak, tanoak, and Douglas-fir. Trilliums are very common here in late winter. Lake Spur Trail heads off to the right, taking the long way around the lake. Continue straight on Lake Trail as it runs within sight of Lake Service Road for a few paces then veers back into the woods. At 1 mile Lake Trail ends at the shore of London Lake. Turn left, walk a few steps, and then turn right onto Mountain Trail. As the fire road swings around the lake, Vineyard Trail departs to the left, with Quarry Trail following in the same direction after a few steps. Continue right (west) on Mountain Trail. The ascent begins an easy but steady climb through redwood, California bay, and madrone.

Unless you're visiting on a particularly busy day, the crowds thin with every step past the lake. The fire road reaches a little sloping meadow known as May's Clearing. Views stretch southeast, as does Old Fallen Bridge Trail on the left. Keep going uphill on Mountain Trail, browsing through a forest crowded with native Bay Area trees: redwood, madrone, coast live oak, bigleaf maple, buckeye, Douglas-fir,

Jack London State Historic Park

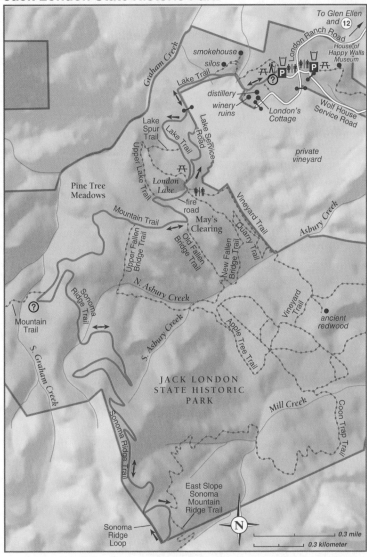

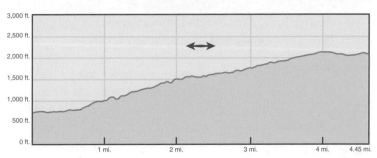

California bay, and Oregon oak. At 1.5 miles Upper Fallen Bridge Trail enters from the left. Keep climbing west on Mountain Trail. The trail winds past Pine Tree Meadows, really more of a grassy patch mostly overtaken by conifers. Just when the ascent seems never-ending, the trail dips to cross a creek and reaches a junction at 2.1 miles. Turn left onto Sonoma Ridge Trail.

Beneath a canopy of California bay, the trail gently ascends through a rocky section. Angling up the side of the mountain, you'll enter a more exposed area where oak, toyon, and manzanita mingle with Douglas-fir. The ascent is easy, initially through dense woods of Douglas-fir, California bay, and madrone.

Where the trail crosses Asbury Creek, redwoods are especially prominent and lovely. On the south side of the creek, the landscape shifts a bit, making a long transition to the grassland you'll see at the ridgeline. Buckeye, black oak, bigleaf maple, and manzanita are common, and wherever there are breaks in the forest, you'll get views extending far to the north, east, and south. The most prominent landform is 4,304-foot Mount Saint Helena, looming to the north. Switchbacks keep the grade nearly effortless, and the climb passes quickly. Before long you'll find yourself bisecting a grassy slope just under the ridgeline at nearly 2,100 feet.

At 4.3 miles, the trail splits into two legs of a loop. Turn left. After less than 0.1 mile, Coon Trap Trail departs downhill on the left. (Using Coon Trap, I turned this out-and-back hike into a loop on my last visit, but I don't recommend it—the trail is steep. Also at this junction, dead-end East Slope Sonoma Mountain Ridge Trail sets off to the south.) Continue right, on Sonoma Ridge Loop, climbing a little, past giant black oaks sprawling through grassland and fences that guard private property on the park boundary to the left. The loop closes at 4.6 miles. Turn left and retrace your steps to Mountain Trail, then turn right and walk downhill to the junction with Lake Trail at 8 miles. This time, keep right on Lake Service Road. With plenty of generous curves, the trail sweeps easily downhill through the woods. If you visit after a rainstorm, look for animal footprints in muddy patches. At 8.4 miles you'll reach the gate and junction with Lake Trail. Continue straight, retracing your steps to the parking lot.

• •

GPS TRAILHEAD COORDINATES N38° 21.381' W122° 32.692'

DIRECTIONS From the Golden Gate Bridge toll plaza, drive north on US 101 about 20 miles, and take Exit 460A for CA 37 E toward Napa/Vallejo. After 7.5 miles, turn left (north) onto CA 121. Drive about 8 miles to the junction with CA 116 and continue on CA 116. Continue 2 miles, then bear right onto Arnold Drive. Continue north 8.4 miles on Arnold into Glen Ellen, then turn left onto London Ranch Road, and drive about 1.3 miles to the park's entrance kiosk. Once past the kiosk, turn right and drive less than 0.1 mile to the parking lot.

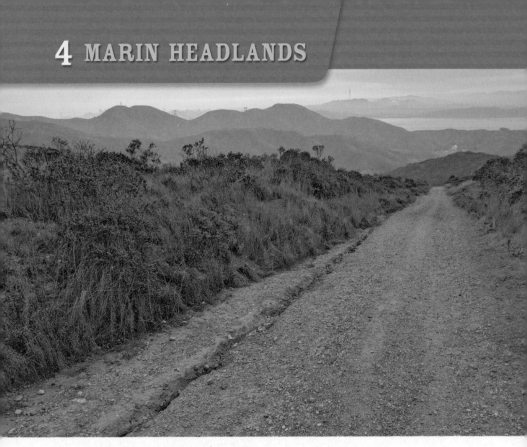

Hikers can see the Golden Gate Bridge towers peeking above a ridge on Miwok Trail.

THE SOFTLY ROLLING hills of the Marin Headlands form a picturesque backdrop for travelers driving north across the Golden Gate Bridge, as well as a perfect platform for San Francisco city views that include the world's most beautiful span. You'll begin this hike at the valley floor, climb through coastal scrub along one side of the valley, and then crest at the ridgeline and return on the other side of the valley. The entire loop sticks to fire roads and is easy to follow, but expect substantial mountain-bike and equestrian traffic.

DESCRIPTION

The Gerbode Valley trailhead is so close to San Francisco that when traffic conditions permit a quick escape, you can make the transition from city mouse to country mouse in 15 minutes. Although the Headlands are a stone's throw from the city and US 101, ridges block traffic noise and trails are peaceful. The Headlands are laced with a handful of trails and lots of fire roads, some of them remnants from the land's military past and others part of a development that never happened.

Just north of the Golden Gate, a military installation occupied the area now known as the Marin Headlands until the 1960s. After the bunkers and batteries were shuttered, a developer planned to build a massive housing complex called Marincello.

DISTANCE & CONFIGURATION: 5.9-mile balloon loop

DIFFICULTY: Moderate

SCENERY: Coastal scrub; views of the Golden Gate Bridge, the Pacific, the downtown San Francisco skyline, and Mount Tamalpais

EXPOSURE: Full sun

TRAIL TRAFFIC: Moderate year-round; includes mountain bikers and equestrians

TRAIL SURFACE: Dirt fire roads

HIKING TIME: 3 hours

DRIVING DISTANCE: 4.6 miles from the Golden Gate Bridge toll plaza

ACCESS: Park is open 24/7, but parking areas are only open daily, sunrise–sunset. No fee.

WHEELCHAIR ACCESS: There are designated handicapped parking spots. Wheelchair users should be able to navigate at least 0.25 mile from the trailhead (note that trails are often muddy).

MAPS: Free National Park Service map available at the Marin Headlands Visitor Center or at tinyurl.com/marinheadlandsmap

FACILITIES: Vault toilets at trailhead; restrooms and water at visitor center

CONTACT: 415-331-1540, nps.gov/goga/marin-headlands.htm

LOCATION: Sausalito, CA (at the north end of the Golden Gate Bridge)

COMMENTS: Dogs are permitted on some Headlands trails but not on every trail in this hike (see Nearby Activities for an alternate dog-friendly excursion). Check at the visitor center for specifics.

Environmental and community activists squelched the development, and the land eventually became part of the Golden Gate National Recreation Area, managed by the National Park Service. It's high-profile open space, exemplifying what Bay Area preservationists and outdoors enthusiasts cherish: broadly accessible land close to urban areas, with tons of elbow room for animals, wildflowers, and people.

Begin from the signed trailhead on Coastal Trail. After about 265 feet, turn left and cross a wide footbridge. Keep an eye open for newts in this area during the rainy season. At the far end of the bridge, you'll cross a creek then reach a T-junction; turn left onto Rodeo Valley Trail. Grassy hills rise to the right, but the broad fire road keeps to a level grade, running along a damp meadow dotted with coyote brush. At 0.3 mile Rodeo Valley Trail ends. Bear right onto Bobcat Trail. Ascending gradually, the wide dirt fire road follows the course of a small creek on the left, where willow and blackberry thrive and red-winged blackbirds flutter around the fringes of the stream. A stand of tall eucalyptus and a few scattered fruit trees suggest an old settlement in this area. The medicinal eucalyptus aroma mingles with the licorice scent of fennel, which grows with abandon along the trail. As the fire road begins to climb at a more moderate grade, views open up across Gerbode Valley, including glimpses of Miwok Trail. With each step, more of the ocean becomes visible back to the west.

The sides of Bobcat Trail are lined with many native plants. Coyote brush, purple bush lupine, poison oak, lizardtail, sticky monkeyflower, coffeeberry, sagebrush, and toyon are common coastal scrub plants, but the fog that is often held in this bowl-shaped valley nourishes some plants usually found in less exposed locations, such as creambush, snowberry, and currant. Flowers you might see in bloom range from late-winter specialists such as hound's tongue and milkmaids to spring favorites, including blue-eyed grass, buttercups, blue dicks, California poppies, iris,

31

Marin Headlands

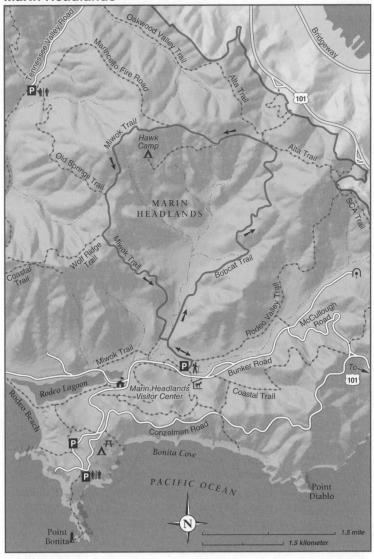

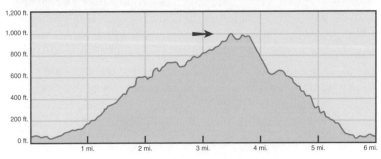

paintbrush, checkerbloom, and fringe cups. In early April, patches of goldfields blaze with color on the highest reaches of the ridge. There are very few trees—just a few clusters of some shrubby coast live oak, Monterey cypress, and a particularly squat Douglas-fir.

After a long, steady ascent, the grade eases and huckleberry shrubs appear on the left. Bobcat Trail climbs until it finally levels out at the ridgeline. At 2.4 miles Bobcat veers left just before a second junction where fire roads split off at a T-junction, with Alta Trail running northwest–southeast. Continue west on Bobcat. Although this is not the highest point on the ridgeline, the sweeping views feel well earned. Gerbode Valley slopes down at your feet, and the ocean sparkles to the west. Bobcat Trail passes under some power lines then takes a dip before rising back to follow the ridge. In spring, California poppies, blue dicks, checkerbloom, blue-eyed grass, and buttercups blossom through the grass along the trail.

At 2.8 miles a trail leading to Hawk Camp breaks off to the left. Continue straight (northwest) on Bobcat, which now makes a final push toward the Headlands' second-highest hill. The northern Golden Gate Bridge tower peeks out from between two hills to the south, and then the entire ridge of Mount Tamalpais comes into view to the north. Marincello Fire Road starts a journey to Tennessee Valley at 3.1 miles, on the right. Continue straight on Bobcat Trail. Still climbing through grassland, the trail finally ends at a junction with Miwok Trail and two fire roads that service a Federal Aviation Administration navigational antenna perched at the hilltop. Turn right onto Miwok. The fire road descends, sweeping around the hill while offering grand views to the north of Tennessee Valley and Mount Tam. After a brief ascent, Miwok crests. But before heading downhill, take a moment to appreciate the views south. The Bay and Golden Gate Bridges are visible, as are downtown San Francisco skyscrapers, Sutro Tower near Twin Peaks, and, farther south, Montara Mountain. If it's not too windy, a little grassy spot off the trail to the left makes a great rest stop. I watched a coyote hide behind a rock here on one winter hike. Where Miwok Trail begins a steep descent, the rest of the journey is downhill.

A gopher played peek-a-boo with me along the trail once, popping out of a hole then diving back down. Although this stretch of trail is closed to cyclists, some riders still brave the harsh descent, so stay alert for traffic. You'll reach a junction with Old Springs Trail on the right at 4 miles; continue straight (south) on Miwok Trail. Trailside vegetation is mostly coyote brush, with lots of mule-ear sunflowers blooming in summer. This is a good trail for raptor-watching, particularly in autumn when migratory birds pass through, and year-round you'll probably see vultures soaring overhead. Jagged Wolf Ridge rises off to the right, and its namesake trail begins at a signed junction at 4.3 miles. Stay left (southeast) on Miwok Trail. The descent is relentless, but I always console myself with the thought that at least it's downhill. If you're a bit rusty, your quads will be hollering.

As the trail drops back into Gerbode Valley, the vegetation on the hillside to the right becomes more lush, with ferns, snowberry, poison oak, purple bush lupine, and sagebrush spread across a hillside of coyote brush. Paintbrush, buttercups, and California poppies are the most common "wild" flowers in early spring, but there's also plenty of non-native Bermuda buttercup, a yellow-blossomed member of the oxalis family related to redwood sorrel. Miwok Trail finally winds its way back to level ground, meeting Bobcat Trail at 5.4 miles. Turn left. The trail crosses over a creek where twinberry, a rather bland shrub most of the year, makes a spectacle of itself in spring, putting forth pairs of orange-red flowers that develop into berries in the summer. After about 300 feet, Bobcat veers left at the start of the Rodeo Valley Trail. Turn right and retrace your steps back to the trailhead.

NEARBY ACTIVITIES

Miwok Trail plays a part in another Headlands loop hike. Start from the Rodeo Beach trailhead at the end of Mitchell Road, and string together Miwok, Wolf Ridge, and Coastal Trails for a 4.3-mile excursion—note that this is one Headlands hike on which dogs are welcome, on leash or under voice control.

• •

GPS TRAILHEAD COORDINATES N37° 49.954' W122° 30.979'

DIRECTIONS From the Golden Gate Bridge toll plaza, drive 2 miles to the far end of the bridge; then, just past the Vista Point exit, take Exit 442 onto Alexander Avenue. Turn right (east) and drive 0.3 mile toward Sausalito, then turn left onto Bunker Road. Drive 0.1 mile to the mouth of a 0.5-mile one-way tunnel (you may need to wait as long as 5 minutes for your turn). From the other side of the tunnel, continue 2.1 miles more on Bunker Road, then turn right into the parking lot (past the horse stables).

Marin Headlands Visitor Center is open Wednesday–Monday, 9:30 a.m.–4:30 p.m. (closed January 1, Thanksgiving, and December 25). From this hike's trailhead, drive west on Bunker Road about 0.4 mile, and where Bunker curves right, turn left onto Field Road. After less than 0.1 mile, turn right into the visitor-center parking lot.

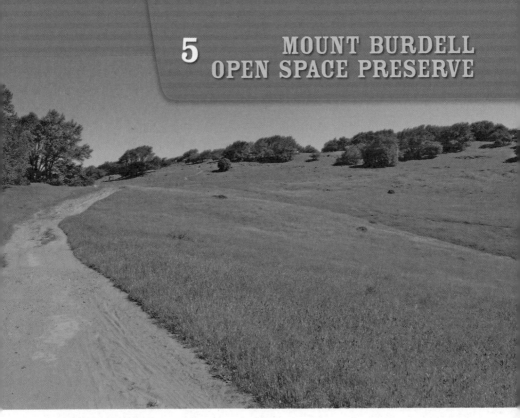

5 MOUNT BURDELL OPEN SPACE PRESERVE

Climbing Cobblestone Fire Road

MOUNT BURDELL IS a big name for a relatively low Marin County peak. This preserve is backyard wilderness for Novato dog walkers and runners and is a great destination for easy to moderate hikes like this one—a loop through oaks and grassland to the high flanks of the mountain and the upper reaches of Olompali State Historic Park.

DESCRIPTION

Two parks occupy the slopes of Mount Burdell: Olompali State Historic Park and Mount Burdell Open Space Preserve. The state park, on the east slope, features a small, reconstructed Miwok village and trails that snake uphill through gorgeous oak woods. Unfortunately, traffic noise from US 101 is pervasive in the state park—the open-space preserve is quieter and offers more options for loops through oak savanna, with good wildflower displays in spring.

From the roadside parking area, veer right, entering the preserve through either the V-shaped stile or the cattle gate. A shortcut path heads right, but follow the access path straight, then begin hiking north, uphill. After 300 feet, San Marin Fire Road begins on the right near a huge coast live oak. Continue north on San Andreas Fire Road, ascending past coast live oaks and California bays at a moderate clip. At 0.2 mile Little Tank Fire Road departs left—stick to San Andreas Fire Road and keep

DISTANCE & CONFIGURATION: 5.1-mile balloon loop

DIFFICULTY: Moderate

SCENERY: Grassland and oaks; nice flowers in late winter and spring

EXPOSURE: Mostly full sun

TRAIL TRAFFIC: Moderate

TRAIL SURFACE: Rocky dirt trails and fire roads and 1 paved fire road

HIKING TIME: 2.5 hours

DRIVING DISTANCE: 26 miles from the Golden Gate Bridge toll plaza

ACCESS: Open 24/7. Good year-round. No fee.

WHEELCHAIR ACCESS: Not recommended for wheelchairs

MAPS: None at trailhead but available at tinyurl.com/mountburdellmap

FACILITIES: None

CONTACT: 415-473-6387, marincountyparks .org/parkspreserves/preserves/mount-burdell

LOCATION: Novato, CA

COMMENTS: Dogs are permitted in the preserve but not the state park (1 short out-and-back segment of this hike). Tour the east slope of Burdell Mountain from Olompali State Historic Park (415-898-4362, parks.ca.gov), accessed off US 101.

climbing. A few black oaks and buckeyes appear; in late winter, look for a good display of Chinese houses on the left (west) side of the trail. San Andreas Fire Road crests at the lip of a bowl-shaped valley at 0.4 mile.

Dwarf Oak Trail heads back downhill on the left—stay to the right (northeast) on San Andreas Fire Road, ignoring a dead-end fire road that heads straight, leading to the park boundary. On one early-April hike, the grass in this valley was completely overtaken by the yellow flowers of blooming johnny-tuck and California buttercup. Two months later the grassy bowl and oak-dotted slopes ascending out of the valley were a sea of dry, blonde grass. San Andreas Fire Road curves right and ascends again, winding past mature valley oak, California bay, and buckeye, then ends at a fork at 0.7 mile. Deer Camp Fire Road, to the left (north), is a longer option—for this hike, continue straight (east), now on Middle Burdell Fire Road.

Blue dicks and popcorn flower bloom along the trail in early spring, preceding a June bonanza of clarkia and elegant brodiaea. Ascending easily, Middle Burdell Fire Road is mostly unshaded, although there is one small grove of California bay, coast live oak, and buckeye. At 1.1 miles you'll reach the edge of Hidden Lake, fenced to keep cows (and dogs) out of this sensitive habitat. In dry months the seasonal pond looks like a damp meadow, but in winter it does hold water. Cobblestone Fire Road begins at 1.2 miles. Turn left (north).

The fire road initially climbs at an easy to moderate grade, but there is one short, rocky, steep stretch. Cobblestones were quarried from the upper slopes of Mount Burdell for San Francisco street construction, and as you progress uphill, the trails and hillsides get increasingly rocky. At 1.5 miles Deer Camp Fire Road enters from the left—stay to the right (east) on Cobblestone Fire Road. The trail ascends through grassland, with buckeyes, California bays, and oaks standing well back on sloping hillsides. In June, look for yellow mariposa lilies blooming along with California poppy, clarkia, and venus thistle. A rough path sweeps off to the right—supposedly a

Mount Burdell Open Space Preserve

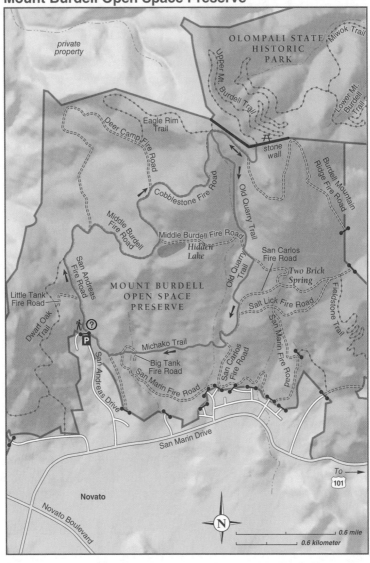

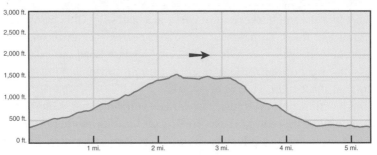

shortcut—but it offers no relief from the climb, so stay left. A microwave relay struc-ture is visible to the left, and off to the right one of the old quarries is conspicuous. Cobblestone Fire Road levels out as it approaches the summit area, then ends at a multiple junction at 2.2 miles. A paved fire road heads west (left) to the micro-wave relay and east to the park boundary. Old Quarry Trail, this hike's return route, departs sharply to the right. Turn right onto Burdell Mountain Ridge Fire Road.

The fire road keeps a level pace as it winds just downslope from the mountain's highest ridge. There's considerable, if distant, noise from US 101, visible downhill to the east. More scenic are views to Big Rock Ridge and Mount Tamalpais to the south. At 2.4 miles veer left (southeast) onto an unsigned dirt road that quickly leads to a fence and entry into Olompali State Park. As you enter the state park, a grassy hillside falls steeply to the east, revealing long views of the Petaluma River, upper San Pablo Bay, and the southern tip of the Sonoma Mountains. Two picnic tables here invite a lingering lunch. Follow the trail off to the left (north) through a sparse, grassy forest of California bay to a stone wall crossing the trail at 2.5 miles. This rock fence and others on the mountain were constructed without mortar by Chinese laborers in the 1800s. If you want to extend this hike, you could continue, winding downhill another 3.5 miles to the next junction. For now, though, retrace your steps back to the junction with Cobblestone Fire Road and Old Quarry Trail at 2.9 miles. Turn left (southeast) onto Old Quarry Trail.

Descending through grassland, the slight path shifts from easy to steep near a pocket of sagebrush and sticky monkeyflower. Coast live oak, California bay, and buckeye nestle in a little creekbed on the right, as the trail descends into a mostly unshaded canyon. Steep, grassy slopes on the left are scored with animal paths, and you may see deer browsing in this area of the park, where mule-ear sunflowers are common in spring. After the steepest section, littered with loose rock, Old Quarry Trail eases up in the middle of a California bay grove then emerges into grassland. At 3.5 miles the trail reaches a T-junction with Middle Burdell Fire Road. Turn left (southeast) onto the fire road.

After about 300 feet of level strolling, turn right (south) onto the continuation of Old Quarry Trail. The descent is steep, but less so than the previous segment, and not nearly as rocky. An expanse of grassland stretches off the sides of the trail, punctuated by oaks and buckeyes. Just past a gate and stile, Old Quarry Trail ends at San Carlos Fire Road. Turn right. The fire road descends easily through coast live oaks, with summer displays of milk thistle. Salt Lick Fire Road sets off to the left at 3.9 miles—stay right on San Carlos Fire Road, curving downhill to the junction with Michako Trail at 4.2 miles. Turn right (west).

At this junction, note the granary tree drilled with holes and stuffed with acorns by birds. At a slight descent, Michako Trail passes through another cattle gate then skips across a small creek. In June large patches of Davy's centaury, a pink flower,

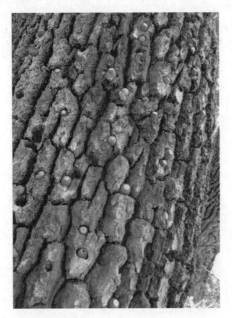

A granary tree, stuffed by birds, at Mount Burdell

bloom in the drying grass, accompanied by sprinkles of elegant brodiaea. The trail forks at another creek crossing—the two legs rejoin shortly—and a fire road crosses the trail, leading left to a water tank. Follow the fire road to the right or continue straight (east) on the trail; the two routes meet at a junction at about 4.8 miles. Veer right, now on San Marin Fire Road.

The green, waxy rock exposed along the trail is serpentine, and this stretch of trail hosts a good display of native flowers in early spring. Nearing the preserve boundary, the trail bends to the right and descends, then levels out as it approaches the trailhead. Officially, San Marin Fire Road continues to its terminus at San Andreas Fire Road, but a well-worn path shortcuts the route to the left, leading to the entrance gate.

• •

GPS TRAILHEAD COORDINATES N38° 07.809' W122° 36.254'

DIRECTIONS From the Golden Gate Bridge toll plaza, drive north 23.5 miles on US 101 to Novato, and take Exit 463, San Marin Drive/Atherton Avenue. At the end of the exit ramp, turn left onto Atherton Avenue. At the junction with Redwood Boulevard, continue straight, now on San Marin Drive, 2 miles. Turn right onto San Andreas Drive.

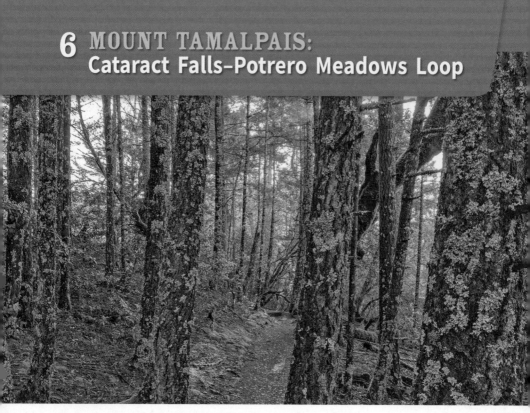

Lichen on tree trunks along Benstein Trail

ONE OF MOUNT TAMALPAIS'S most compelling assets is its broad variety of possible hikes. You can order up your hike like a San Francisco burrito: hot or mild, small or *grande*, with just rice and beans or the works. This 6.3-mile loop is one of the mountain's wildest, with only two short segments on fire roads and the rest on narrow and rocky hiking-only trails.

DESCRIPTION

This entire loop is a tour de force of the mountain's magic: you'll experience dense forests, aromatic chaparral, rushing creeks, waterfalls, and flower-dotted meadows. In fact, the hike begins at a meadow, just off the Rock Spring parking lot. Here Cataract Trail starts a long journey from Tam's high ridges down to the shores of Alpine Lake. Follow Cataract Trail 0.1 mile north to a junction with Simmons Trail, and continue to the left (west) on Cataract. At a slight descent, the narrow trail skirts a grassy meadow where patches of blue and white lupine are common in spring, then begins to follow its namesake creek, here just a trickle. Huge Douglas-firs line the trail and creek, mixed in with huckleberry, tanoak, California bay, and madrone. Old trail segments are occasionally visible on the opposite bank, but this trail crosses Cataract Creek only on a series of small footbridges—if you're stymied, look for a bridge; don't cross the creek without one.

DISTANCE & CONFIGURATION: 6.3-mile loop with 2 short out-and-back segments

DIFFICULTY: Moderate–strenuous

SCENERY: Grassland, woods, chaparral, and waterfalls

EXPOSURE: Back and forth through shade and sun

TRAIL TRAFFIC: Moderate on Cataract Trail; otherwise light

TRAIL SURFACE: Dirt fire roads and trails

HIKING TIME: 4 hours (includes lunch break)

DRIVING DISTANCE: 16 miles from the Golden Gate Bridge toll plaza

ACCESS: Daily, sunrise–sunset (Pantoll gate opens at 7 a.m.). Good year-round but muddy in winter. No fee at this trailhead.

WHEELCHAIR ACCESS: Not recommended for wheelchairs

MAPS: None at trailhead but available at tinyurl.com/mounttammarin. I highly recommend Redwood Hikes Press's *Mount Tamalpais* map ($10.95; redwoodhikes.com/Store/MtTam.html).

FACILITIES: Pit toilets at trailhead and Laurel Dell

CONTACT: 415-945-1180, marinwater.org/188/visiting-watershed-lands

LOCATION: Mill Valley, CA

COMMENTS: Leashed dogs are welcome on this hike (on Marin Municipal Water District land) but are prohibited in the adjacent state park.

Although the grade is easy, the trail is quite rocky in places, and some big boulders loom beside the path. Where Cataract Trail steps out into grassland, we saw gorgeous orange leopard lilies near the creekbed one Fourth of July weekend, and hundreds of swallowtail and California sister butterflies, dragonflies, and damselflies drifted lazily over the meadow. Back in the woods on this same hike, a powerfully sweet smell led our noses to an azalea bush in full bloom right at the trail's edge. As Cataract Trail continues downhill into a canyon, the tree cover becomes thicker and the creek swells with water feeding in from side streams. Once, on a February hike here, I saw a giant salamander eating a mouse.

At 1 mile, signed Ray Murphy Trail crosses the creek toward Laurel Dell Fire Road. Continue straight (northeast) on Cataract Trail. This is a good stretch to look for little pink Calypso orchids in late winter. Mickey O'Brien Trail departs on the right at 1.3 miles—stick to the left on Cataract Trail as it continues toward Laurel Dell. The trail passes some pit toilets and reaches a junction with Laurel Dell Fire Road at 1.4 miles. Cross the fire road and remain on Cataract Trail. Once past a few picnic tables, the trail begins to descend again along the north bank of Cataract Creek. In winter and early spring the water flows swiftly, and you'll pass the first cascade. Bigleaf maples intersperse with California bay, redwood, and Douglas-fir in the forest, where birding is often sublime. On one winter hike I caught the orange flash of a varied thrush flitting through the woods and watched a brown creeper earn its name—this little brown bird scrambles up tree trunks, looking for insects. At 1.6 miles, Cataract Trail meets High Marsh Trail at a signed junction. Continue west on Cataract downhill a short distance to the waterfall viewpoint. After winter storms, water crashes down over huge boulders here—this is one of the most scenic waterfalls in the Bay Area. The trail (and creek) continue steeply

41

Mount Tamalpais: Cataract Falls–Potrero Meadows Loop

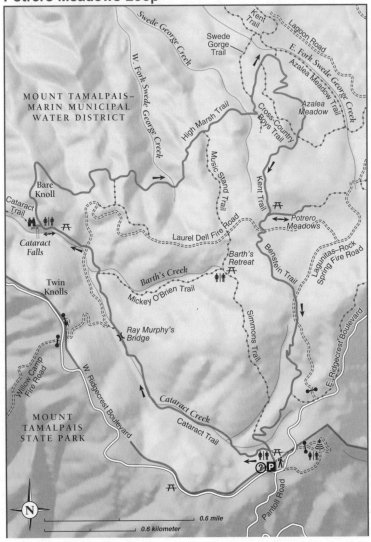

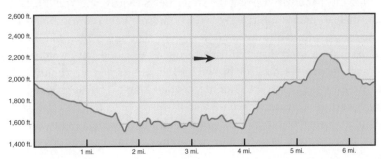

downhill toward Alpine Lake, but for this hike, retrace your steps back uphill and turn left (north) onto High Marsh Trail.

The trail descends through woods away from Cataract Creek, then begins to contour across steeply sloped Bare Knoll. As the name suggests, the open, sunny knob is grassy, with only a few Douglas-firs here and there. Views north are the best you'll get on High Marsh Trail, which from here on is mostly wooded and passes through no other grassland. Pass Bare Knoll Trail heading uphill to Laurel Dell Fire Road at 2.3 miles, and as High Marsh Trail prepares to head back into the woods, look on the left side of the trail for canyon live oaks. These evergreen trees are easy to pick out—their glossy, oval leaves are dusted with golden powder on their undersides. Once under tree cover again, High Marsh Trail begins a campaign of rolling ups and downs, with some level interludes. From time to time the trail crests and steps out into sunny chaparral dominated by manzanita, but the majority of the time, you'll be hiking beneath California bay, madrone, tanoak, redwood, and Douglas-fir.

At around 3.1 miles, Music Stand Trail heads uphill on the right—continue straight on signed High Marsh Trail. As the trail drops into a canyon surrounding Swede George Creek, look for irises in May. This part of High Marsh Trail is moist and almost completely shaded—it can be chilly here in winter, but in the summer you'll be glad for the shelter. High Marsh Trail steps across the creek (transformed into a waterfall in winter), and at 3.3 miles you'll reach a two-part junction with Swede George Trail (also known as Willow Trail). The first leg of Swede George Trail is unsigned and doubles back to the right, then climbs along the creek. To the left, Swede George and High Marsh Trails run together briefly before Swede George Trail departs to the left (the High Marsh part of this junction is signed). Continue on High Marsh Trail. The trail begins to climb at this point, then levels out—High Marsh, on the left, is a tiny pond ringed with cattails, coyote brush, and Douglas-fir. In winter the trail becomes a bit swamped here, but by summer the trail (and sometimes the marsh) is dry. Cross Country Boys Trail departs to the right at the edge of the marsh, at 3.5 miles; continue straight (northeast). The trail heads back into the woods. At 3.6 miles, you'll reach a junction with Kent Trail. Turn right (southeast) and begin a moderate climb alternating between quiet dark woods and patches of chaparral. This narrow path is very rocky in stretches. Kent Trail meets Cross Country Trail at 4.1 miles—continue straight (southwest). We encountered a coiled and rattling rattlesnake here on a summer hike. Because it showed no interest in moving, we took a wide path around it. Kent Trail emerges from the woods and passes through a big patch of manzanita dotted with towering Douglas-fir. Here views extend far to the north. As the trail continues uphill, native bunchgrasses line the way in places.

At 4.5 miles Kent Trail ends at the Potrero Meadows picnic area, on the right. In hot weather, the shaded tables make perfect lunch stops. Another option is Potrero

Meadows proper: Turn left (east) and, at a level grade, pass along the edge of a small, flat, grassy spot (this is the lesser of the two meadows). Once through a pocket of woods, the trail emerges to a wide, open meadow. This is one of Mount Tam's special places. On a winter weekday it can be surprisingly lonely, but in the thick of spring you'll likely see plenty of people. (The area's name may annoy grammar sticklers—it's redundant, as *potrero* means "meadow" in Spanish.) Little carpets of flowers brighten the grass in May, when you might see buttercups, goldfields, California poppies, and linanthus in bloom. When ready, retrace your steps to the picnic area, then turn left onto a wide, unsigned dirt service road. Look for azaleas in bloom on the left in early summer, as the road climbs briefly then ends at a T-junction with Laurel Dell Fire Road. Turn left and walk about 50 yards to the junction with Benstein Trail. Turn right.

The trail begins to climb. The initial section is very rocky and can be slippery when wet. Nestled in the woods is a little chaparral pocket of Sargent cypress and manzanita. As Benstein Trail ascends, it becomes enveloped by a very dense forest of tanoak, chinquapin, Douglas-fir, and madrone—so thick that there is little understory vegetation. The going is steep, but the trail soon levels out a bit to the left of a manzanita thicket.

At 5.4 miles Benstein feeds into Lagunitas–Rock Spring Fire Road. Go with the flow to the right briefly, then abandon the fire road for the path as Benstein veers off to the right. This well-cared-for segment of trail is delightful. At an easy descent, Benstein drifts downhill through madrone, Douglas-fir, and live oak. Some switchbacks drop the trail away from a fragile serpentine meadow. Milkmaids, shooting stars, and hound's tongue are common late-winter flowers along the trail. You may hear Ziesche Creek rushing in winter; you'll cross two tiny streams that head downhill to the bigger creek.

At 5.8 miles a signed path heads left toward Ridgecrest Boulevard. Bear right (southwest), remaining on Benstein. The descent through madrones is still easy. Look left for a peek at a huge serpentine swale—a conspicuous greenish-blue swath of rock in a sloping, grassy meadow. Benstein Trail ends at 6.1 miles. Turn left onto Simmons Trail, which sweeps across a meadow back toward Rock Spring. At 6.2 miles, turn left onto Cataract Trail and retrace your steps back to the trailhead.

• •

GPS TRAILHEAD COORDINATES N37° 54.652' W122° 36.765'

DIRECTIONS From the Golden Gate Bridge toll plaza, drive north about 5.5 miles, then take Exit 445B, CA 1/Mill Valley/Stinson Beach, and drive about 1 mile on Shoreline Highway to the junction with Almonte Boulevard (look for the CA 1 sign). Turn left to stay on CA 1, and drive about 2.5 miles to the junction with Panoramic Highway. Turn right on Panoramic and drive about 5.5 miles to the junction with Pantoll Road. Take a right onto Pantoll and drive another 1.5 miles to the Rock Spring trailhead, at the junction of East and West Ridgecrest Boulevards.

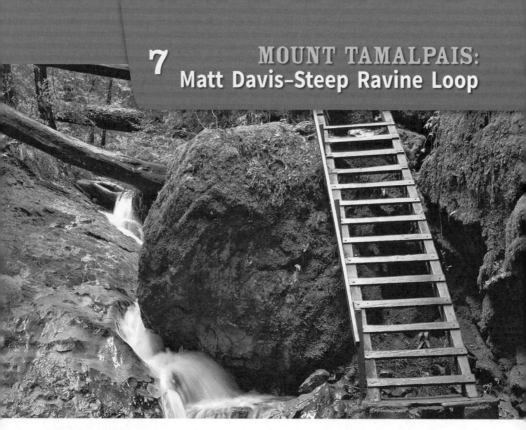

Steep Ravine Trail's famous ladder

THIS LOOP SHOWCASES the best of the Bay Area. While a number of other parks have a more pronounced wilderness vibe, Mount Tamalpais is a short drive for most, and San Francisco residents flock to the mountain, particularly on sunny weekends in spring.

DESCRIPTION

On weekends in the heart of summer, there are so many visitors on the trails around Mount Tamalpais's Pantoll area that you might feel like a shopper trying to enter Best Buy on Black Friday. Travel is sluggish, particularly on Steep Ravine Trail, a narrow route that doesn't tolerate crowds well. Try to plan this hike for a weekday or early in the day during the off-season. The best possible time may be the thin overlap between late winter and early spring, particularly if it's been a wet winter. During that window, wildflowers bloom everywhere and the waterfalls are plump with runoff.

Steep Ravine Trail departs from a signed trailhead at the southern edge of the parking lot. Without any prelude, the narrow trail begins to drop into a canyon. After a few switchbacks across a steep hillside, Steep Ravine Trail hooks up with Webb Creek and follows the stream as it makes its way through a lush forest of redwood, California bay, ferns, tanoak, and Douglas-fir. Little bridges channel hikers back and forth

45

DISTANCE & CONFIGURATION: 6.5-mile loop

DIFFICULTY: Moderate

SCENERY: Grassland, woods, and waterfalls

EXPOSURE: Equal parts sun and shade

TRAIL TRAFFIC: Heavy on trails near Pantoll Ranger Station; otherwise moderate

TRAIL SURFACE: Dirt fire road and trails

HIKING TIME: 4 hours

DRIVING DISTANCE: 14.5 miles from the Golden Gate Bridge toll plaza

ACCESS: Daily, 7 a.m.–sunset. Good year-round, but late winter (for waterfalls) and spring (for flowers) are best. Pay $8 fee at ranger station.

WHEELCHAIR ACCESS: Not recommended for wheelchairs

MAPS: At the ranger station (when open) and parks.ca.gov; Redwood Hikes Press *Mount Tamalpais* map ($10.95; redwoodhikes.com /Store/MtTam.html)

FACILITIES: Restrooms and drinking water at trailhead

CONTACT: 415-388-2070, parks.ca.gov

LOCATION: Mill Valley, CA

COMMENTS: This trailhead packs 'em in, particularly in summer, so arrive early. If you don't want to tote a lot of stuff with you, plan for lunch in Stinson Beach, where you can either eat at a café or pick up supplies. No dogs allowed.

across the creek a few times along the route. Spring wildflowers here include plants that adore moist environments, such as trillium, coast fairy bells, and stream violets.

At 0.8 mile you'll reach the famous ladder. The wood can be slippery, so take it slow—I prefer to descend facing the ladder rather than facing out. Beside the ladder, a little waterfall—one of a couple along the trail—burbles soothingly. Trailside vegetation seems to become even more lush. Redwoods uprooted or snapped off by winter storms lie across the trail and in the streambed in places; some are notched for passage.

At 1.5 miles the first of two junctions with Dipsea Trail departs on the left. Continue straight another 0.1 mile past an old dam on the left, then bear right, following the sign toward Stinson Beach. As Dipsea Trail begins a slight climb, a connector back to Steep Ravine veers left—keep straight. The trail climbs through some young Douglas-fir and toyon, then reaches a junction where you'll continue straight and emerge at the edge of a sloping meadow and another junction with a fire road. Cross the fire road, remaining on Dipsea, and watch as incredible views unfold to the north. On a clear day you'll see Stinson Beach, Bolinas Lagoon, and the forested hills of the Point Reyes peninsula.

While it's hard to top the enchantment of Steep Ravine, a spring hike through here boasts pockets of verdant grass dotted with orange California poppy, pink checkerbloom, and blue and white lupine in spring. Dipsea Trail descends steadily through coastal scrub and then a pocket of woods stretching along a creek. Gnarled moss-covered buckeyes are the star here, although California bays are more common. At 2.6 miles Dipsea reaches Panoramic Highway. Carefully cross the road and pick up the trail on the other side.

On the descent toward the town of Stinson Beach, traffic and neighborhood noise are abundant. At 2.7 miles, where Dipsea Trail meets CA 1, you can add an

Mount Tamalpais: Matt Davis–Steep Ravine Loop

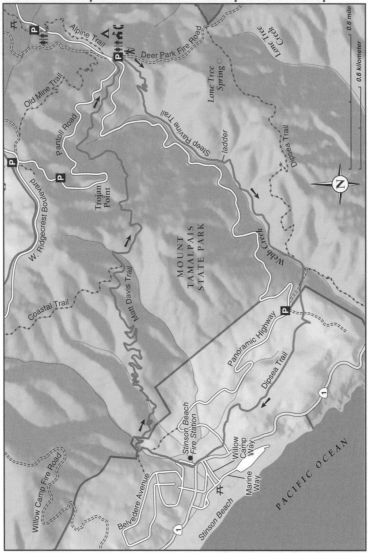

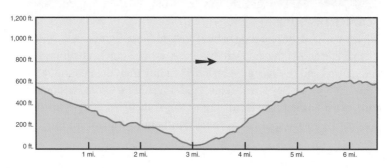

optional out-and-back by continuing across the highway and walking on city streets to Dipsea Trail's terminus at the beach. Otherwise, carefully turn right and walk along the side of CA 1. (The other side of the street may be a better option, but you'll have to cross the road twice. If you're looking for lunch or a place to buy water, walk past the firehouse to Stinson's commercial district.) After less than 0.1 mile turn right at the firehouse onto Belvedere Avenue. Walk up this street and, just past the WRONG WAY sign, turn right onto signed Matt Davis Trail.

Back in the woods, this narrow trail winds uphill. When you reach a signed T-junction, turn left, then cross a creek on a bridge and, at a second (slight) junction, bear right. This is the last junction for the next 2.2 miles. The hum of town life quickly fades away, replaced by the sounds of murmuring creek and crashing surf as the trail rises through a forest of buckeye and California bay. A bridge crosses a descending stream with less gush than Webb Creek, but the setting is incredibly pretty year-round.

After a series of switchbacks, Matt Davis Trail bisects a patch of coastal scrub. Glance over purple-flowered lupine and sagebrush bushes and already you'll have views to the ocean. The sunny interlude is short, and soon you'll ascend through a shaded woodland. The trail climbs relentlessly, but at a moderate pace. Just past another bridge, a long series of steps may be the toughest stretch of the trail, especially if you have short legs.

With Table Rock Creek tumbling downhill on the left, the trail skirts a huge boulder. California bays mix through a forest of massive Douglas-firs, and ferns are a perennial star of the understory, with trilliums, irises, forget-me-nots, and milkmaids making appearances in spring. Next: more switchbacks and occasional sets of steps. Still ascending, negotiate a few broad switchbacks. The woods thin slightly and brighten. Look for huckleberry along the path. Finally, you'll step out of the woods into grassland. The transition is startling, particularly in late winter, when the grass is so green it practically throbs with life.

Matt Davis Trail ascends gently downslope from the ridgeline, through grassland and little pockets of trees that linger in hillside creases. Framed by tall Douglas-firs, views west take in the ocean. In late winter and spring, peruse the sides of the trail for blue-eyed grass, California buttercups, California poppies, and blue dicks. At 5 miles Coastal Trail swings sharply left from a signed junction—bear right to remain on Matt Davis Trail.

With the worst of the climbing behind you, this next segment is a pleasurable stroll at a gentle incline across the grassy hillside. Bypass two quick junctions, the first with an ascending trail and the second with a descending trail; then continue straight, following the symbols for Bay Area Ridge Trail. Prepare for more sweeping views, this time south, extending past the Headlands to San Francisco and the San Mateo County coast. You may be able to spot northern harriers hunting from overhead.

Matt Davis Trail leaves the grassland for woods once more. Dense stands of California bay, redwood, Douglas-fir, and live oak filter the sun, creating shade that sustains a little flower favored by native-plant enthusiasts: the Calypso orchid. I saw dozens of the delicate purple flowers along the trail on one late-March hike, along with red larkspur, hound's tongue, and milkmaids.

The trail's elevation remains nearly level through here, and although trees block any views, they fail to screen the sound of traffic on Pantoll Road, just uphill to the left. You will probably cross paths with a steady flow of hikers on this part of the trail, a signal that the trailhead is growing closer with each step. Pass through an open, rocky area marked with soaring Douglas-firs, where ceanothus and chamise line the trail. Matt Davis Trail breaks off to the left, continuing toward Mountain Home Inn. Bear right, descend a few steps, and carefully cross the street to the Pantoll parking lot.

• •

GPS TRAILHEAD COORDINATES N37° 54.195' W122° 36.250'

DIRECTIONS From the Golden Gate Bridge toll plaza, drive north on US 101 about 5.5 miles, then take Exit 445B, CA 1/Mill Valley/Stinson Beach, and drive about 1 mile on Shoreline Highway to the junction with Almonte Boulevard (look for the CA 1 sign). Turn left to stay on CA 1 and drive about 2.5 miles to the junction with Panoramic Highway. Turn right on Panoramic and drive about 5.5 miles to the junction with Pantoll Road. Using caution, turn left into the parking lot.

A view from Dipsea Trail north to Bolinas Bay

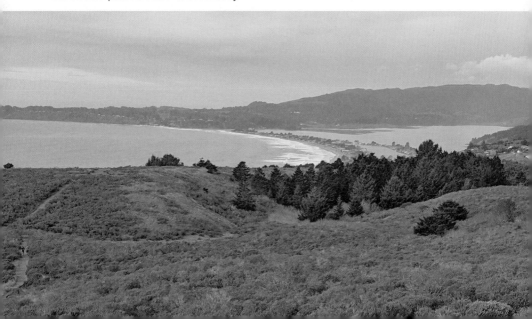

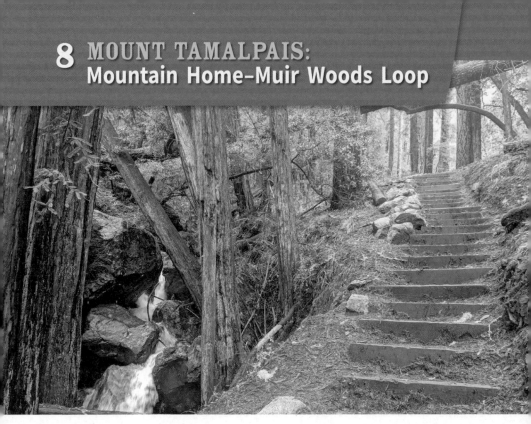

8 MOUNT TAMALPAIS: Mountain Home–Muir Woods Loop

Steps drop down along Bootjack Creek.

THIS HIKE STARTS across from Mountain Home Inn, descends on a paved service road, and then winds through woods on a narrow footpath. At Van Wyck Meadow, you'll begin a steep descent following creeks into Redwood Canyon and Muir Woods, where you'll mingle with the crowds on the park's main trail. The hike then veers off into Fern Canyon and relative solitude. A long set of steps ascends through woods into grassland, and a nearly level path makes for a quick return to the trailhead.

DESCRIPTION

Steep-sloped Redwood Canyon escaped the flying axes of the Bay Area's gold rush and today preserves some of the oldest and most majestic redwoods in the Bay Area. To prevent logging, William Kent began buying canyon property in 1905, then donated the land to the federal government for protection. The woods became a national monument in 1908, named in honor of conservationist John Muir. Although Muir Woods proper is quite small, the land is surrounded by Mount Tamalpais State Park and Golden Gate National Recreation Area property, forming a huge greenbelt of protected redwood canyons, creeks, coastal grassland, and mixed woodland that stretches from the Golden Gate Bridge to the northern flanks of Mount Tam.

DISTANCE & CONFIGURATION: 4.5-mile loop

DIFFICULTY: Moderate

SCENERY: Redwoods, forested canyons, and creeks

EXPOSURE: Mostly shaded

TRAIL TRAFFIC: Moderate around trailhead; very heavy in the heart of Muir Woods

TRAIL SURFACE: 2 short paved sections, dirt trails, and lots of steps

HIKING TIME: 3 hours

DRIVING DISTANCE: 11.7 miles from the Golden Gate Bridge toll plaza

ACCESS: Daily, 7 a.m.–sunset. Good year-round, but summer is busiest; fall is gorgeous. No fee at this trailhead; entrance to the main Muir Woods trailhead requires a $15 day-use fee and advance reservations.

WHEELCHAIR ACCESS: Not recommended for wheelchairs

MAPS: None at trailhead but available at parks .ca.gov. The best map for the area is Redwood Hikes Press *Mount Tamalpais* ($10.95; redwood hikes.com/Store/MtTam.html).

FACILITIES: Vault toilets and drinking water at trailhead

CONTACT: 415-388-2070, parks.ca.gov

LOCATION: Mill Valley, CA

COMMENTS: No dogs allowed. Arrive very early for parking in summer.

Whether you're a Bay Area visitor or a permanent resident, a trip to Muir Woods is mandatory—everyone should visit this awesome redwood monument at least once. With so many people pouring into one small canyon, Muir Woods always seems crowded, but there are ways to tour the park and still have a few quiet moments; this hike makes the most of an alternate trailhead.

Begin at the north end of the parking lot on Trestle Trail, entering Mount Tamalpais State Park. This little path drops down a flight of steps, then ends at Alice Eastwood Road. Turn right. Descending easily, the paved road, which accesses a group camp, winds through sun-drenched slopes where bush poppy and chaparral pea bloom in spring. Broom, chamise, toyon, and manzanita are common, but as the trail drops into a cool canyon, redwood, California bay, and Douglas-fir take over. At 0.4 mile, where the road crosses Fern Creek and swings left, turn right onto Troop 80 Trail.

The narrow trail, built by Boy Scouts in 1931, ascends along Fern Creek, then veers left and climbs at an easy pace. Redwoods, Douglas-firs, and tanoaks completely shade the trail. At 0.7 mile Sierra Trail heads downhill on the left, but continue straight on Troop 80 Trail. Running downslope from Panoramic Highway, the forest screens views of the road, but traffic noise is common, especially on summer weekends. Troop 80 Trail crosses creeks and damp seeps on a series of pretty bridges, winding through huckleberry patches, woods, and a few sunny stretches of chaparral, where you might see pitcher sage and chaparral pea in bloom in spring, accompanying manzanita, coffeeberry, and chinquapin. Occasional views south encompass forested hillsides rising from Redwood Canyon.

The trail forks at 1.6 miles, with the path on the right heading uphill to the Bootjack trailhead. Continue straight/left another 0.1 mile, through a display of false lupine (in spring) to Van Wyck Meadow. *Meadow* is a big word for this little grassy spot, but

Mount Tamalpais: Mountain Home–Muir Woods Loop

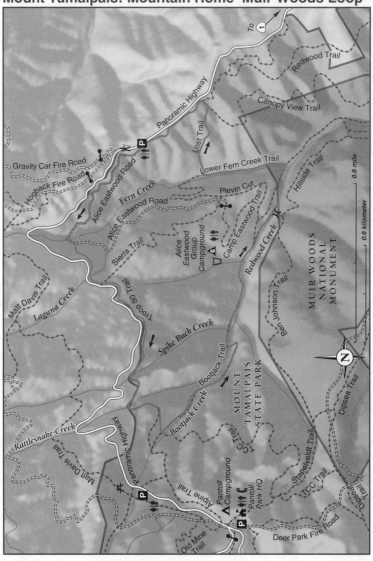

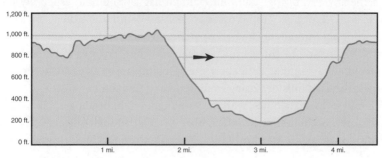

everyone seems to get a kick out of the VAN WYCK MEADOW POP. 3 STELLER'S JAYS sign. The meadow is a good place for a short rest before continuing into the canyon. When you're ready, head downhill to the left, on Bootjack Trail.

Stone steps begin the descent, dropping the narrow trail to the side of Bootjack Creek. Redwoods tower overhead, mixed through a lush forest of Douglas-fir and tanoak, with ferns in the understory. Look for trilliums and starflower blooming in spring. Some sections are nearly level, but the overall trend is quite steep and somewhat rocky in areas. Deer are common in this quiet part of the park, and you might see them clinging to the steeply sloped canyon walls like mountain goats, calmly munching vegetation. Bootjack Creek joins Rattlesnake Creek, plumping the stream with added water, which cascades merrily downhill.

As Bootjack Trail progresses down into the canyon, you may notice bigleaf maple, elk clover, and thimbleberry along the creekbed. The trail sweeps left and crosses a confluence of streams on a curving bridge, supported in the middle by a large boulder. Still following the creek, the grade slackens to a slight descent. At 2.8 miles a path breaks off on the left, on the way to Alice Eastwood Group Campground. Continue straight, following the sign toward Muir Woods. Trail traffic picks up and increases to a fever pitch as Bootjack Trail leaves the state park and ends at 2.9 miles at the main Muir Woods trail. Stay left, on the wide paved path, as it meanders beneath huge redwoods on the canyon floor. Another trail to the group camp bends left at 3.1 miles, but continue a bit farther, to the signed junction with Fern Creek Trail. Turn left.

With a course along the banks of Fern Creek, the trail gets quieter with every step, weaving slightly uphill through redwoods and ferns, with redwood sorrel a common understory plant. At 3.5 miles, you'll reach a junction with a third trail to the left leading to Alice Eastwood Group Campground; turn right onto Lost Trail.

The trail starts out on an easy grade, ascending out of the canyon, but the climb soon stiffens. On a long sequence of steps, you might come to the conclusion that Lost Breath Trail would be a more appropriate name for this route. Redwoods give way to live oak, Douglas-fir, and California bay; then Lost Trail ends at 3.9 miles. Turn left onto Canopy View Trail.

Now keeping to an easy uphill grade, Canopy View Trail departs the wooded canyon and emerges in grassland just below Panoramic Highway. There are views north to Tam's peaks and west toward the Pacific Ocean; this path's name used to be Ocean View and was changed to reflect the reality of the vista—a sea of trees. Stay left, near a boulder, and when Canopy View Trail ends at 4.1 miles, turn left onto Panoramic Trail.

The nearly level trail winds through grassland dotted with broom and acacia, two non-native plants, and coyote brush, one of the most common native shrubs in the Bay Area. Western fence lizards scamper along the path in summer. At 4.3 miles

Panoramic Trail ends at the top of Alice Eastwood Road. You can return to the parking lot by heading down Alice Eastwood Road to Trestle Trail, or by simply walking (with caution) 0.2 mile along the side of Panoramic Highway to the left.

NEARBY ACTIVITIES

Instead of visiting the redwood canyons of Muir Woods, you can hike to the top of Mount Tam from this trailhead, via easily graded fire roads that follow the route of an old railroad. Gravity Car Grade begins across the street from the parking lot, and Old Railroad Grade makes the final push to the top, although you can take alternate routes on several minor footpaths.

• •

GPS TRAILHEAD COORDINATES N37° 54.612' W122° 34.633'

DIRECTIONS From the Golden Gate Bridge toll plaza, drive north on US 101 about 5.5 miles. Take Exit 445B for CA 1, and drive about 1 mile west on CA 1 to the junction with Almonte Boulevard (look for the CA 1 sign). Turn left to stay on CA 1 and drive about 2.5 miles. Turn right on Panoramic Highway and drive about 2.5 miles to a parking lot on the left, across from the Mountain Home Inn.

Just some of the 235 ascending steps on Lost Trail

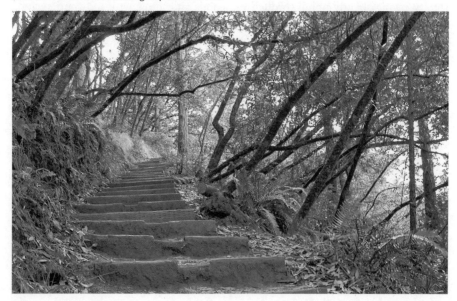

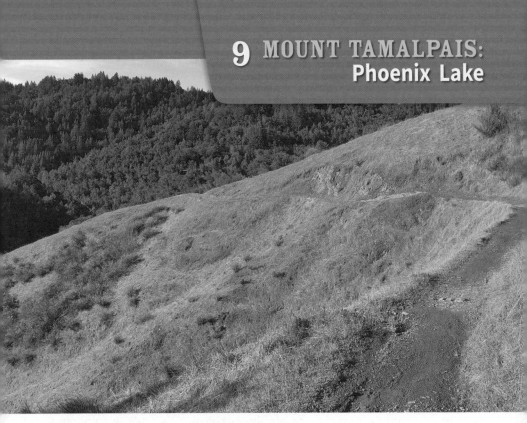

Hidden Meadow drops through grassland into the woods.

HOW DO I LOVE THEE? Let me count the trails. Mount Tamalpais has many trailheads and a lifetime's worth of paths. The options for hikes here are staggering, and you can't really take a wrong step, but this gorgeous route through woods and grassland, with great views to Tam's summit, thrills me each time.

DESCRIPTION

This northern flank of Mount Tam is Marin Municipal Water District land, preserved for the primary purpose of storing and providing water to Marin County residents. The hiker's benefit is a network of many trails and fire roads that connect to Mount Tamalpais State Park and a few small Marin County Open Space District preserves. I've loved this hike from my first visit, and it's a particularly good choice for late winter and spring, when wildflowers bloom everywhere.

From the parking lot, begin walking uphill on a broad fire road. This trail provides access to many destinations farther up the mountain and is heavily used by cyclists and runners. It ascends at an easy grade through a mixed woodland of madrone, coast live oak, buckeye, and California bay. Early spring flowers include California buttercups and milkmaids. In winter months, the water rushing downhill from Phoenix Lake is a melodious accompaniment.

DISTANCE & CONFIGURATION: 4.8-mile balloon loop

DIFFICULTY: Easy

SCENERY: Grassland, woods, and lake

EXPOSURE: Nearly equal parts shade and sun

TRAIL TRAFFIC: Moderate–heavy

TRAIL SURFACE: Dirt fire roads and trails

HIKING TIME: 2.5 hours

DRIVING DISTANCE: 14.2 miles from the Golden Gate Bridge toll plaza

ACCESS: Daily, sunrise–sunset. Good year-round, although trails are muddy in winter. No fee.

WHEELCHAIR ACCESS: Not recommended for wheelchairs

MAPS: None at trailhead but available at tinyurl .com/mounttammarin. Map also available from Redwood Hikes Press (*Bay Area Trail Map: Mount Tamalpais*, $10.95, redwoodhikes.com/Store /MtTam.html).

FACILITIES: Pit toilets at trailhead and Phoenix Lake. Water available at the junction of Worn Springs and Phoenix Lake Trails.

CONTACT: 415-945-1180, marinwater.org/188 /Visiting-Watershed-Lands

LOCATION: Ross, CA

COMMENTS: Dogs welcome

The fire road passes the spillway and crests at 0.3 mile. Another fire road, the return route for this hike, heads off to the left, but you continue straight. After one last little hill, the fire road levels out. On the left Phoenix Lake stretches its arms into the creases of a wooded canyon. Mature buckeye, black oak, coast live oak, and California bay provide partial shade but still permit views to the lake. Worn Springs Fire Road departs from a small cluster of redwoods on the right at 0.4 mile, offering a steep route to Bald Hill. Continue on the tour around Phoenix Lake to the next junction, at 0.6 mile, then turn right onto Yolanda Trail.

This diminutive trail begins to climb at a moderate grade along a creekbed, through madrone, black oak, coast live oak, and California bay. Wildflowers emerge in these woods as early as January, when you might see hound's tongue, milkmaids, and shooting stars. In early spring, blue dicks, buttercups, and irises are common. Yolanda crosses the creek and winds uphill into a more grassy area somewhat overgrown with a young forest of broom. On one morning hike here, I got a little wakeup jolt when a jackrabbit came barreling down the trail toward me.

At 0.8 mile, after you pass a spur doubling back to the right and signed only with a NO HORSES symbol, the trail levels out for a few feet in a saddle between two hills, then skirts a knoll and begins a slight ascent across the flanks of Bald Hill to the right. Pockets of shaded California bay, coast live oak, buckeye, and madrone are interspersed with long sunny stretches through grassy chaparral, with chamise, sticky monkeyflower, sagebrush, toyon, and coyote brush enjoying the western exposure.

After rainstorms in winter, mini-waterfalls gush down the slopes of Bald Hill at nearly every little fold in the hillside. A March or April hike on this stretch of Yolanda Trail is usually a very good choice for wildflower-viewing. In early spring I've seen larkspur, blue dicks, shooting stars, paintbrush, popcorn flower, California poppy, blue and white lupine, and blue-eyed grass. During those soft days of late spring, grassy knolls, which extend off the trail on the left, invite a sunny snooze.

Mount Tamalpais: Phoenix Lake

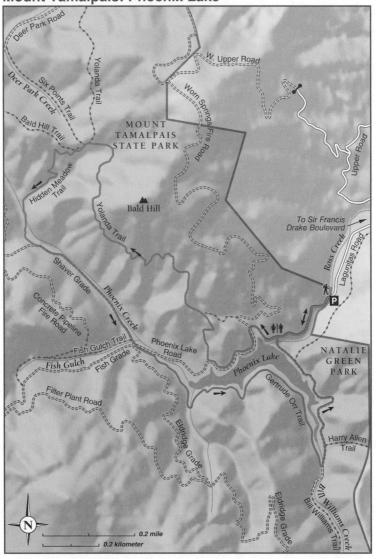

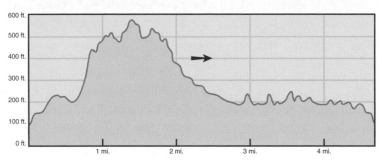

As the trail travels northwest, you have unobstructed views of Tam's summit ridgeline. Yolanda Trail then descends a bit through cool woods where a pint-size waterfall flows well into spring. It's such a spectacular journey that I always feel a little sad to reach Six Points Junction at 1.9 miles. Yolanda Trail continues right; then, moving counterclockwise, there's Six Points Trail, Bald Hill Trail, and Hidden Meadow Trail. Take Hidden Meadow Trail, to the left. As it starts to descend through oaks and then grassland, the panorama revealed on the left is one of my favorite Tam vistas. From Bald Hill to East Peak and everything in between, it's all beautiful. After a foray through grassland, the trail descends into a mixed woodland. A few short, tight switchbacks descend to cross a creek as the trail enters Hidden Meadow, a small, level, grassy shelf running between a creek on the left and an ascending hillside on the right. A forest of buckeye, California bay, and oak surrounds the meadow, and the trail winds among a few large oaks and buckeyes. Great colonies of hound's tongue linger at the fringes of the meadow in late winter.

The trail crosses another creek then turns to accompany the water flow toward Phoenix Lake. Some young redwoods are mixed through the forest. At 2.5 miles Hidden Meadow Trail ends at a junction with Shaver Grade. Turn left onto the fire road, which follows Phoenix Creek at an easy downhill grade. Be alert for bicycle traffic along this well-traveled route. The surrounding forest, where I've heard turkeys yodeling back and forth, is mostly California bay, redwood, madrone, bigleaf maple, and buckeye. At 2.9 miles Shaver Grade ends at a multiple junction. Fish Gulch Trail and Fish Grade climb off to the near right, and Eldridge Grade sets off to the far right. Continue straight; then, after about 300 feet, veer right onto Gertrude Orr Trail (signed with generic water-district HIKING ONLY symbols but not named at this junction). Tall hazelnut shrubs tower above the trail, welcoming visitors into a redwood forest. The trail follows Phoenix Creek about 150 feet, then reaches a junction just before a bridge. Turn right and cross the creek.

Gertrude Orr Trail runs along Phoenix Creek, which soon empties into the lake. Redwoods are common in the fingerlike extensions of the lake, accompanying ferns, hazelnut, creambush, and trilliums and milkmaids that bloom in early spring. In slightly sunnier stretches uphill from the shoreline, you might notice madrone, California bay, coast live oak, bigleaf maple, and black oak. The trail alternates level sections with some undulating areas where steps keep the path stable. Just past an area heavily colonized by tanoak, the trail rises, drops on a graceful flight of curving stairs, and then ends at 4.0 miles.

Bill Williams Trail heads deeper into the mountain, to the right. Turn left onto a fire road, ascending at a barely noticeable rate along the east shore of Phoenix Lake. On the right, look for a short but pretty waterfall that's active during the rainy season; redwood, bigleaf maple, madrone, and California bay line the trail. At 4.1 miles Harry Allen Trail sets off on the right, but continue on the fire road. Blossoms on broom and ceanothus shrubs draw hordes of bees in early spring, filling the air with a drowsy buzzing sound. Look for brilliant displays of red ribbon clarkia on the right in late spring. A bench a short distance off the trail to the left is a good spot to enjoy views that stretch across the lake to the crest of Bald Hill.

The fire road levels out above the dam, and a path leading back to Lagunitas Road departs on the right at 4.5 miles. The shallows to the left of the trail host many somewhat-tame ducks that often waddle over to quack for snacks along the shoreline. At 4.55 miles, you'll return to a familiar junction, above the spillway. Turn right and walk back downhill on the fire road.

• •

GPS TRAILHEAD COORDINATES N37° 57.473' W122° 34.348'

DIRECTIONS From the Golden Gate Bridge toll plaza, drive north on US 101 about 10 miles, then take Exit 450B, Sir Francis Drake/San Anselmo. Stay left, toward San Anselmo, and drive west on Sir Francis Drake Boulevard about 3 miles to the intersection with Lagunitas Road (at the Marin Art and Garden Center). Turn left onto Lagunitas Road and drive about 1 mile to the parking lot at the end of the road.

Milkmaids, a common winter wildflower

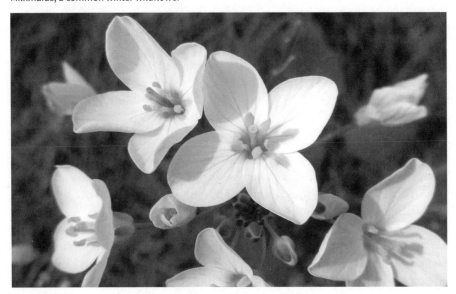

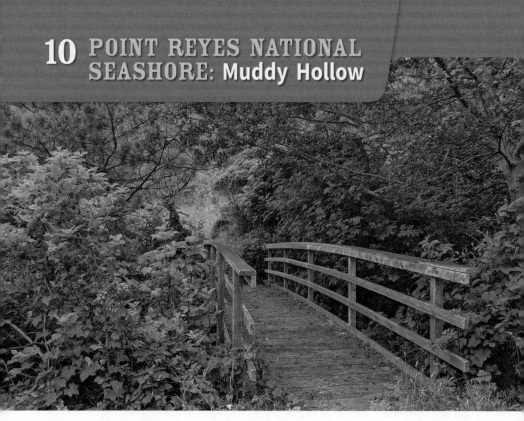

Bridge over Glenbrook Creek

THE AREA AROUND Muddy Hollow offers exceptional wildlife-viewing. You may see tule elk, as some of the herd from Tomales Point have been relocated to this part of the seashore. Songbirds and hawks are common, and rabbits (and rabbit fur) may be glimpsed throughout the coastal scrub. Foxes, coyotes, bobcats, and even mountain lions also roam these lands. Berry enthusiasts hiking in summer may find themselves in purple-stained-finger heaven. Blackberry brambles sprawl across hillsides, thimbleberries hide in the shade on Estero Trail, and salmonberries—rare in the Bay Area—line Muddy Hollow Trail.

DESCRIPTION

Most Point Reyes visitors know that Limantour Road leads to the hostel and is a quick route to a gorgeous beach. A number of the seashore's lesser-known and most primitive trailheads are reached from the Limantour area as well, like this loop from Muddy Hollow.

From the parking area at the trailhead, start in front of the trail markers at the junction of Muddy Hollow Road and Muddy Hollow Trail. Walk north on Muddy Hollow Road (toward Bayview Trail), which is open to equestrians and hikers only. After a few steps on the wide trail, you'll cross a creek then step into coastal scrub. At 0.1 mile Bayview Trail heads uphill to the right at a signed junction. Continue

DISTANCE & CONFIGURATION: 7.4-mile loop with other options (see Nearby Activities, page 63)

DIFFICULTY: Moderate

SCENERY: Coastal scrub and ocean views

EXPOSURE: Full sun except for a few pockets of shade

TRAIL TRAFFIC: Light

TRAIL SURFACE: Dirt fire roads and trails

HIKING TIME: 3 hours

DRIVING DISTANCE: 39 miles from the Golden Gate Bridge toll plaza

ACCESS: Daily, sunrise–midnight. Muddy in winter; otherwise wonderful year-round. No fee.

WHEELCHAIR ACCESS: Not recommended for wheelchairs

MAPS: Pick up the free official Point Reyes trail map at the Bear Valley Visitor Center, or download it at nps.gov/pore/planyourvisit/upload/map_trailsnorth.pdf.

FACILITIES: None at this trailhead

CONTACT: 415-464-5100; nps.gov/pore

LOCATION: Inverness, CA

COMMENTS: No dogs allowed

straight on Muddy Hollow Road. Some cypresses, bush lupines, ceanothus, and Bishop pines grow near the junction; coyote brush is the dominant trailside plant. Muddy Hollow Road climbs gently, with a forest of Bishop pines continuing to march across the hillsides burned in the Mount Vision fire of 1995. Look right for a rocky outcrop on the side of the hill. At 0.9 mile Muddy Hollow Road meets Bucklin Trail at a signed junction. Continue straight/left on Muddy Hollow Road.

The trail bends right and begins to descend gently through coastal scrub. This segment replaces the old fire road, shifting traffic away from Glenbrook Creek's damp upper basin, instead traveling across hillsides to the north of the old section. This is a very quiet part of the park. You are likely to see wildflowers blooming in every month of the year, from ceanothus in winter to monkeyflower in autumn. Muddy Hollow Road (here a narrow path) crosses a bridge and begins an easy climb through grassland and pine. The trail crests and then meets Glenbrook Trail at a signed junction at 2.3 miles. Turn left on Glenbrook.

The trail, closed to cyclists, climbs easily through coyote brush and pines. You might see pussy ears, clover, iris, California buttercup, and blue-eyed grass in spring. As Glenbrook levels out and heads south toward the ocean, on a clear day look back to the north for views of Mount Vision, and east to recap the hike so far. Glenbrook is straight and the trail surface is grassy. Hawks and harriers swoop overhead, searching for cottontails. I'd say from the amount of rabbit fur along the trail, the hunters are frequently successful. At 3.0 miles Glenbrook Trail ends at a signed junction with Estero Trail. Remain straight, now on Estero Trail.

From here it's a lonely near-4-mile stretch to the next trail junction. Estero continues, descending slightly. Limantour Estero is visible to the right. You might hear sea lions or harbor seals beached on Limantour Spit. Ignore any side paths as Estero turns left, away from the ocean, and heads back north. Estero Trail descends gently, passes a few eucalyptus trees, and then turns and crosses Glenbrook Creek on a bridge. Meandering through an enchanting little pocket of alder, thimbleberry,

Point Reyes National Seashore: Muddy Hollow

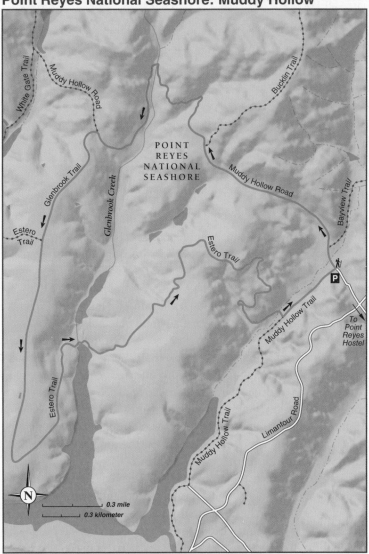

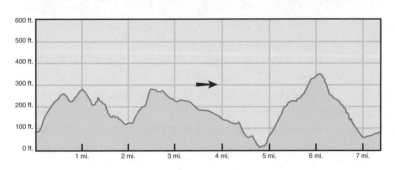

nettle, and salmonberry, look for huge cow parsnips towering over 5 feet, while miner's lettuce and candy flower nestle close to the damp ground. After passing through the pocket of green near the creek, Estero Trail, now shrunken to a narrow path, steps back out into coastal scrub. Spring flowers include iris, blue-eyed grass, paintbrush, lupine, and checkerbloom—watch out for poison oak here. Elk are now common in this part of Point Reyes, and you may see them (usually in herds) or at least their scat. On an October hike I startled a herd that were munching at the edge of the marsh. They ran off in a hurry, with aquatic plants streaming from their heads like green wigs. The trail bends left (the old trail segment that went south to Muddy Hollow is fenced off and closed) and begins to climb along the slope of a long hill. Bishop pines line the trail, but grassland still dominates here. (But for how long? The trees grow fast!) Irises are gorgeous in spring, and in summer you may see a variety of butterflies, including buckeyes, checkerspots, and mylitta crescents. Estero Trail keeps climbing, but the grade is easy, and before long you'll be cresting the hill. A bench on the left offers great views past sloping grassland and coastal scrub north to Chimney Rock. Now the sandy path descends, bisecting a crowded Bishop pine forest. If these young trees thin themselves, a new understory may fill in, including huckleberry and salal. Once through the forest, the trail drops into Muddy Hollow and ends at 7.0 miles. Turn left onto Muddy Hollow Trail. The wide alder-lined fire road offers an easy return to the trailhead—it's just 0.4 mile back to the parking lot.

NEARBY ACTIVITIES

Lonely Muddy Hollow is the starting point for a number of loop hikes. You can trek up Bucklin Trail and return via Drakes View Trail, a 7-mile loop. For a 9-mile loop, string together Bayview, Laguna, and Coast Trails, finishing up on the gravel road past the hostel and down to Muddy Hollow. Or extend the featured hike by remaining on Muddy Hollow Road at the junction with Glenbrook. Turn left on White Gate Road, left on Estero, and then right at the junction with Glenbrook, and continue the featured hike.

• •

GPS TRAILHEAD COORDINATES N38° 02.884' W122° 52.157'

DIRECTIONS From the Golden Gate Bridge toll plaza, drive north on US 101 about 10 miles, and take Exit 450B, Sir Francis Drake Boulevard/San Anselmo. Stay left toward San Anselmo and drive west about 20 miles on Sir Francis Drake Boulevard to the junction with CA 1. Turn right and drive 0.1 mile, then turn left onto Bear Valley Road. Drive 1.8 miles, then turn left onto Limantour Road. Continue about 6 miles, then turn right onto the signed road accessing Muddy Hollow. Drive 0.2 mile to the parking lot at the end of the road.

11 POINT REYES NATIONAL SEASHORE: Tomales Point

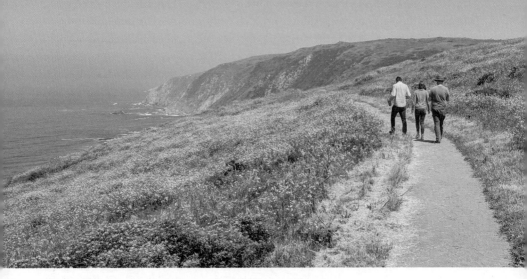

On an early-morning hike, fog may conceal some of the coastal scenery.

ANIMAL SIGHTINGS ARE not uncommon in the Bay Area, but at a few locations you are nearly assured of a peek at wild creatures. One of the best spots is Point Reyes' Tomales Point. This hike is an out-and-back trek on a remote peninsula where tule elk roam through coastal scrub and birds paddle in the ocean and soar through the skies. Bring binoculars, a hat, and a windbreaker.

DESCRIPTION

At its northwestern edge, Point Reyes tapers to Tomales Point. Pierce Point Ranch occupied the area until 1973, and the farm buildings, now historically preserved, stand near the Tomales Point trailhead. A self-guided tour through the ranch is a fine way to begin (or end) a hike. In 1978, 10 tule elk were reintroduced to the point, which was then fenced off from the rest of Point Reyes. Other creatures you might see on the point are a variety of birds, coyotes, bobcats, and (although sightings are rare) mountain lions.

The weather plays a big part in enhancing (or ruining) hikes along the coast, and Tomales Point is no exception. Attempt a hike during one of the Bay Area's famous foggy summer days, and not only will the views be completely obscured, but the wind can also chill you thoroughly. Spring and autumn are the best seasons for

DISTANCE & CONFIGURATION: 7.6-mile out-and-back

DIFFICULTY: Moderate

SCENERY: Coastal scrub, grassland, and coastal views

EXPOSURE: Full sun

TRAIL TRAFFIC: Heavy

TRAIL SURFACE: Broad, sandy fire road and meandering paths, with some loose sand

HIKING TIME: 4 hours

DRIVING DISTANCE: 48 miles from the Golden Gate Bridge toll plaza

ACCESS: Daily, sunrise–midnight. Spring and autumn are best. No fee.

WHEELCHAIR ACCESS: Wheelchairs can access the trail from the parking lot, but the trail is sandy and narrow, so wheelchairs are not recommended.

MAPS: Pick up the free official Point Reyes trail map at the Bear Valley Visitor Center, or download it at nps.gov/pore/planyourvisit/upload /map_trailsnorth.pdf.

FACILITIES: None at trailhead; pit toilets at nearby McClures Beach

CONTACT: 415-464-5100; nps.gov/pore

LOCATION: Inverness, CA

COMMENTS: No dogs allowed. From this trailhead (or from a second parking lot 0.1 mile west), it's a 1-mile round-trip hike to McClures Beach.

a visit; note that when the elk rut (July–November), males are more aggressive and you should give them an extra-wide berth.

The trail starts at a level grade, skirting the ranch buildings before heading into a grassy community of coastal scrub plants, dominated by coyote brush. In early spring, wild radish covers the knoll on the left, presenting a lavish display of white and lavender blossoms. Northern harriers seem to favor the point, and you might see one or two fluttering in place above the ground, looking for a meal. As the trail travels north it offers views of the coastline, which past McClures Beach gradually ascends to steep, rocky bluffs. Tomales Point Trail drifts downhill to aptly named Windy Gap. The sloping valley on the right is a favorite spot for elk. A brief moderate ascent brings the trail up to the grassy ridgeline, dotted in some spots with wind-sculpted coyote brush. Look left for ocean views and right to take in the hills of Bolinas Ridge rolling up from Tomales Bay. The trail descends to Lower Pierce Point Ranch, a site now marked by a handful of cypress trees often occupied by raptors. Salmonberry shrubs mingle through stinging nettles in a damp spot on the right.

Once again the trail begins to climb, but here vegetation begins to crowd the route. Somewhat abruptly, the path dissolves to sand at about 3 miles—some firmer patches are ahead, but this is the trend for the rest of the trail. Navigating becomes a bit tricky, as elk paths score the area, so try to stick close to the ridgeline and keep heading northwest. Elk scat is common everywhere, and you stand a good chance of observing tule elk if you keep your noise level down. On the other hand, if you're *too* quiet, you might come across a loner mostly camouflaged by the tall, thick stands of lizardtail and yellow bush lupine. Even if you don't see them, you'll hear them—elk bellows are unlike any other animal vocalization I've ever heard. I can only describe the sound as similar to a loud, high-pitched door squeak.

Point Reyes National Seashore: Tomales Point

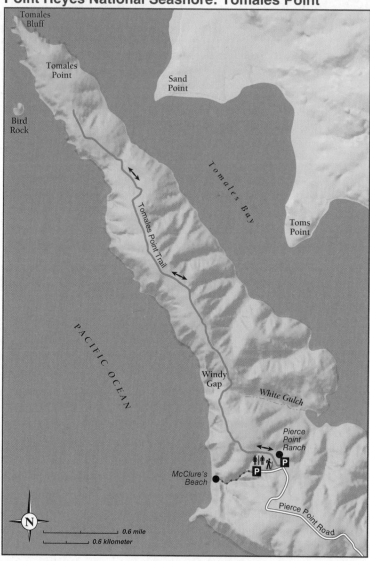

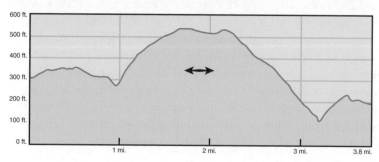

The trail finally begins to descend slightly, signaling that the first leg of the hike is near its end. *Warning:* Be careful of unannounced sheer drop-offs on the left—the views are incredible, but the ground can be unstable near the edge. This is one of the most isolated and quietest hiking destinations on the coast, where the only sounds are the crash of the surf, the cries of the birds, and the peal of a buoy near the mouth of Tomales Bay. At about 3.8 miles a bare spot—kind of a sandy bowl that's a bit sheltered from the wind—makes a decent rest stop, especially if you're in a group. Beyond that, a tiny path drops straight down to the tip of the point, but I don't recommend this option. After you've had your fill of this coastal gem, backtrack to the trailhead.

• •

GPS TRAILHEAD COORDINATES N38° 11.348' W122° 57.248'

DIRECTIONS From the Golden Gate Bridge toll plaza, drive north on US 101 about 10 miles, then take Exit 450B, Sir Francis Drake Boulevard/San Anselmo. Stay left toward San Anselmo and drive west about 20 miles on Sir Francis Drake Boulevard to the junction with CA 1. Turn right and drive 0.1 mile, then turn left onto Bear Valley Road. After about 2 miles, Bear Valley Road ends at Sir Francis Drake Boulevard; turn left. Continue on Sir Francis Drake about 5.5 miles, then veer right onto Pierce Point Road. Drive about 9 miles on Pierce Point Road to the signed Tomales Point trailhead, a short distance from McClures Beach at the end of the road.

Elk at Tomales Point

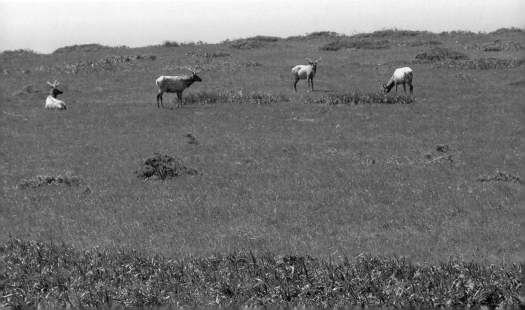

12 RING MOUNTAIN OPEN SPACE PRESERVE

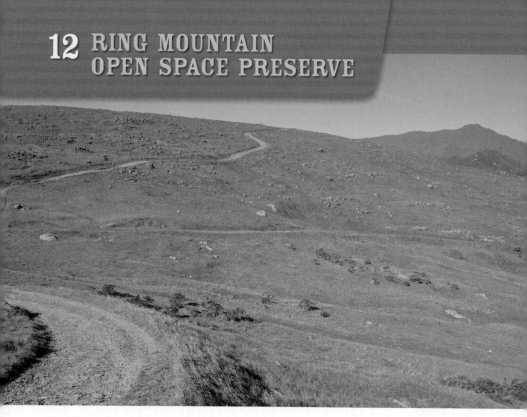

Mount Tamalpais seen from Ring Mountain

THERE'S A DRAMATIC backdrop to the spectacular views hikers enjoy on Ring Mountain. Although small and contained by Tiburon residential neighborhoods, the preserve hosts an incredibly rare flower.

DESCRIPTION

This small preserve sits on ultraprime real estate. A short drive from US 101, Ring Mountain offers views of San Pablo Bay, Mount Tamalpais, and San Francisco. The property was never developed because of a single flower: the Tiburon mariposa lily, which grows in a small section of Ring Mountain and nowhere else in the world. Access the preserve from an open-space gate, and stop at the information signboard for a map, which also contains the key for the self-guided tour.

Beginning on Phyllis Ellman Loop Trail, you'll skirt a marshy area then climb through rocky grassland, coyote brush, and poison oak. These lower reaches of Ring Mountain are dominated by a damp basin fed from little streams. In winter, near Post 1, look for osoberry, a slight deciduous shrub that produces clusters of little white nodding flowers. At 0.2 mile the trail splits; you can hike the loop in either direction, but to follow the self-guided tour and these directions, turn left. Maintaining an easy grade, the trail travels laterally across the hillside. Toyon, coyote brush, young California bays, and some poison oak dot the grassland. Wildflowers are

DISTANCE & CONFIGURATION: 1.9-mile balloon loop

DIFFICULTY: Easy

SCENERY: Rock-strewn grassland and views

EXPOSURE: Mostly unshaded

TRAIL TRAFFIC: Moderate

TRAIL SURFACE: Dirt fire roads and trails

HIKING TIME: 1 hour

DRIVING DISTANCE: 10.7 miles from the Golden Gate Bridge toll plaza

ACCESS: Daily, sunrise–sunset. Good year-round; Tiburon mariposa lilies usually bloom mid-May–early June. Trails are muddy in winter.

No fee. There's no parking lot but plenty of street parking along Paradise Drive.

WHEELCHAIR ACCESS: Not recommended for wheelchairs

MAPS: Available at an information signboard inside the preserve and tinyurl.com/ringmtn ospmap

CONTACT: 415-473-2816, marincountyparks .org/parkspreserves/preserves/ring-mountain

LOCATION: Corte Madera, CA

COMMENTS: Because of the rare plants that thrive here, take special care to stay on the trails. Leashed dogs welcome.

sprinkled across these sloping, grassy hillsides from February through late summer. The first arrivals are often milkmaids and buttercups, followed by blue-eyed grass, lupine, Ithuriel's spear, and, later still, tarweed.

Where the trail crosses the creek, look right for ninebark, a shrub with leaves that resemble blackberry and currant. Like those edible, berry-producing plants, ninebark is a member of the rose family and prefers a moist yet exposed environment. Ninebark's bracts of red flowers set it apart from its kindred berry plants.

Just past Post 7 stay right, avoiding a well-trampled path that heads left and steeply uphill toward the ridge. At the next unsigned split, at 0.7 mile, stay left or you'll shortcut the loop—you should be continuing uphill. The trees get bigger and more impressive on this part of the mountain, despite the exposed location. Post 8 points out a massive coast live oak, and near Post 9 the trail winds through an incredible multitrunked California bay—one of the magical spots on the mountain.

As the trail presses on uphill, Mount Tamalpais's east peak pops up to the west. Past the creek's headwaters, the trees fade away and grassland returns, although you'll wind through one last cluster of bays and oaks near the crest. Where the first leg of Phyllis Ellman Loop Trail ends at a junction with a fire road at 0.9 mile, you'll surely want to pause and savor the views south, which extend past Richardson Bay to San Francisco. The big hunk of a rock just off the trail on the left is Turtle Rock. Turn right onto Ring Mountain Fire Road.

As the fire road follows the bare ridgeline, there are dead-on views to Mount Tam. After a brief downhill stretch, and when you reach a saddle where trails stretch out in each direction at 1 mile, turn right on Phyllis Ellman Loop Trail. Returning downhill, the long views north may distract you from the trailside display of flowers. The rocky soil along the trail sustains native wildflowers, including the Tiburon mariposa lily. These unusual flowers bloom when the grassland fades from green to tan, so they blend into the landscape. Find just one and then you'll likely see dozens.

Ring Mountain Open Space Preserve

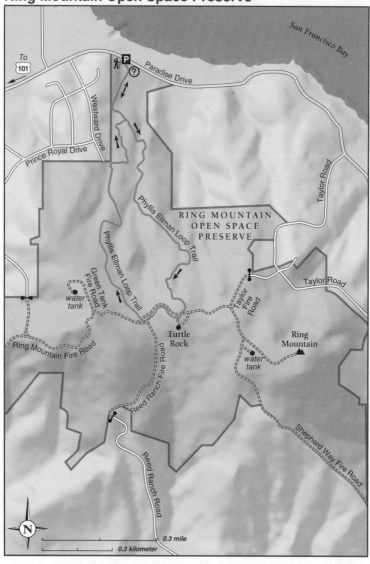

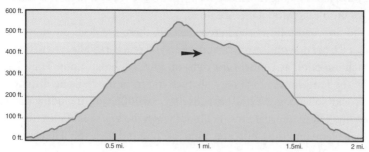

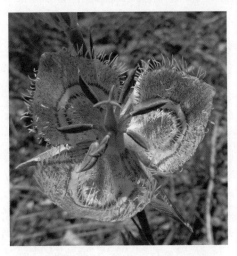

The beautiful and unusual Tiburon mariposa lily

As you continue downhill, San Quentin State Prison is visible, perched on the edge of its namesake point. A gracefully canopied buckeye tree sits alone in the grassland on the right. A trail heads right and bisects the loop at 1.4 miles. Continue downhill to the left, following the route highlighted by a couple of arrow signs. In winter, before rains transform the hillsides into a verdant canvas, toyon shrubs loaded with cheerful red berries are a favorite of small birds. Where the loop closes at about 1.7 miles, stay left and retrace your steps back to the trailhead.

• •

GPS TRAILHEAD COORDINATES N37° 55.254' W122° 29.657'

DIRECTIONS From the Golden Gate Bridge toll plaza, drive north 9 miles on US 101 and take Exit 449, Paradise Drive/Tamalpais Drive. Turn right onto Tamalpais, drive east a short distance, and bear right onto San Clemente Drive (before The Village shopping center). After a few blocks, San Clemente dumps into Paradise Drive. Continue on Paradise 0.9 mile, past Westward Drive to the preserve gate, on the right side of the road.

Fiddleneck and California poppies on the upper reaches of Barnabe Peak

FROM AN EASE-OF-HIKING STANDPOINT, this 6.2-mile Barnabe Peak loop is close to perfect—like taking the escalator up and the elevator down. An easily graded path starts along a creek where salmon spawn some winters, makes a short detour to a waterfall, and then ascends through wooded canyons to the high, grassy slopes of Barnabe Peak. From a viewpoint with sweeping vistas of Point Reyes, Mount Tamalpais, and Bolinas Ridge, you'll return downhill on a moderately steep fire road through grassland and back into woods.

DESCRIPTION

Samuel P. Taylor State Park's Barnabe Peak hides in plain sight. Although the 1,466-foot mountain is bare at the summit, the lower reaches are heavily forested, obscuring views from the bottom to the top. The park's campground, picnic sites, and ranger station sit in a canyon alongside Lagunitas Creek, where hillsides covered with redwood and Douglas-fir ascend to Bolinas Ridge (out of the park, but part of the Golden Gate National Recreation Area). Across Sir Francis Drake Boulevard on the low slopes of Barnabe Peak, redwood groves thrive near the creek, while Douglas-fir, California bay, and coast live oak woods fill steep-sided canyons where small waterfalls run in winter and spring. At the top, near a Marin County fire lookout, wildflower displays brighten the grassland in spring.

DISTANCE & CONFIGURATION: 6.2-mile balloon loop

DIFFICULTY: Moderate

SCENERY: Douglas-fir, California bay, bigleaf maple, and coast live oak woods; creek; waterfall; grassland; and views

EXPOSURE: Start and finish are shaded; middle section is exposed.

TRAIL TRAFFIC: Light from autumn to spring; moderate during summer camping season

TRAIL SURFACE: Dirt fire roads and trails

HIKING TIME: 3.5 hours

DRIVING DISTANCE: 27 miles from the Golden Gate Bridge toll plaza

ACCESS: Daily, 8 a.m.–sunset. Best in winter for the waterfall and in spring for the flowers. Muddy after rains. No fee at this trailhead.

WHEELCHAIR ACCESS: Usually unobstructed (a vehicle gate is sometimes closed—call to check), and folks with wheels should be able to navigate at least 0.15 mile on Devil's Gulch Road. There is no designated handicapped parking at this trailhead, and you must cross Sir Francis Drake Boulevard to access Devil's Gulch Road.

MAPS: Available at ranger station (when staffed), 1 mile back down Sir Francis Drake Boulevard, or tinyurl.com/samtaylorsp

FACILITIES: None at trailhead; pit toilets at Devil's Gulch Horse Camp

CONTACT: 415-488-9897, tinyurl.com/sam taylorsp

LOCATION: Lagunitas, CA

COMMENTS: No dogs allowed. From the park-headquarters trailhead, you can make a 3-mile loop through redwoods on Pioneer Tree Trail.

From the pullout, carefully cross Sir Francis Drake Boulevard, and begin walking up a paved, gated service road signed for Devil's Gulch Horse Camp. This nearly level road runs along one of the feeder streams for the largest waterway in the park, Lagunitas Creek. The sides of the trail are lined with buckeye, California bay, redwood, Douglas-fir, bigleaf maple, and California nutmeg, with wild rose, poison oak, hazelnut, and blackberry in the understory. After 0.1 mile veer right onto a path signed with NO DOGS/BIKES/HORSES icons. The first of two interpretive signs explains that coho salmon and steelhead trout arrive in this creek when the water level is high enough for them to spawn, generally October–March. I've never visited when the creek was full, but in early spring I always scan the water, just in case. The little path weaves around California bays and coast live oaks and then, at 0.3 mile, reaches a junction I call Redwood Fork, for the huge tree just off the trail. A path to the left leads to the horse camp. Cross the bridge to a T-junction, then turn left onto Bill's Trail.

Now on the opposite bank of the creek, the multiuse trail starts a slight climb. In spring look for columbine, woodland star, fringe cup, iris, starflower, and bleeding heart peeking out from a lush landscape of ferns, hazelnut, Douglas-fir, and California bay. This sheltered canyon is home to some very large, old trees, including some graceful mature bigleaf maples. At 0.9 mile the trail forks. Veer left to visit Stairstep Falls.

The path descends gradually at first, just barely clinging to the hillside. In the wettest months you'll hear the gush of water long before the path curves right and ends at the falls at about the 1-mile mark. Stairstep Falls, as the name suggests, is a tiered waterfall with three drops totaling about 35 feet. When ready, return to Bill's Trail and turn left.

Samuel P. Taylor State Park

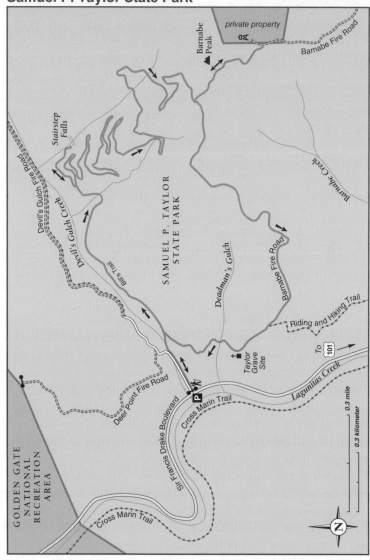

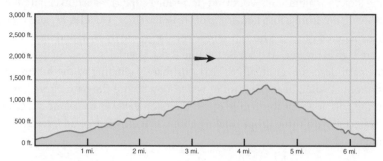

A long series of drawn-out switchbacks begins, keeping the grade incredibly easy. The first time I hiked this loop, it was so windy that tree branches crashed to the ground continuously, and I felt lucky to escape without a beaning. Usually these woods are almost totally quiet, except for the sound of the wind through the trees and birdsong. Wildflowers begin to bloom along the trail as early as February, when the first blossoms on pink-flowering currant and milkmaids appear. Hound's tongue and checker lily are usually the next to bloom, in March; later still, you might see varieties of iris, lots of woodland star, fringe cup, starflower, and California larkspur. Banana slugs creep across the trail, in the shade of Douglas-fir, coast live oak, bigleaf maple, and California bay. Evergreen California nutmegs are common and easy to identify by their fleshy, olive-shaped arils (eaten by birds, but not edible for humans)—much different from redwood and Douglas-fir cones. Beware of poison oak, which crowds the trail in many areas.

As the trail ascends you'll cross pretty bridges and pass through woods and a few small grassy knolls. Near the end of the trail, the grassy patches are more common and bigger. Finally, at 3.8 miles, Bill's Trail emerges from the woods and ends at Barnabe Fire Road. Turn left.

After miles of easy hiking, the moderately steep uphill grade of the fire road is less than ideal, but the setting makes up for the climb. To the west, rolling grassy hills, dotted in spring with California poppy, buttercup, and clarkia, drift downhill and meet, on the other side of the canyon, a forest of evergreens, thickly covering the ascending slope. Ahead, the fire lookout at the mountaintop is conspicuous, so with the goal in sight, trudge on uphill, winding through grassland and small pockets of California bay. At 4.1 miles you'll reach a junction at a fenceline and the park boundary. Ridge Trail continues right, descending steeply along a grassy ridge to a redwood forest.

The fire lookout sits on private property, so mind the NO TRESPASSING signs while enjoying outstanding views—particularly to the northwest—of Tomales Bay, the entire Point Reyes Peninsula, and Bolinas Ridge. Gaze south here for a rare glimpse of Kent Lake's spillway, most evident when the runoff is heavy.

When I hiked here one May, I found a sheltered spot on the slope of the peak and lunched alongside a nonplussed western fence lizard while bees browsed the huckleberry blossoms. If you're here in spring, you may want to look through the grass downhill near the junction for creamcup, California poppy, clover, fiddleneck, clarkia, and checkerbloom, with the best displays occurring in early May. When you're ready, retrace your steps back downhill past the junction with Bill's Trail, continuing on the fire road.

Barnabe Fire Road drops moderately steeply, with the upper reaches of a forested canyon on the right and grassland on the left, then swings left away from the canyon into grassland and coyote brush. In spring look for paintbrush, sticky monkeyflower, blue-eyed grass, and buttercup. Other than one short uphill stretch, this is a quad-working downhill segment. At 5.4 miles Riding and Hiking Trail departs left; continue straight. The trail continues to descend. A white-picket-fenced plot is visible ahead; this is the grave site of the park's namesake, and the path leading to it breaks off to the left at 5.5 miles, a 0.1-mile out-and-back spur. Samuel P. Taylor, a gold rush entrepreneur, bought the area now preserved as this park and built a paper mill along the creek. It's widely reported that he named the tallest peak on his property after his mule Barnabe. (Bet his wife loved that!)

Past the grave-site path, Barnabe Fire Road returns to woods in Deadman's Gulch, an area that's often very muddy after rains. The trail bends left and sweeps around the base of a hill. On my May hike, butterflies fluttered everywhere, landing on buttercups and blue-eyed grass flowers strewn through the grass. The fire road commences its moderately steep descent through the woods. At 5.9 miles you'll reach the first bridge and junction with Bill's Trail again. Turn left and retrace your steps back to the trailhead.

• •

GPS TRAILHEAD COORDINATES N38° 01.783' W122° 44.207'

DIRECTIONS From the Golden Gate Bridge toll plaza, drive north on US 101 about 10 miles, then take Exit 450B, Sir Francis Drake Boulevard/San Anselmo. Stay left toward San Anselmo and drive west on Sir Francis Drake Boulevard 15 miles, then continue past the main park entrance 1 more mile to a dirt pullout on the left, just past the DEVIL'S GULCH sign on the right.

A snarl of old trees along Devil's Gulch Creek at Samuel P. Taylor State Park

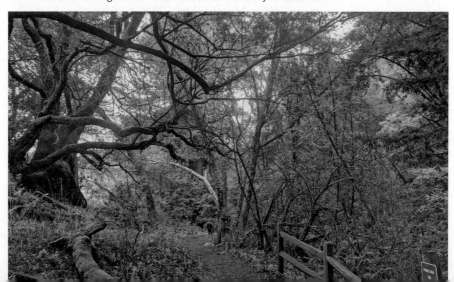

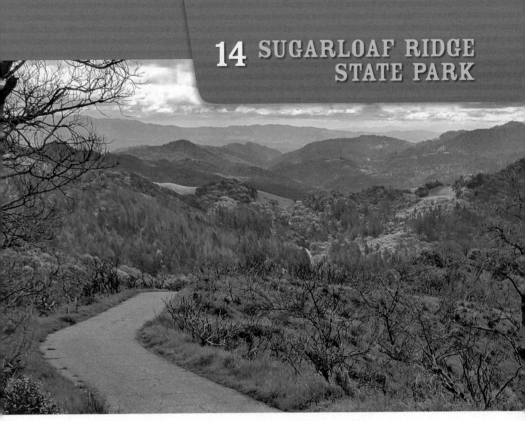

A landscape recovering from wildfires at Sugarloaf Ridge State Park

SUGARLOAF RIDGE'S BALD MOUNTAIN holds bragging rights to one of the prettiest and most serene viewpoints in the Bay Area. From a relatively diminutive height of 2,729 feet, views include every significant wine-country peak and valley. This hike starts at the edge of a sloping meadow, climbing steadily through a mixture of grassland, chaparral, and woodland for 2.5 miles to the summit. The return route travels along a quiet ridge, drops steeply through gray pines and chaparral to cross Sonoma Creek, and then wanders across a meadow on the way back to the trailhead.

DESCRIPTION

At Sugarloaf Ridge, every step seems like a gift. From the get-go, the trails are quiet and the scenery is gorgeous—views from the top of Bald Mountain are icing on the cake. There's so much variety at Sugarloaf that every season has its charm. Sonoma Creek's headwaters originate here, and in winter, streams gush downhill at such a rate that you may feel transported from dry California to a more lush locale. Spring flowers are pretty, and the temperatures are hospitable. Summer (if you can endure the heat) brings hillsides stacked with fragrant blooming chamise. In autumn, foliage on black oaks and bigleaf maples is stunning. The tragic fires of October 2017 burned more than 75% of the park, but Sugarloaf is recovering—park staff and volunteers

DISTANCE & CONFIGURATION: 6.4-mile loop, with a shorter option

DIFFICULTY: Moderate

SCENERY: Grassland, oaks, views, chaparral, and creeks

EXPOSURE: Mostly full sun

TRAIL TRAFFIC: Light

TRAIL SURFACE: Dirt fire roads, rocky trails, and 1 paved fire road

HIKING TIME: 3.5 hours

DRIVING DISTANCE: 53.8 miles from the Golden Gate Bridge toll plaza

ACCESS: Daily, 6 a.m.–8 p.m. Spring is best;

muddy after rains and hot in summer. Pay the $8 fee at the entrance kiosk.

WHEELCHAIR ACCESS: Not recommended for wheelchairs

MAPS: Available at visitor center or entrance kiosk (when staffed) or tinyurl.com/sugarloaf parkmap

FACILITIES: Portable toilet at trailhead

CONTACT: 707-833-5712, tinyurl.com/sugar loafridgesp, sugarloafpark.org

LOCATION: Kenwood, CA

COMMENTS: Dogs are not permitted on park trails. After rains, you'll get your feet wet crossing Sonoma Creek.

have rebuilt bridges, benches, and trail signs. The flames scorched chaparral and trees, actually improving views from most of the trails. Visit often to observe the changing natural restoration.

Begin from the parking lot on Lower Bald Mountain Trail. At an easy grade, the rocky path begins to ascend from the valley floor, winding through grassland past a few coast live oaks, Douglas-firs, and manzanitas. Look for goldfields, buttercups, shooting stars, irises, blue dicks, and blue-eyed grass in spring. A few small ceanothus shrubs growing close to the ground suggest the presence of serpentine soil—while it may not be obvious in this part of the park, significant serpentine swales are visible off Bald Mountain and Gray Pine Trails.

After a short foray through some trees, Lower Bald Mountain Trail returns to grassland and reaches a junction with Meadow Trail at 0.3 mile. Stay left on Lower Bald Mountain Trail. The grade picks up as the path climbs into an open woodland composed mostly of madrone, coast live oak, California bay, and manzanita. On an April hike, I saw jackrabbits hopping up the trail. Switchbacking uphill between two creekbeds, the trail gradually transitions to chaparral, where chamise, toyon, scrub oak, ceanothus, sticky monkeyflower, and poison oak are the most notable plants. The deep umber color of the trail surface is adobe clay. This rocky segment ends at a T-junction at 0.9 mile. Turn right onto Bald Mountain Trail.

The trail—a wide, paved road used to access communications equipment atop Red Mountain—ascends at a moderate, steady pace. Vegetation ranges from chamise, manzanita, toyon, monkeyflower, and poison oak to coast live oak and madrone. In spring, flowering purple bush lupine brightens the sides of the trail. At the 1.2-mile mark, Vista Trail departs on the right, offering an early out for hikers who are discouraged by the grade or want a shorter hike. Continue uphill on Bald Mountain Trail.

Sugarloaf Ridge State Park

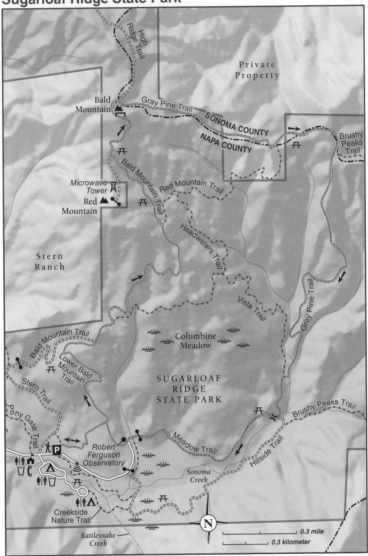

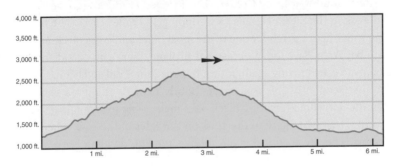

In winter and early spring, the sound of running water from a creek out of sight on the right will probably accompany your hike. Bald Mountain Trail sweeps uphill through an open area where ceanothus and coyote brush are common. At one corner, water spills downhill from the left then drops into a ravine where buckeyes nestle. California poppies, blue and white lupine, and scorpionweed bloom along the trail in May. As the trail climbs, trailside vegetation reflects the change in elevation and exposure—there's lots of chamise, ceanothus, cercocarpus, and scrub oak. At about 1.7 miles, if the day is clear, pause and look south to see Mount Diablo and Mount Tamalpais. Red Mountain Trail breaks off to the right at 1.9 miles, headed toward Gray Pine Trail. Continue straight on Bald Mountain Trail.

In the shadow of Red Mountain, the trail is lined with black oak, bigleaf maple, California bay, and live oak. After a swing into grassland, you'll reach a junction and saddle at 2.2 miles. Straight ahead, the hillside drops then gradually rises to the flanks of Mount Hood. The pavement curves left on a dead-end spur to Red Mountain. Turn right, remaining on Bald Mountain Trail.

Now a dirt fire road, the trail adopts a moderately steep course uphill through grassland. You may notice bluish serpentine, exposed on a rock cut on the left. The grassy hillside on the right gently slips away, offering expansive views south. On an April visit, blooming popcorn flowers painted huge white swaths in spring's still-green grass. As you follow Bald Mountain Trail, sweeping around the very top of the mountain, ignore any side trails and persist to a signed junction at 2.5 miles. Here High Ridge Trail heads left on a dead-end journey. Turn right onto Gray Pine Trail. After just a few feet, Gray Pine veers left. Turn right and walk uphill a few more feet to the summit. Interpretive signs assist you in identifying the surrounding sites: In the immediate area you can see Napa Valley, Sonoma Valley, the steep hillsides of Jack London State Historic Park, and the more gently graded hillsides of Trione-Annadel State Park. On one April hike, the top of Mount Saint Helena, to the north of Sugarloaf, hid in a puffy white cloud.

When visibility permits, you may also see Mount Wittenberg, the highest peak on Point Reyes (33 miles west); Snow Mountain (65 miles north and, because it's well named, easy to pick out); Mount Diablo (51 miles southeast); Mount Tamalpais (37 miles southwest); the Golden Gate Bridge (44 miles southwest); and even Pyramid Peak in the Sierra Nevada (a whopping 129 miles east). The bench at the grassy summit offers a perch for one of the most quiet and gorgeous lunch breaks in the entire Bay Area. Save for an occasional airplane, there's no outside noise. When you're ready to start moving again, return to Gray Pine Trail and begin to descend.

The first section of this trail seems poorly named, as there's nary a pine in sight. On the left, some towering black oaks make a big foliage impact in autumn, but in spring, train your gaze to the grass on the sides of the trail, where bird's-eye gilia blooms. The fire road just about follows the line dividing Napa and Sonoma

Counties as it descends, generally along the ridgeline. You'll see more manzanita, California bay, Douglas-fir, coyote brush, chamise, and toyon. In early April, blue-blossom ceanothus flowers are followed a bit later by clematis, a trailing vine with white flowers, which drapes itself over shrubs. Although the route is downhill, there is one short uphill section. At 3.3 miles Red Mountain Trail ventures off to the right—you could make an alternate return on Red Mountain, Headwaters, and Vista Trails. For this hike, continue straight on Gray Pine Trail.

As you descend at a slightly steep pitch, look for woodland star, buttercups, and blue-eyed grass in spring. Black oaks, chaparral, and grassland continue to line the trail, but the first of the gray pines appears as well. After one last hill climb, you'll reach the junction with Brushy Peaks Trail at 3.7 miles. Turn right, remaining on Gray Pine Trail.

By now the trailside blend of chamise, cercocarpus, ceanothus, scrub oak, manzanita, and monkeyflower should be familiar. Tall and spindly gray pines (also known as ghost pines) tower above the trail here and there—if you're hiking when it's a bit breezy, you may want to pause and enjoy the sound of the wind whispering through them. Descending off the ridge, the grade is steep, and some sections are very rocky. Gray Pine Trail leaves its namesake trees behind and arcs through a grassy area, where wet-weather runoff flows down the hillsides and muddies the trail.

With your path now following a branch of Sonoma Creek, still descending but at an easy grade, madrone and coast live oak appear. After a sharp left, you'll cross another feeder creek. Look along the sides of the trail for golden fairy lanterns in late April and early May. Wandering through this flat creek basin during a spring hike with the sounds of rushing water everywhere, I felt like I was on an alpine vacation. Gray Pine Trail makes its first creek crossing; in the warmest months of the year, you can hop over whatever water is left in the creekbed, but from winter through spring, the water level is high enough that your feet (and ankles) will likely get wet. I took off my shoes and socks and waded across the cool water, and my feet felt like they'd been given a new lease on life. Buckeye, alder, and California bay stand near the creek, enjoying the reliable water source.

At 5 miles Vista Trail feeds in from the right. Continue left on Gray Pine to the second creek crossing, with generally even deeper water to ford. A gorgeous mature bigleaf maple graces the stream here—if you're here in spring when the tree is clothed in fresh green leaves, you'll have to imagine it lit up with autumn foliage. Gray Pine Trail ends at 5.1 miles. Turn right onto Meadow Trail.

From here on out, the grade is easy—a relaxing stroll, really. You'll cross Sonoma Creek once more (this time on a bridge), then pass through groves of maples. A curious SATURN sign on the left is part of the Planet Walk interpretive hike that originates at Ferguson Observatory. The creek veers off to the left, continuing its journey toward Sonoma Valley, but the trail leaves the streamside to make its way through a meadow. Some chaparral thrives in a serpentine patch on the right, but grassland soon overtakes the landscape. The meadow is yet another superscenic Sugarloaf spot. This would be a good location for a bench, since both grass and trail are often damp in winter and spring.

At 5.9 miles Hillside Trail breaks off to the left, heading back over Sonoma Creek toward the park's campground. Continue straight, through or around a gate, where you'll emerge in a parking lot. Veer right, passing Ferguson Observatory, and pick up the continuation of Meadow Trail. On a slight ascent through a rocky area, another feeder creek descends on the left. Goldfields make a big impact along the trail in spring, when they form sunny carpets in the grass. In patches of serpentine with sparse grass, you'll likely see more bird's-eye gilia. Here, on my April hike, I had another jackrabbit sighting.

At 6 miles, you'll reach a junction with Lower Bald Mountain Trail. Stay left and retrace your steps back to the trailhead.

NEARBY ACTIVITIES

Sugarloaf abuts **Hood Mountain Regional Park and Open Space Preserve** (707-539-8092, parks.sonomacounty.ca.gov), a Sonoma County park with a peak 1 foot higher than Sugarloaf's Bald Mountain.

• •

GPS TRAILHEAD COORDINATES N38° 26.280' W122° 30.851'

DIRECTIONS From the Golden Gate Bridge toll plaza, drive about 20 miles north on US 101, then take Exit 460A onto CA 37 E. Drive east for 7.5 miles, then turn left onto CA 121/Arnold Drive. Continue north on CA 121 for 6.5 miles, then continue straight on CA 116 W. Drive north on CA 116/Arnold Drive 6.6 miles, then turn right onto Aqua Caliente Road W. Continue 0.8 mile, then turn left onto CA 12 W. Drive north on CA 12 W for 8 miles, then turn right onto Adobe Canyon Road. Drive east for 3 miles to the entrance kiosk, pay the fee, and then continue a short distance to the parking lot on the left.

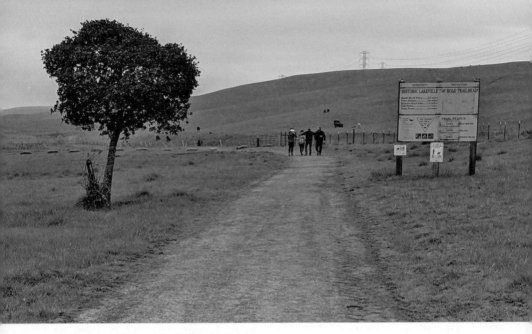

Hikers set out on Historic Lakeville Road Trail.

TOLAY LAKE IS a damp basin held by soft rolling hills. Miwok tribes considered the area a sacred spiritual center, and the Federated Indians of Graton Rancheria celebrate their heritage through cultural demonstrations at the annual Tolay Fall Festival. The Sonoma County Regional Parks department clarifies that Tolay Lake is not a recreation lake; don't show up with your Jet Ski and bathing suit. Do bring binoculars for bird-watching. This 3-mile trek over low hills above San Pablo Bay leads to a viewpoint, one of four at this park.

DESCRIPTION

I was charmed by Tolay Lake even before arriving at the trailhead. Sheep were grazing in the vineyard along Cannon Lane. A grove of olive trees graces a hillside, and the road is narrow and winding. The journey to the park is like a mini–Mediterranean vacation.

The atmosphere is bucolic at the park too. Stash your car on the historic ranch grounds, then begin walking to the right of a green barn on Historic Lakeville Road Trail. The wide, flat multiuse trail passes a trail heading right at 0.1 mile, then crosses through a cattle gate. We saw goldfinches flitting about on a winter hike, and cattle graze on the hillsides to the right. As you travel farther from the ranch area, look back for views to Tolay Lake. At 0.6 mile Historic Lakeville Road Trail meets Burrowing Owl Trail at a junction. Historic Lakeville Road Trail continues straight

DISTANCE & CONFIGURATION: 3-mile balloon

DIFFICULTY: Easy

SCENERY: Grassland and views

EXPOSURE: One stretch of shade; otherwise full sun

TRAIL TRAFFIC: Moderate

TRAIL SURFACE: Dirt trails and fire roads

HIKING TIME: 1.5 hours

DRIVING DISTANCE: 34 miles from the Golden Gate Bridge toll plaza

ACCESS: Daily, 7 a.m.–sunset. Lovely in late spring. Muddy in winter. Pay $7 entrance fee at electronic pay station.

WHEELCHAIR ACCESS: There are designated handicapped parking spots. If trails are dry, folks in wheelchairs may be able to navigate some of the trails here, although assistance will be needed to open cattle gates. The hike described below is not recommended for wheelchairs.

MAPS: Under glass at trailhead and at parks.sonomacounty.ca.gov

FACILITIES: Portable toilets at trailhead. No drinking water.

CONTACT: 707-539-8092, parks.sonomacounty.ca.gov

LOCATION: 5869 Cannon Lane, Petaluma, CA

COMMENTS: Leashed dogs welcome

another 0.75 mile, and Farm Bridge begins on the left. You can make a loop of these trails and/or continue on Pond Trail to Tolay Creek Vista. Note that these trails can be swamped in winter and temporarily closed then. For our hike, turn right onto Burrowing Owl Trail.

This narrow ribbon of a path winds uphill through grassland then ends at a signed junction at 0.9 mile. Views of the park from this ridge are wonderful. Turn left onto West Ridge Trail. High-tension power lines run parallel to the wide multiuse trail. On a late-February hike, we saw hundreds of Fremont's star lily blooming in the short grazed grass. At 1.2 miles turn right from a signed junction onto South Creek Trail. The path dips, then rises and ends at the Petaluma Marsh Vista at 1.5 miles. On a clear day, views include Mount Burdell to the west, and Mount Tamalpais and San Pablo Bay to the south. Even though cows graze the area, wildflowers thrive here. I noticed a bunch of Johnny-jump-ups, little yellow violets, hunkered down in trim grass. When ready, retrace your steps back to the junction with Burrowing Owl Trail, and continue straight on West Ridge Trail.

It's an easy stroll on the nearly flat trail as it travels along the ridgeline. We saw a northern harrier hunting over the grassland on a February hike, and some juncos flashed off the trail to a safer perch on the fence. At 2.7 miles West Ridge Trail ends at a signed junction. Turn right onto Cardoza Road Trail.

The wide trail is lined with eucalyptus trees. After a gentle descent, a path breaks off to the right at 2.9 miles, heading back to Historic Lakeville Road Trail, but continue straight, back to the ranch area and the trailhead.

NEARBY ACTIVITIES

The longest hike at Tolay Lake Regional Park is the 6.9-mile out-and-back trek to **Bay View Vista.** That hike offers views and terrain similar to the hike described above.

Tolay Lake Regional Park

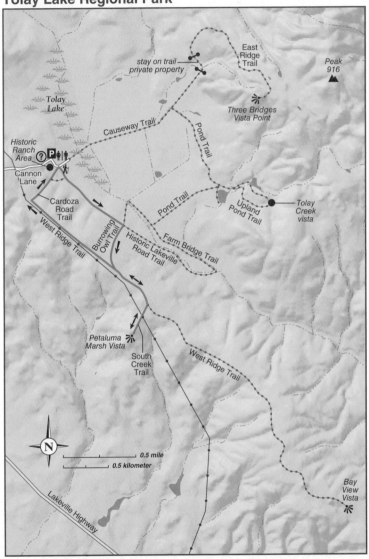

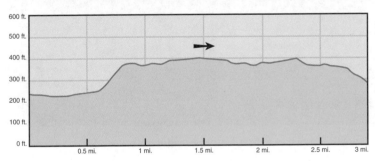

For a different experience, depart the ranch area and head east over the "lake" on Causeway Trail, then pass through an easement and climb through pockets of woods on East Ridge Trail to the **Three Bridges Vista Point.** Backtrack to the trailhead or add on Pond Trail for more variety. When Tolay Lake really resembles a lake, trails east of Historic Lakeville Road Trail can be flooded and closed, so check trail conditions when planning a hike.

• •

GPS TRAILHEAD COORDINATES N38° 12.295' W122° 31.256'

DIRECTIONS From the Golden Gate Bridge toll plaza, drive north on US 101 about 20 miles, then take Exit 460A onto CA 37 toward Napa/Vallejo. Drive east about 6 miles, then turn left onto Lakeville Highway. Drive north 5.7 miles, then turn right onto Mangel Ranch Road/Cannon Lane. Drive uphill 2 miles to the park entrance, then continue to the parking area at the ranch.

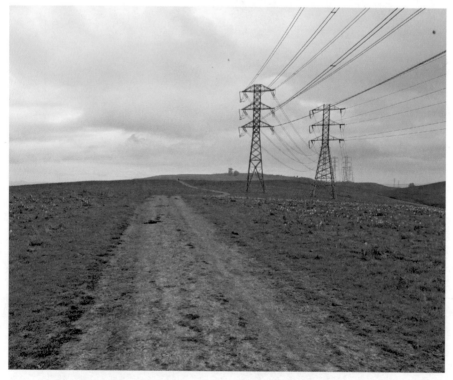

Fremont star lilies bloom under high-tension power lines at Tolay Lake.

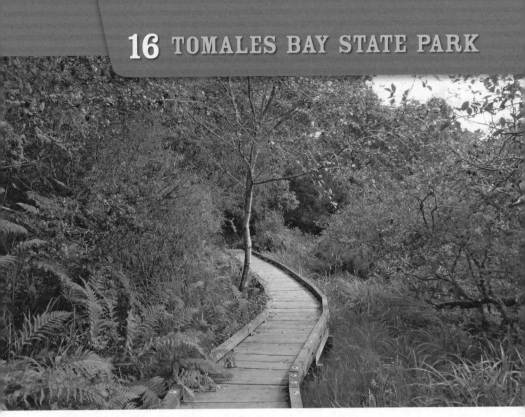

A boardwalk keeps boots dry and helps preserve the habitat on Johnstone Trail.

MOST PEOPLE ARE drawn to Tomales Bay in summer, particularly to Heart's Desire Beach, which sits just off one of the state park's parking lots. Three other beaches can be reached only by foot. Hike to one busy and one quiet beach on this 2.6-mile loop through a gorgeous woodland along the bay.

DESCRIPTION

This little park, largely ignored by tourists who flock to the Point Reyes peninsula, is no secret with locals, who favor it for beach parties, picnics, and hikes.

Tomales Bay, a body of water that separates Point Reyes from the rest of West Marin, sits directly above the San Andreas Fault. The beaches here, more sedate than the Pacific coastline, appeal to families with kids. With beaches this pretty, it's tough to tear yourself off the sand. Perhaps that's why the park trails can be a quiet refuge even when the beaches are crowded.

Begin the hike at the signed Jepson Trailhead, about midway through the upper parking lot. Immediately the scenery is incredibly lush, with huge coast live oaks covered in moss, and ferns, huckleberry, hazelnut, and California coffeeberry crowding the narrow trail. The ascent is steady but easy. You may hear deer tramping through the woods, but the foliage is so thick that it's hard to see more than a few feet into the forest.

DISTANCE & CONFIGURATION: 2.6-mile loop with 2 short out-and-back segments

DIFFICULTY: Easy

SCENERY: Woods and beaches

EXPOSURE: Mostly shaded

TRAIL TRAFFIC: Light during off-season; moderate in summer; heavy near Heart's Desire Beach

TRAIL SURFACE: Dirt trails

HIKING TIME: 1.5 hours

DRIVING DISTANCE: 42 miles from the Golden Gate Bridge toll plaza

ACCESS: Daily, 8 a.m.–sunset. Good year-round; peaceful autumn–spring. Pay $8 entrance fee at ranger-station kiosk using a credit or debit card only—no cash is accepted.

WHEELCHAIR ACCESS: Not recommended for wheelchairs

MAPS: At ranger station and tinyurl.com /tomalesbaysp

FACILITIES: Restrooms and drinking water at trailhead

CONTACT: 415-669-1140, tinyurl.com /tomalesbaysp

LOCATION: 1100 Pierce Point Road, Inverness, CA

COMMENTS: No dogs or bicycles allowed

In late spring look for tiny white flowers on yerba buena, a native herb that creeps close to the ground. Gradually Bishop pines and madrones muscle their way into the woods. In the understory, a variety of berry-producing native plants provide food for birds and small mammals. Some of these berries, such as thimbleberries, huckleberries, and currants, are palatable for humans as well. If you notice masses of a glossy-leaved shrub that seems familiar yet out of place, that's salal, a plant often used in floral arrangements; in April, you might catch it in bloom. At 0.7 mile a path heads off to the right toward a parking area on Pierce Point Road—continue straight on Jepson Trail.

Although there's a break in the tree cover, dense stands of toyon, coyote brush, and coffeeberry still obscure any views. At 0.75 mile Jepson Trail crosses a paved road that leads to a private beach. Continue straight. The same familiar vegetation lines the trail, although poison oak seems especially assertive. Honeysuckle vines dangle from shrubs, producing fragrant pink blossoms in June and pretty red berries in autumn. Jepson Trail ends at 0.85 mile. Turn left onto Johnstone Trail.

The grade remains close to level as Johnstone Trail winds through Bishop pine, coffeeberry, huckleberry, coast live oak, hazelnut, and tanoak. At 1.1 miles the trail crosses the private road for the last time and begins to descend easily. A bench on the left offers somewhat screened views of the bay. Madrones and manzanitas grow together in one area, inviting a comparison between these two related plants of the heath family that are common throughout the Bay Area. Manzanitas usually grow no larger than other chaparral shrubs, while madrones can attain stately heights. Both feature reddish, peeling bark; white, urn-shaped blossoms; and red, berrylike fruit. Because height comparisons can be deceiving (some manzanitas can reach 30 feet), a crucial difference is the leaves. While manzanita leaves average about 1 inch in length, the madrone's are much larger, about 5 inches long.

Johnstone Trail reaches the slopes of a little canyon that drains to a creek, and you may notice moisture-loving plants along the trail, including alder, chinquapin,

Tomales Bay State Park

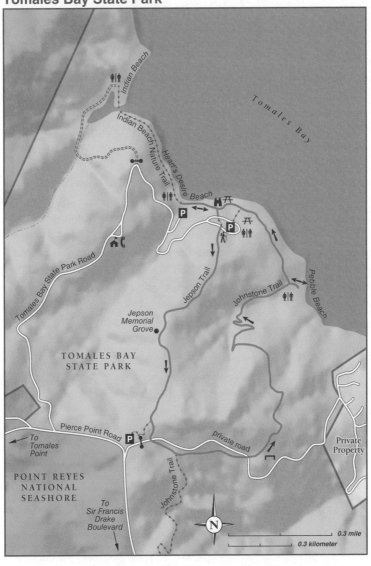

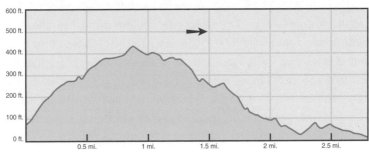

ferns, huckleberry, and salmonberry. Labrador tea, a shrub that looks a bit like azalea, blooms in June. A few switchbacks ease the descent, and a series of three gorgeous elevated boardwalks keep your feet dry. Where Johnstone Trail levels and reaches a junction with a path to Pebble Beach at 2 miles, turn right. The path descends briefly then ends at the beach. Not surprisingly, given the name, Pebble Beach is rocky, but it's also much quieter than sandy Heart's Desire Beach. Look across the bay for views of a series of low, rolling, grassy hills. Return to the previous junction and turn right, back onto Johnstone Trail.

Back on the main trail, California bay, coast live oak, madrone, huckleberry, ferns, and creambush line the path. At 2.3 miles Johnstone Trail steps out of the woods at the restrooms near the trailhead. If you don't want to make the trip to Heart's Desire Beach, turn left and walk back to the parking lot; otherwise continue straight.

After passing under some huge coast live oaks, the trail bisects a pretty group picnic area. When it is vacant, you can have your pick of tables, but I prefer to snack at a wooden bench overlooking the bay on the right. Keep hiking and drop down a set of steps to reach Heart's Desire Beach at about 2.5 miles. When you're ready, retrace your steps back to the junction near the restrooms, then turn right and return to the parking lot.

NEARBY ACTIVITIES

If you want to check out a nearby ocean beach, try **Abbotts Lagoon.** From the Tomales Bay State Park turnoff on Pierce Point Road, continue another 2 miles north on Pierce Point Road to the signed trailhead on the left. From the parking lot, a nearly level path travels west along a butterfly-shaped lagoon. After 1 mile, in a gap between the two lagoon wings, the trail disintegrates in loose sand, leaving the route to the ocean up to you.

• •

GPS TRAILHEAD COORDINATES N38° 07.887' W122° 53.492'

DIRECTIONS From the Golden Gate Bridge toll plaza, drive north on US 101 about 10 miles, then take Exit 450B, Sir Francis Drake Boulevard/San Anselmo. Stay left toward San Anselmo and drive west on Sir Francis Drake Boulevard about 20 miles to the junction with CA 1; turn right and, after 0.1 mile, make the first left onto Bear Valley Road. After about 2 miles Bear Valley Road ends at Sir Francis Drake; turn left. Continue on Sir Francis Drake about 5.5 miles, then turn right onto Pierce Point Road. Drive about 1.2 miles to the park entrance, on the right. Turn right and drive down the park road about 0.7 mile to the ranger station; stop and pay the fee, then continue about 0.7 mile to the parking lot at the end of the road (past the Heart's Desire lot).

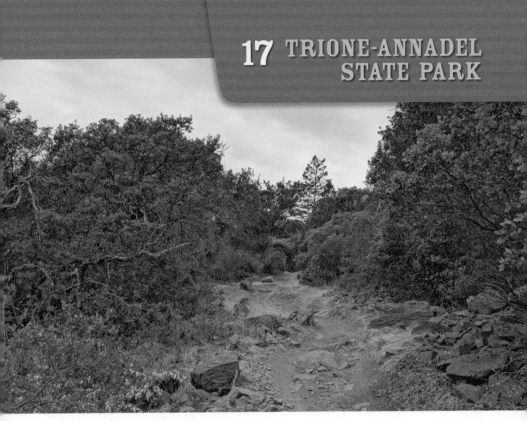

A rocky and rugged stretch of North Burma Trail

IF HIKES WERE marketed like new cars, I'd say that this Trione-Annadel loop has the most meadow views per mile. This hike climbs through a forest, loops around a meadow, and skirts the shore of Lake Ilsanjo before returning through woods to the trailhead.

DESCRIPTION

Trione-Annadel's grassy expanses are at their best in spring, when carpets of flowers bloom at the feet of mature oaks. The park is situated at the north end of the Sonoma Mountains, a long series of rolling hills that run from the eastern outskirts of Santa Rosa to the flats of San Pablo Bay. Like Jack London State Historic Park a few miles south (see Hike 3, page 26), Trione-Annadel has pretty woods and good views, but it also offers lakeside picnic spots, big sweeps of grassland, and oak savanna. Because Trione-Annadel is surrounded by residential communities, there are quite a few trailheads, many paths and trails, and lots of loop opportunities. Note that all the legitimate routes are signed and appear on the map; there are many social trails in the park, but major junctions are signed. As you hike you'll surely notice rocks and boulders all over the place, evidence of the cobblestone quarrying that took place in the area before the 1920s.

DISTANCE & CONFIGURATION: 6.2-mile figure eight

DIFFICULTY: Moderate

SCENERY: Woods, grassland, oaks, and lake

EXPOSURE: First and last section shaded; the rest mostly full sun

TRAIL TRAFFIC: Moderate

TRAIL SURFACE: Rocky dirt fire roads and trails

HIKING TIME: 3 hours

DRIVING DISTANCE: 56 miles from the Golden Gate Bridge toll plaza

ACCESS: Daily, 8 a.m.–sunset. Spring is best;

muddy after rains and hot in summer. Pay $7 entrance fee at ranger station.

WHEELCHAIR ACCESS: Not recommended for wheelchairs

MAPS: At ranger station and tinyurl.com /annadelmap

FACILITIES: Pit toilets and drinking water at trailhead

CONTACT: 707-539-3911, tinyurl.com/annadelsp

LOCATION: Santa Rosa, CA

COMMENTS: Dogs are not permitted on park trails. All trails but one are multiuse.

Begin from the middle of the parking lot, uphill on Warren Richardson Trail. After about 0.1 mile on the fire road, turn right onto Steve's "S" Trail. The park's sole hiking-only path begins a mostly easy climb through an open forest of California bay, Douglas-fir, coast live oak, and black oak. You might see woodland star and iris in spring. Views are obscured by the forest, and noise from the surrounding neighborhoods is steady, but the hubbub fades as the trail progresses uphill. Look for shiny black shards of obsidian on the trail—American Indians used the rock for arrow points and spearheads. In some spots, there's so much obsidian directly on the trail that you might initially mistake it for broken glass. As the trail makes its way across the wooded flanks of the hillside, boulders loom in the shadows, beneath Douglas-fir and California bay. Steve's "S" Trail crosses a little creek then bends sharply left. On one spring hike I saw a deer moving through the woods out of the corner of my eye and heard turkeys yodeling in the distance. At 0.8 mile the trail ends near a picnic table, at a junction with Warren Richardson Trail. Turn right.

The fire road ascends slightly, leaving the forest for a grassy savanna where deciduous black and Oregon oaks mingle with evergreen coast live oak and manzanitas. Spring wildflowers include linanthus, lupines, blue-eyed grass, popcorn flower, goldfields, blue dicks, and hound's tongue. At 1.2 miles turn right onto North Burma Trail.

The setting, with oaks sprinkled through grassland, is incredibly scenic, but stay alert for mountain bikes on the narrow path. North Burma Trail descends briefly along a sloping hillside then veers left into a young forest (an old closed trail to the right leads back toward Steve's "S" Trail). At 1.5 miles Louis Trail heads left. Continue straight on North Burma Trail. Douglas-fir and madrone crowd the rocky, level trail, giving way to manzanita, ceanothus, and poison oak. Among the small boulders strewn about the trail, look for shooting stars and blue-eyed grass in late winter and a generous amount of golden fairy lanterns in mid- to late April. The left side of the trail opens up to a descending meadow dotted with oaks, where lupines,

Trione-Annadel State Park

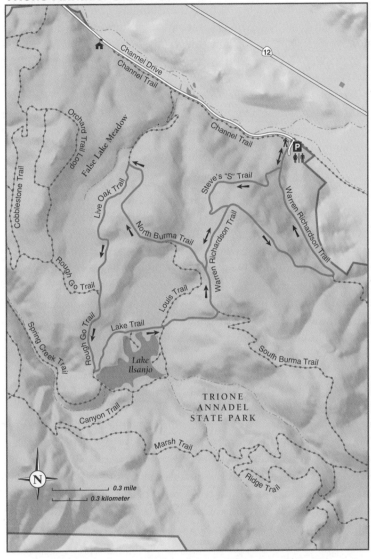

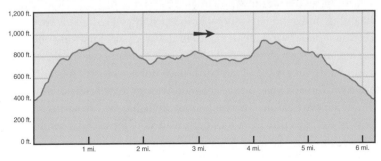

popcorn flower, linanthus, and goldfields were blooming on one midspring hike. As the trail proceeds slightly downhill, ceanothus, poison oak, coyote brush, manzanita, and toyon close off views, and Douglas-fir, black oak, and madrone provide occasional shade. At 2.1 miles North Burma Trail bends left to a junction. Turn left onto Live Oak Trail.

The narrow path runs parallel to False Lake Meadow, a short distance downhill to the right, mostly screened by an assortment of young Douglas-fir and coast live, Oregon, and black oak. Because trees line Live Oak Trail at a distance, grassy patches abound where you might see false lupine, blue-eyed grass, lupines, blue dicks, irises, shooting stars, and linanthus in spring. Rocks and small boulders are strewn all over the place. As the trail travels slightly downslope from a little knoll, you'll pass through a pocket of woods where California bay and buckeye blend into the other trees, and will then emerge on the western side of a meadow (apparently unnamed, although it's one of the park's largest). To the right are unobstructed views down to False Lake Meadow. Expect big patches of lupines along the trail in April, along with some California poppies and blue larkspur. The trail winds past an old, sprawling coast live oak then ends at 2.9 miles. Bear left onto Rough Go Trail.

Oaks and manzanita are common along the trail, which descends very gently through rocky grassland. Although Rough Go is heavily trafficked, this is a quiet part of the park, far from the trappings of suburban Santa Rosa. Two rugged Sonoma County peaks, Mounts Hood and Saint Helena, loom in the distance on the left. Just past a bench, Rough Go Trail ends at 3.3 miles. Turn left onto Lake Trail. (If you want to take the long way around the lake, continue past this junction, then turn left at the junction with Spring Creek Trail.)

Lake Ilsanjo is the heart of the park and a regular destination for many visitors who enjoy picnicking on the shores of the little reservoir, so you'll likely cross paths with plenty of runners, equestrians, and cyclists in this part of Trione-Annadel. This level segment of Lake Trail skirts the northern shoreline at a distance. Even when you can't see the water, cries from red-winged blackbirds indicate that it is close by, off to the right, and the trail is often muddy in all but the driest months of the year. Native bunchgrasses thrive beneath oak, manzanita, and California bay, in an understory where California buttercups, shooting stars, and irises bloom in spring. At the south edge of the meadow, you might see johnny-tuck and concentrated clusters of linanthus and goldfields blooming in April. If you're looking for a good spot for lunch, you'll find several picnic tables in the area—try following one of the side paths veering off to the right or left. At 3.8 miles Lake Trail sweeps right, continuing its loop around the lake. Louis Trail heads back uphill to North Burma Trail, on the left. Make a soft left and you're once again on Warren Richardson Trail.

This stretch starts as an easy climb along a small creek. In spring, red larkspur and yellow buttercups provide a nice contrast to the ferns and creambush beneath

Douglas-fir and California bay. South Burma Trail heads right at 4.2 miles—continue left on Warren Richardson Trail. The fires that devastated Santa Rosa in 2017 scorched parts of Trione-Annadel, and you may notice some dead-looking trees uphill to the south. As these trees die and fall, they will become an important part of the healthy park ecosystem, providing habitat for many wild creatures.

The surface of the fire road may be scored with tracks made by one of the most commonly spotted animals at Annadel, the wild turkey. I've seen or heard turkeys on every Annadel visit, either shuffling through oak woods, searching through the fallen leaves for insects, or tootling down the trails—these big birds make a substantial racket, gobbling back and forth to each other, and although they seem ungainly, they can move surprisingly fast. Wild turkeys can be feisty, too, especially the males (called toms), who keep a close watch on females (hens) during breeding season.

As Warren Richardson Trail makes its way north, look left for a last view of the meadow and Lake Ilsanjo. At 4.4 miles you'll once again reach the junction with North Burma Trail. Stay right on the fire road and retrace your steps back to the junction with Steve's "S" Trail at 4.8 miles. Continue right and downhill on Warren Richardson Trail.

The fire road begins a moderate descent, through a forest of redwood, Douglas-fir, California bay, and coast live oak. At a hairpin turn at 5.5 miles, Two Quarry Trail departs on the right, heading into the eastern part of the park. Continue left on Warren Richardson Trail, which runs at the edge of the woods, presenting nice views of a little egg-shaped hill on the right. A few bigleaf maple trees call attention to themselves in autumn, when they show off their foliage. As the trail descends, traffic and household noise filters through the trees. At 6.1 miles you'll return to the junction with Steve's "S" Trail. Retrace your steps back to the parking lot.

• •

GPS TRAILHEAD COORDINATES N38° 26.669' W122° 36.945'

DIRECTIONS From the Golden Gate Bridge toll plaza, drive about 50 miles north on US 101, then take Exit 488B on CA 12. Drive east toward Sonoma/Napa 1.5 miles, then turn left onto CA 12 E/Farmers Lane. After 0.7 mile turn right onto Montgomery Drive. Drive east 2.7 miles, then turn right onto Channel Drive. In less than 0.1 mile, continue straight where the road makes a sharp turn right toward Spring Lake. Drive into the park, stop and pay the entrance fee at the ranger station, then continue 1.1 miles to the parking lot at the end of the road.

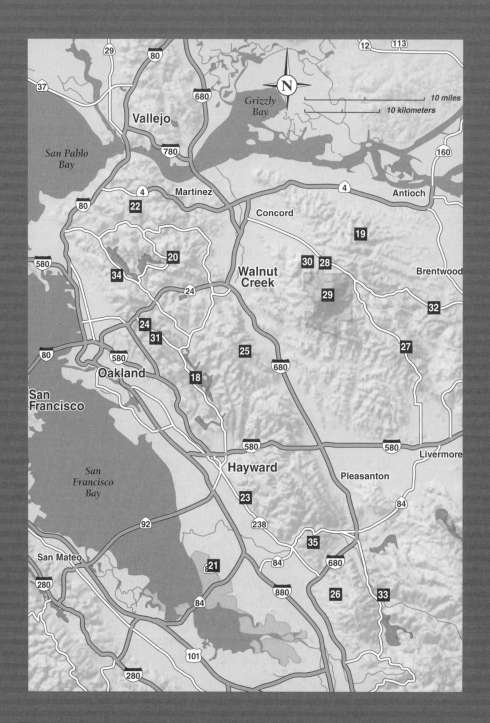

EAST BAY

(Including Alameda and Contra Costa Counties)

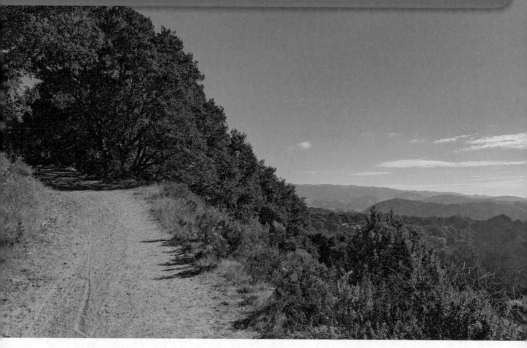

View of rolling East Bay hills from Goldenrod Trail

THIS LOOP IS a circuit through the heart of Chabot, bisecting Grass Valley, climbing to a ridge, and then descending into Bort Meadow through quiet woods. I've enjoyed Chabot hikes in every season, but the park really shines in spring when the wildflowers are blooming. If you're a novice flower enthusiast, this is a good, accessible place to start, with plenty of common blossoms best seen in April and early May.

DESCRIPTION

Anthony Chabot Regional Park is shaped like a foot, with long, thin toes pressing against Redwood Regional Park, and Lake Chabot settled near the ankle. The East Bay Municipal Water District defines the entire eastern border of Chabot, and the western boundary is mostly residential, but a ridge blocks the bulk of the noise.

If you're unfamiliar with the area, it would be easy to consider Chabot and neighboring Redwood as one, but it's remarkable how different two adjoining parks can be—Redwood is heavily forested, while Chabot boasts extensive grassland. The area around Lake Chabot is a warren of paths, leading to and from a golf course, picnic areas, and campsites, but the rest of the park has an undeveloped feel.

DISTANCE & CONFIGURATION: 6.3-mile loop

DIFFICULTY: Moderate

SCENERY: Grassland and woods

EXPOSURE: Mostly full sun

TRAIL TRAFFIC: Moderate

TRAIL SURFACE: Dirt fire roads and trails

HIKING TIME: 3 hours

DRIVING DISTANCE: 13.7 miles from the Bay Bridge toll plaza

ACCESS: Daily, 5 a.m.–10 p.m. Summer is often hot; late winter and spring are best; trails are usually muddy through winter and early spring. No fee.

WHEELCHAIR ACCESS: Not recommended for wheelchairs

MAPS: At trailhead's information signboard and tinyurl.com/chabotrpmap

FACILITIES: Pit toilets at Bort Meadow

CONTACT: 888-327-2757, ebparks.org/parks/anthony_chabot

LOCATION: 9999 Redwood Road, Castro Valley, CA

COMMENTS: Dogs welcome

Begin from the trailhead on a paved, gated road near the information signboard. As the service road sweeps downhill, there are views past the coyote brush and poison oak along the trail to Grass Valley on the left. At 0.1 mile you'll reach a three-way junction. The road to the right continues to Bort Meadow, and the middle path leads to Brandon Trail, which runs parallel to Grass Valley Trail on the far side of Grass Valley Creek. Turn left onto Grass Valley Trail.

Once through a cattle gate, you'll begin a nearly level stroll along the length of Grass Valley, a narrow meadow where wildflowers are common in spring. Some oaks, coyote brush, and poison oak shrubs dot the valley, but grassland dominates the landscape, where in early April suncups, blue-eyed grass, and buttercups bloom in clusters and tiny-blossomed filaree makes a huge impact, overtaking hillsides with a purple hue. At 1 mile Redtail Trail sets off uphill on the left. Continue on Grass Valley Trail, winding slightly downhill into a grove of eucalyptus companionably mixed through some redwoods. At 1.5 miles Grass Valley Trail swings left toward Lake Chabot. Turn right and pass over Grass Valley Creek on Stone Bridge to a second junction, with Cascade Trail on the left and Brandon Trail on the right. Continue straight, now on Jackson Grade.

At a moderate pace, the fire road climbs through a mélange of vegetation, including eucalyptus, bigleaf maple, creambush, hazelnut, blackberry, wild rose, toyon, coast live oak, and coffeeberry. In spring you're likely to see purple bush lupine and sticky monkeyflower blooming. The ascent ends at a junction with Goldenrod Trail at 1.9 miles. Turn right.

A short distance from the park boundary, the fire road runs downslope of a hillside, within audible range of Skyline Boulevard, and you'll likely hear some vehicle and residential noise. Chaparral favors this sunny area, although eucalyptus trees have extended their range out of the canyon on the right. In spring you might see bluewitch nightshade, checkerbloom, California poppy, blue-eyed grass, and blue dicks blooming beneath poison oak, toyon, broom, blue elderberry, and sticky monkeyflower.

Anthony Chabot Regional Park

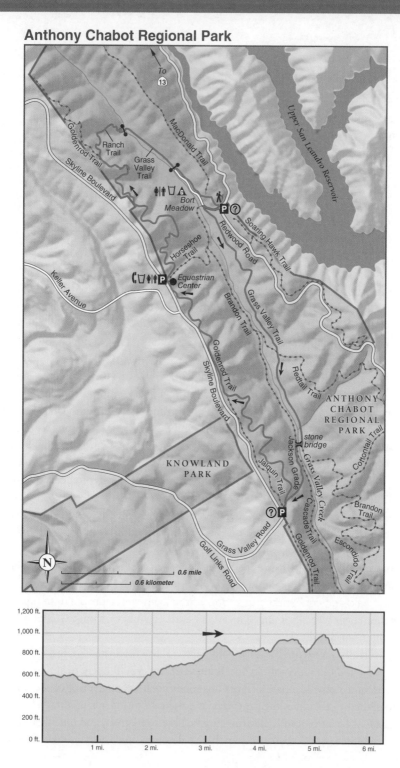

As Goldenrod Trail veers right at the 3-mile mark, a spur trail heads back left; continue right. Now, following close to Skyline Boulevard, eucalyptus trees are mostly replaced with some pines. Good views range across Grass Valley to the Upper San Leandro Reservoir watershed, managed by the East Bay Municipal Water District. At 3.6 miles you'll approach the grounds of Chabot Equestrian Center. Follow the trail signs as a skimpy path leads left, crosses an access road, and heads back into chaparral. Horseshoe Trail sets off downhill on the right. Continue on Goldenrod Trail.

This is a good section for wildflowers, ranging from delicate, wispy woodland star to giant, sturdy cow parsnip. In May you might see owl's clover. The trail alternates between chaparral and shade, with little substantial elevation change. California poppies occupy some grassy knolls just off the trail on the right. When you reach a T-junction with a paved service road at 4.5 miles, turn right. The road skirts a water tank then returns to dirt. Creambush, a deciduous shrub, puts forth froths of white flowers in late spring and early summer, brightening the sides of the trail. You might also notice some bigleaf maple and hazelnut. If it's a clear day, you should be able to make out Las Trampas Ridge to the east. At 4.8 miles you'll reach a junction with Buckeye Trail (which is closed and no longer on the official park map). Continue straight on Goldenrod.

After a short climb, the trail mostly levels out and passes through pockets of coast live oaks and California bays. At 5.2 miles turn right from a signed junction onto Ranch Trail.

Narrow Ranch Trail (closed to bikes) begins a sharp descent. At first the path is well shaded by California bays and coast live oaks, with thimbleberry, ferns, poison oak, and even a little huckleberry in the understory. About halfway downhill, Ranch Trail steps out into grassy chaparral and adopts a series of switchbacks, at still quite a steep grade. Finally the trail flattens across an area muddy in spring and reaches a gate at 5.6 miles. Once through the gate, turn right.

You'll now be back on Grass Valley Trail, passing through a damp meadow on a wide track. Gradually the trail narrows to a nearly flat single path cut through coyote brush. Some tall eucalyptuses loom ahead, and coast live oaks join the party. In late summer, red berries dangle from honeysuckle vines, shining like jewels in the sun. At 5.9 miles you'll reach the eucalyptus and another gate. Bort Meadow is to the right (with drinking water and pit toilets). Turn left onto a small path (easy to miss) running parallel to the paved road.

This slip of a trail passes through coyote brush, poison oak, and eucalyptus. There are quite a few plum trees along the trail, and when the fruit is ripe you might see animals, ranging from birds to coyotes, gorging on the sweet plums. In spring California buttercups and blue-eyed grass draw your attention to their colorful petals. At 6.1 miles the trail forks at a signed junction; Grass Valley Trail goes right. Stay left and continue uphill. At 6.2 miles, at the crest of a hill, the spur ends at a signed T-junction with MacDonald Trail. Turn right and walk the few remaining steps to the gate at the edge of the parking lot.

NEARBY ACTIVITIES

The park's main trailheads surround **Lake Chabot** (888-327-2757, ebparks.org/parks /lake_chabot), around which you can hike or bike on a 12.4-mile loop; you can also spend the night at one of several campsites.

• •

GPS TRAILHEAD COORDINATES N37° 46.653' W122° 07.501'

DIRECTIONS From the Bay Bridge toll plaza, drive east about 0.5 mile and bear right onto I-580 E. Drive 5.7 miles, then take Exit 24, 35th Avenue. Turn left on 35th Avenue and drive about 2.5 miles to the junction with Skyline Boulevard. Continue straight on Redwood about 4 miles to the trailhead, on the right.

Looking south down the length of Grass Valley

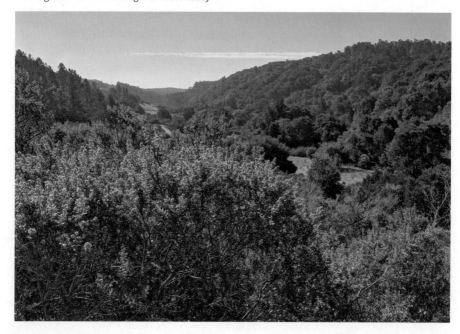

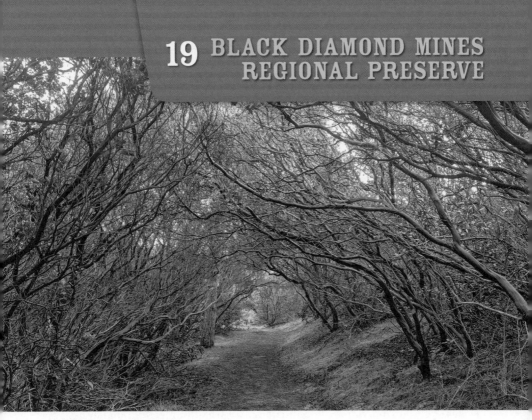

Manzanita bower on Chaparral Loop Trail

WANT TO RAMBLE through grassland and chaparral on one hike? This loop is a perfect tour through grassy, rolling hills as well as slopes covered with chamise, black sage, and manzanita. You'll begin in the heart of the park, climb through grassland dotted with blue oaks, follow an undulating course through chaparral, climb some more back into grassland, and then descend steadily back to the trailhead.

DESCRIPTION

Have you heard the one about the coal mine in Contra Costa County? It's no joke. From 1860 to 1906, the property we now know as Black Diamond Mines was the largest coal-mining district in California. Nearly 4 million tons of coal (black diamonds) were mined, with as many as 900 miners populating five towns in the area. When coal-mining operations ceased, underground sand mining continued until the late 1940s. The East Bay Regional Park District has preserved Black Diamond Mines as a recreational and historical park, with miles of trails laced across more than 6,000 acres of land and remnants from the mining era accessible in several locations. Although almost all the mine shafts, portals, and tunnels are shuttered, 200 feet of Prospect Tunnel are open for exploration, and the Greathouse Visitor Center occupies the original opening to the sand mine.

DISTANCE & CONFIGURATION: 3.7-mile loop

DIFFICULTY: Easy–moderate

SCENERY: Grassland, chaparral, and rock formations

EXPOSURE: Mostly full sun

TRAIL TRAFFIC: Mostly moderate; can get busy near visitor center

TRAIL SURFACE: Dirt fire road and trails; 1 very short paved segment

HIKING TIME: 2 hours

DRIVING DISTANCE: 35 miles from the Bay Bridge toll plaza

ACCESS: Opens daily at 8 a.m.; closing hours vary by season (check website). Summer is often very hot; late winter and spring are best. Pay the

$5 fee (cash or check only) at entrance kiosk, when staffed.

WHEELCHAIR ACCESS: There are designated handicapped parking spots, and trails are wheelchair accessible, but most are steep, and some present barriers; thus, wheelchairs are not recommended.

MAPS: At trailhead and tinyurl.com/black diamondminesmap

FACILITIES: Vault toilets and drinking water at trailhead

CONTACT: 888-327-2757, ebparks.org/parks /black_diamond

LOCATION: 5175 Somersville Road, Antioch, CA

COMMENTS: Dogs welcome ($2 fee)

Begin from the parking lot on paved Nortonville Trail. The broad fire road ascends gently toward the visitor center. After just 315 feet, turn left onto Stewartville Trail. Still gaining elevation, the fire road cuts through grassland and then reaches a gate and junction with Railroad Bed Trail at 0.1 mile. Continue straight on Stewartville Trail. The trees that tower above the trail here—tree of heaven, black locust, eucalyptus, and pepper tree—were planted during the mining era. At 0.3 mile Pittsburg Mine Trail begins on the right, but continue straight on Stewartville Trail. A long, steady climb begins through grassland where you might see fiddlenecks and lupines in March. The trail crests at 0.7 mile, reaching a multiple junction. Look back to the west for views of the park's prominent bald peak, 1,506-foot Rose Hill. Turn right onto Ridge Trail.

In the distance to the southwest, you'll get a peek at the top of Mount Diablo. At a nearly level grade, the trail skirts a knoll on the left. Buckeye and blue oak sprawl through grassland along the trail—this is a good spot for wildflowers all spring long. Early in the season, smatterings of shooting stars, blue dicks, lupines, and buttercups are common, but an even better display occurs in late April, when Ithuriel's spear, California poppy, and owl's clover heavily freckle the grassland like rainbow sprinkles. Sticking downslope from the ridgeline, the trail rises a bit steeply into a dramatically different landscape of manzanita, Coulter pine, yerba santa, and sagebrush. At 1.2 miles the trail crests at a little bare spot on the left—a wonderful place for a break, offering good views of Mount Diablo and a pretty valley downhill to the left. On a mid-May hike here, I admired a bountiful display of gorgeous mariposa lilies mixed through paintbrush. Ridge Trail begins to descend, enclosed by thick stands of chaparral. When the trail bends left, views open up to the north, encompassing rock formations in the foreground and Antioch in the distance. Quite

Black Diamond Mines Regional Preserve

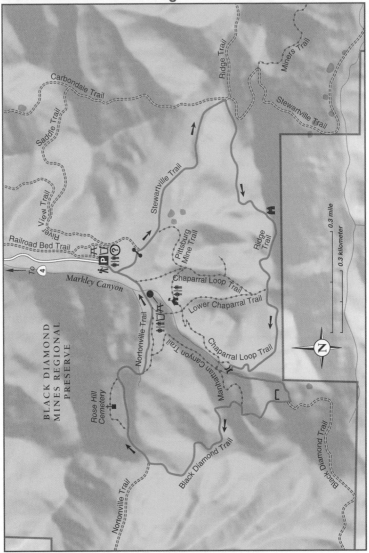

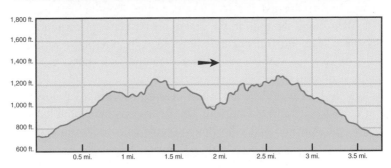

a few bush poppy shrubs are mixed through chamise and manzanita—look for bush poppy's bold yellow flowers in spring. Ridge Trail descends somewhat steeply over slippery bare sandstone then ends at a junction at 1.4 miles. Lower Chaparral Trail sets off to the right, skirting a rock formation on the way downhill toward the visitor center area. Continue straight on Chaparral Loop Trail.

To the west, past a low-slung sandy knoll, a prominent reeflike hill rises, with rocks jutting out at an angle. The trail rises to a power tower then begins a descent. A few long, straight stretches are aromatic alleys, with sweet smells wafting from manzanita blossoms in winter, black sage and pitcher sage flowers in spring, and a froth of chamise blooms in summer. Some live oaks mingle with pine and yerba santa as Chaparral Loop Trail drops on steps and some steep grades into Manhattan Canyon. In mid-May, I've seen dozens of fairy lanterns blooming along the trail. Just after a bridge crosses the canyon at 1.8 miles, you'll reach a junction, with the trail to the right closing Chaparral Loop. Turn left, following the sign toward Manhattan Canyon Trail.

After a brief, winding climb through chamise and 6-foot-tall manzanitas, you'll reach a second junction, with Manhattan Canyon Trail. To the right, it leads uphill then downhill back toward the trailhead. Turn left.

On a slope just uphill from the canyon floor, the narrow trail ascends through live oaks, pine, sticky monkeyflower, toyon, and manzanita. Somewhat abruptly, the canyon widens into a grassy bowl near the park boundary. Blue oaks dot the hillsides as Manhattan Canyon Trail veers right and climbs steeply, ending at a junction with Black Diamond Trail at 2.1 miles. A bench to the right just before the junction is a good place to catch your breath. Turn right onto Black Diamond Trail.

Trailside vegetation is a mixture of grassland, pine, manzanita, and blue and live oak. Look off to the right for views back to Chaparral Loop and Ridge Trails. After a brief level interlude, the fire road begins to descend easily into chaparral, where you might see ceanothus, black sage, yerba santa, chamise, and pitcher sage. At 2.3 miles the connector to Manhattan Canyon Trail departs on the right. Continue straight on Black Diamond Trail, ascending at a moderate grade back into grassland. On the far side of a cattle gate beneath a power tower, you get sweeping views to Stewartville Trail. By mid-May, the tips of high hills rising up to the northeast begin to fade from green to dull brown, drained of color. In early spring, shooting stars bloom in staggering numbers along the trail, in the grassy breaks between clusters of blue and live oaks. Black Diamond Trail begins to descend easily, offering views northwest to Suisun Bay on clear days. At 2.9 miles Black Diamond Trail ends at a junction with Nortonville Trail; turn right.

Nortonville Trail loses elevation at a moderate grade, dropping along the side of a sloping valley to the right of Rose Hill. Owl's clover is common in the short grass of early spring, but by mid-May billowing mustard plants and thistles take over. You may see and hear red-winged blackbirds in this part of the park.

At 3.0 miles a path departs on the left, leading to Rose Hill Cemetery, the final resting place for some of the residents of the mining era. This is an optional detour— a path returns to Nortonville Trail less than 0.1 mile downhill. Nortonville Trail sweeps right and begins a return to the main park area, with tree of heaven lining the route. At 3.3 and 3.5 miles, two forks of Manhattan Canyon Trail depart on the right. Continue straight on Nortonville Trail to a junction at 3.6 miles. Turn right if you'd like to tour the visitor center (open on weekends). Otherwise, turn left and follow Nortonville Trail another 0.1 mile back to the parking lot.

• •

GPS TRAILHEAD COORDINATES N37° 57.500' W121° 51.797'

DIRECTIONS From the Bay Bridge toll plaza, drive east about 0.5 mile and bear right onto I-580 E. Drive 1.5 miles, then take Exit 19B onto CA 24. Drive 13 miles east on CA 24, then at the I-680 junction, use the middle lane to exit Ygnacio Valley Road. Drive east on Ygnacio Valley Road 7.5 miles to the junction with Clayton Road. Continue straight, now on Kirker Pass Road, 5.3 miles to the junction with Buchanan Road. Turn right and drive 2.8 miles, then turn right onto on Somersville Road. Drive south on Somersville 1 mile to the junction with James Donlon Boulevard. Continue straight into the park, 1 mile to the entrance kiosk, and then drive a little less than a mile to the parking lot at the end of the road.

Nortonville Trail winds up the side of Rose Hill.

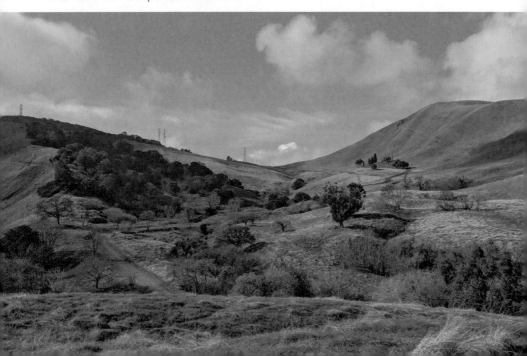

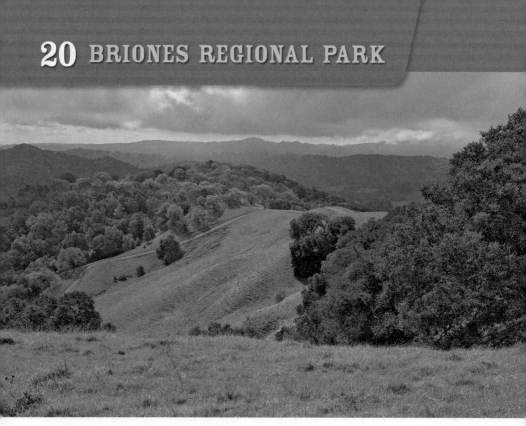

Black Oak Trail drops through oaks and grassland.

THIS HIKE REMINDS me of Goldilocks and the Three Bears: it's not too long and not too hard, but just about right for most people. Briones is a happy combination of rolling hills, grassy valleys dotted with oaks, seasonal lagoons, and tree-lined creeks. Visiting the heart of the park, this loop climbs along an old ranch road to a viewpoint and then descends past black oaks on the way back to the trailhead.

DESCRIPTION

How can a park with so many cows have so many flowers? The meeting of lush flora and hungry bovids seems a contradiction, but it somehow works at Briones, home to one of the best spring wildflower displays in the Bay Area. I also love the park in autumn, when a riot of orange black-oak leaves complements the tall, tawny-colored grass. Is there a bad time to visit? Not really, although the trails do get muddy after a typical winter storm's deluge.

Start from the parking area on Old Briones Road, initially a paved route. Along the flat, wide trail, the vegetation is a mix of young coast live oak, blue elderberry, and coyote brush. At 0.1 mile Seaborg Trail breaks off to the right. Continue straight on Old Briones Road, now pavement-free. Once through a gate, you'll enter a cattle range, skirting a hill on the left. On one hike, I noticed a little cow figurine nestled in

DISTANCE & CONFIGURATION: 4.3-mile balloon loop

DIFFICULTY: Easy

SCENERY: Grassland

EXPOSURE: Full sun

TRAIL TRAFFIC: Moderate

TRAIL SURFACE: Dirt fire roads

HIKING TIME: 2.5 hours

DRIVING DISTANCE: 16.4 miles from the Bay Bridge toll plaza

ACCESS: Opens daily at 8 a.m.; closing hours vary

by season (check website). Late winter and spring are best. Pay $3 fee at entrance station.

WHEELCHAIR ACCESS: Unobstructed; folks with wheels should be able to navigate at least 0.25 mile on Old Briones Road.

MAPS: At trailhead's information signboard and tinyurl.com/brionesrpmap

FACILITIES: Pit toilets and water at trailhead

CONTACT: 888-327-2757, ebparks.org/parks /briones

LOCATION: 1611 Bear Creek Road, Lafayette, CA

COMMENTS: Dogs welcome ($2 fee)

the grass along the trail—an homage or an ironic statement? Either way, it made me laugh. The trail rises slightly, following a creekbed on the right into a little shaded woodland of California bay and coast live, valley, and black oak. Great yellow drifts of California buttercups sprawl beneath the trees in early spring.

Black Oak Trail sets off uphill on the left at 0.7 mile. This trail is your return route, much more steeply pitched than easy Old Briones Road, so continue straight. A grassy valley on the left gently rises toward Briones's highest peaks. You'll pass a corral as the trail sticks to an easy grade, but Old Briones Road begins to climb just past a junction with Valley Trail on the right, at 1.0 mile.

You might find a variety of flowers along the trail in late winter and spring, with buttercups often the first to bloom, blazing the way for fiddlenecks, lupines, California poppies, and blue dicks. Buckeye and California bay are common, particularly in the damp creases of the hillsides. Old Briones Road climbs at an easy grade, offering pretty views down into the valley and up to grassy hills on the left. At 1.7 miles the trail approaches a junction, fence, and crest. Just before a gate, veer left on a slight path, and walk uphill a few yards to a bench.

This bench is perhaps the perfect lunch destination if you're alone or with one other person (no one volunteers to sit on the grass in a cow-grazed park), with 360-degree views of the park and the surrounding area, including Mount Diablo to the southeast. In late April and early May, the hillsides just downslope from the bench show off dense, colorful patches of creamcups, California poppy, and lupine. If the flowers aren't blooming, you could easily while away some time watching hawks and kestrels soaring over the valley below.

When you're ready, walk back down the path, then turn left, pass through the gate, and make another left. After a few steps the trails fork again, this time at one end of a big triangular junction. Stay left, on Briones Crest Trail. At a level grade, the wide fire road skirts a knoll on the left. You might notice small ponds downhill on the right—those are the Sindicich Lagoons, important sources of water for the park's

Briones Regional Park

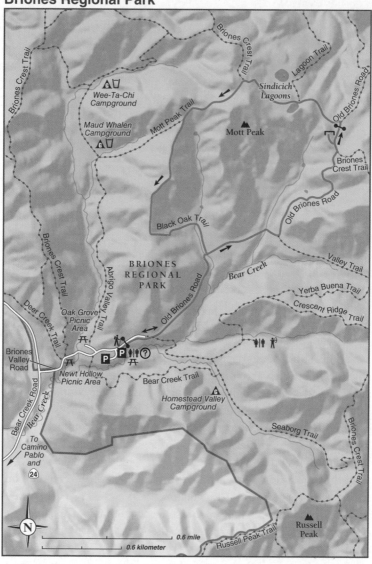

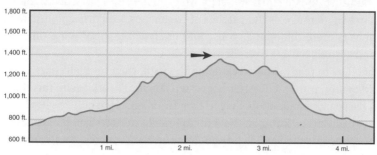

birds, mammals, and newts. Buttercups bloom like crazy along Briones Crest Trail in April, tinting entire hillsides lemon yellow. A cluster of coast live oaks lines the right side of the trail, interrupting the sea of grass.

Lagoon Trail begins on the right at 2.0 miles, across from one of the Sindicich Lagoons. Continue straight on Briones Crest Trail. As the trail ascends easily, good views open up downhill, to the right, of another lagoon. When it's full and the sun is shining, the water makes a nice mirror, reflecting puffy white clouds drifting across the bluest skies. At 2.3 miles, Briones Crest Trail continues off to the right. Turn left onto Mott Peak Trail. After a short ascent, the fire road crests and begins to descend, skirting its namesake peak through grassland with a few lonely oaks sprinkled here and there. On spring hikes in this part of the park, I've seen orange patches of California poppy that were so vivid and colorful I wondered if Mother Nature played paintball. Fiddlenecks are a late-winter fixture along the trail.

Where Mott Peak Trail reaches a junction at 2.7 miles, veer left onto Black Oak Trail, which roller-coasters along the ridgeline past displays of blue and white lupine in spring. Up close in late winter's short green grass, the blooms really pop, but from a distance they make the hillsides look bruised. On a spring hike I watched a group of three coyotes traveling downslope on the left—I had heard them calling earlier. Black Oak bends left as the descent sharpens. In the driest months of the year, loose stones on the trail can make the descent a bit scary. I've taken the steepest section in a zigzag pattern more than once to keep from sliding. The trail runs between a beautiful oak forest on the right and a sloping, grassy hillside on the left, where a few buckeyes line a creekbed. Although they blend into the woods in spring and summer, the trail's namesake trees are easy to pick out in autumn when their leaves turn orange. Black Oak Trail levels out on the valley floor then ends at 3.6 miles at Old Briones Road. Turn right and retrace your steps back to the trailhead.

• •

GPS TRAILHEAD COORDINATES N37° 55.627' W122° 09.350'

DIRECTIONS From the Bay Bridge toll plaza, drive about 0.5 mile and bear right onto I-580 E. Drive 1.5 miles, then take Exit 19B onto CA 24. Drive 7 miles east on CA 24, then take Exit 9, Orinda/Moraga. Turn left and drive north on Camino Pablo about 2 miles, then turn right onto Bear Creek Road. Drive on Bear Creek about 4.4 miles to the park entrance on the right. After passing the entrance kiosk, continue straight to the parking lot.

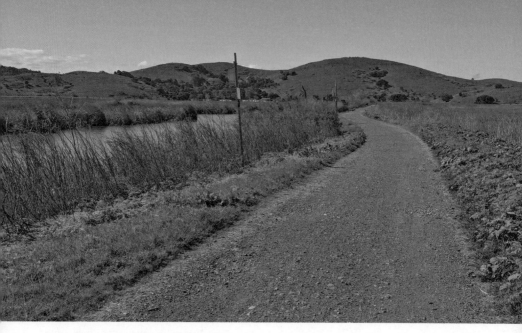

Coyote Hills: a park with flat and hilly paths

A NUMBER OF PARKS perch on the shores of San Francisco Bay, but Coyote Hills is the whole enchilada: excellent wildlife-viewing, extensive facilities, and trails that explore not only marsh and coastline but grassland as well. You can choose an easy hike through Coyote Hill's marsh or stretch your legs a bit on a few short but steep paths that roller-coaster up and down grassy hills fronting the bay. This 5-mile loop does both, starting in the marsh and then traversing the hills.

DESCRIPTION

Coyote Hills is a small collection of grassy, rolling knolls rising above the bay just north of Dumbarton Bridge. The Ohlone, original inhabitants of the Bay Area who settled here more than 10,000 years ago, found this area particularly bountiful, leaving a shell mound and other historical artifacts in the marsh. The park is popular with kids, who tour Coyote Hills on school trips guided by park staff or visit on weekends for family bird-watching. Because Coyote Hills offers many flat trails and is a short drive from communities around Fremont, locals use the park for daily exercise. The steady foot traffic seems not to bother the park's wildlife—I've seen a fox, a pheasant, jackrabbits, and many birds here.

DISTANCE & CONFIGURATION: 5-mile loop

DIFFICULTY: Easy

SCENERY: Grassland, marsh, and bay views

EXPOSURE: Full sun

TRAIL TRAFFIC: Moderate

TRAIL SURFACE: Dirt fire roads and trails; 1 paved trail

HIKING TIME: 2.5 hours

DRIVING DISTANCE: 36 miles from the US 101/I-280 junction in San Francisco

ACCESS: Opens daily at 8 a.m.; closing hours vary by season (check website). Good year-round, but marsh trails can flood in winter. Pay $5 fee at entrance kiosk.

WHEELCHAIR ACCESS: There are designated handicapped parking spots, and visitors in wheelchairs should be able to navigate most of the trails in the marsh (conditions permitting).

MAPS: At visitor center and tinyurl.com/coyotehillsmap

FACILITIES: Restrooms and drinking water at visitor center

CONTACT: 888-327-2757, ebparks.org/parks/coyote_hills

LOCATION: 8000 Patterson Ranch Road, Fremont, CA

COMMENTS: Dogs are permitted on most trails ($2 fee) but aren't allowed in the marsh, so leave them at home for this hike.

If the visitor center is open, take a quick prehike tour through exhibits highlighting Ohlone settlements and native flora and fauna. Then walk back to the parking area and cross the street to a multiple-trail junction at the edge of the marsh. Bayview Trail, on the right, runs along the road back toward the park entrance. A boardwalk and Chochenyo Trail split off straight ahead into the marsh. Turn right onto the raised boardwalk section of trail (Chochenyo Trail, to the left, is the optional route if the boardwalk and marsh are flooded).

This boardwalk path, open to hikers and cyclists, passes through the marsh, with cattails and reeds lining the way. Birdsong fills the air, and at the marsh's edge shy groups of geese, grebes, and mallards may swim or fly away quickly if they feel threatened by your presence. At 0.2 mile you'll reach a junction with Muskrat Trail; turn left. After a short, level stretch, turn right onto Chochenyo Trail.

Dock, pickleweed, and New Zealand spinach thrive along the trail, along with thick stands of marsh plants that mostly block water views. Even if you can't see them, you may hear ducks and waterfowl splashing. At 0.5 mile the trail splits at an unmarked junction. Bear left. The trail loops around the Tuibun Village Site, which is fenced.

This former Ohlone village site is usually closed to the public, though tours can be arranged and the park often hosts shell-mound "open houses." Unless you're visiting on one of those days, you'll have to peer through the fence. At 0.65 mile, near a pit toilet, the trail splits again at an unsigned junction; bear right. At 0.8 mile you'll reach a previously encountered junction; bear left and retrace your steps to the connector between Chochenyo and D.U.S.T. (Demonstration Urban Stormwater Treatment) Trail, at 1.0 mile. Turn right, then right again, onto D.U.S.T. Trail.

The marsh surrounding D.U.S.T. Trail was engineered to filter polluted storm runoff before it reaches the bay. A bonus benefit is wildlife habitat for ducks, geese, and more "wild" birds like herons and egrets. Plants along D.U.S.T. Trail range from

Coyote Hills Regional Park

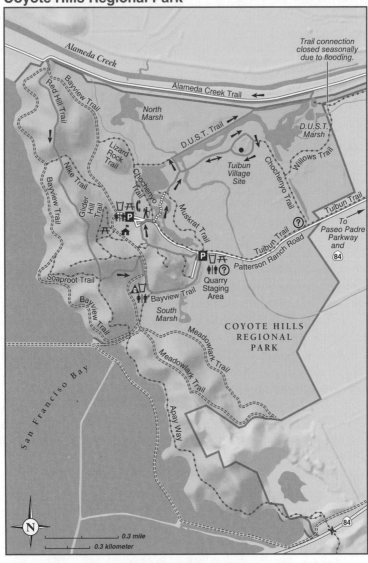

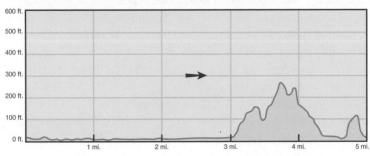

wispy mustard, poison hemlock, and wild radish to sturdy bushes of poison oak. In the summer, after the plant blossoms have dried out, you might see scores of tiny birds such as bushtits and goldfinches feeding on seeds of all these plants. After a long, straight stretch, D.U.S.T. Trail gently curves right (a very short unnamed spur heads off to the left) as the flatlands of Fremont stretch east to a series of low, rolling hills. Where D.U.S.T. Trail ends at 1.8 miles, turn left onto Alameda Creek Trail.

This flat, wide, paved levee trail runs along the shore of the East Bay's longest creek as it makes its way to the bay. Although the creek is really a less-than-natural managed flood channel here, Canada geese are common in and around the creek and in the skies above the channel, and you might see birds of prey, including harriers, hawks, and kestrels. A cluster of eucalyptus trees on the left punctuates the landscape and provides a little oasis of shade. Pickleweed, a ground cover often found in marshes, draws attention to itself in autumn, when it flushes a rusty red. At the hike's 2.9-mile mark, just past an Alameda Creek interpretive display, you'll reach a junction. Bear left, cross paved Bayview Trail, and start uphill on Red Hill Trail.

Climbing moderately through grassland, the trail quickly crests. In March, orange California poppies contrast nicely with vivid green grass and blue sky—an eye-popping late-winter color palette. A steep descent commences, and at 3.4 miles Nike Trail crosses Red Hill Trail. Continue straight on Red Hill Trail.

After another sharp climb you'll reach the park's highest elevation, a mere 291 feet, where big boulders of crimson chert jut up from the grassland. Beware of poison oak nestled among the outcrops. Red Hill Trail descends slightly to a level saddle, where a barely noticeable path, Glider Hill Trail, heads downhill to the left. Proceed uphill on Red Hill Trail to yet another beautiful view, this one located on top of Glider Hill. True to its name, the hill is a good place to fly a kite or model airplane; for those without such accessories, the wind can detract from a hilltop rest break. On clear days, you can enjoy views of the Bay, Dumbarton Bridge, Mission Peak, the Santa Cruz Mountains, and Mount Diablo. As Red Hill Trail steeply descends one last time, look for jackrabbits bounding through the grass and hawks hunting overhead. At 3.9 miles you'll reach a T-junction; turn left onto Soaproot Trail.

As the trail descends easily, look for the trail's namesake plant along the path. Soaproot has long, wavy leaves and narrow stalks that resemble asparagus (both soaproot and asparagus are members of the lily family). Ohlones dug soaproot bulbs and used them not only to make soap but to stupefy fish for easy gathering. The plant blooms May–June, but its blossoms don't open until late in the afternoon. After a sharp curve right, Soaproot Trail ends at 4.2 miles. Turn left on Bayview Trail, and almost immediately turn right to remain on Bayview.

Paved Bayview Trail sweeps past Dairy Glen, a group campsite at right (vault toilets are here if needed). Just before South Marsh, another path veers right, while Bayview Trail bends left and runs parallel to the marsh. Stay on Bayview, skirting a rocky hill on the left, to the fringes of Quarry Staging Area. There are a few well-worn short-cuts, but continue on Bayview almost all the way to the park road at 4.6 miles; then turn left, cross the parking lot, and head uphill on signed Muskrat Trail.

Poison oak, sagebrush, coyote brush, sticky monkeyflower, and toyon mix with grass along the narrow trail. Bush lupine is a pretty accompaniment in spring, when its sweet-smelling, purple-blue flowers emerge. Near a rock outcrop, a path (not shown on the park map) doubles back to the left, but Muskrat continues straight. Veer right in front of a massive boulder, then begin a descent, with one last opportunity to gaze at the marsh as the trail drops down a set of steps. In March you might see shooting stars in bloom beside the trail. At 5.0 miles, the path ends within steps of the parking lot.

• •

GPS TRAILHEAD COORDINATES N37° 33.221' W122° 05.418'

DIRECTIONS From the US 101/I-280 split in San Francisco, drive south 25 miles on US 101, then take Exit 406, CA 84 E/Dumbarton Bridge. Follow CA 84 about 7 miles to the eastern end of the Dumbarton Bridge, then take Exit 36 onto Paseo Padre Parkway/Thornton Avenue (the first exit after the toll plaza). Turn left and drive north on Paseo Padre about 1 mile, then turn left onto Patterson Ranch Road. Drive about 1.5 miles, past the entrance kiosk and Quarry Staging Area, to the trailhead at the end of the road (near the visitor center).

Boardwalk through the marsh at Coyote Hills

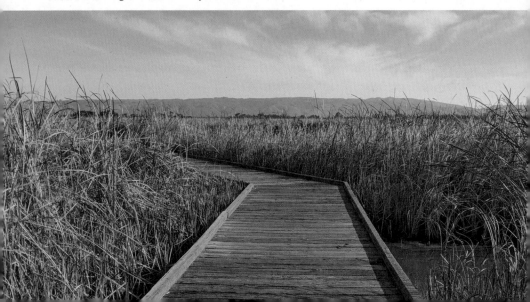

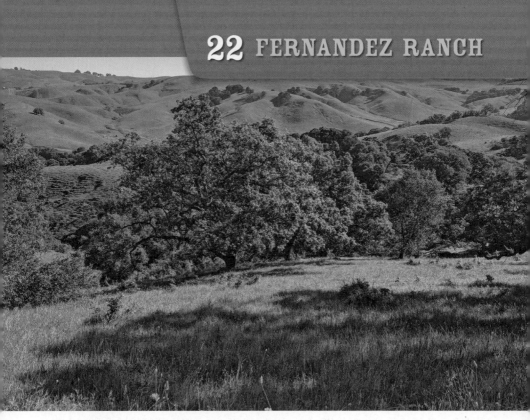

Oaks, wildflowers, and rolling hills at Fernandez Ranch

FERNANDEZ RANCH IS only 7 miles outside Hercules, but the area is remote and undeveloped. Reaching the trailhead requires good navigation skills (the exit from CA 4 is unsigned) and a bit of brave driving on a narrow road. Luckily the ranch entrance is well signed and the trailhead is a welcoming spot, with a gravel parking lot, a vault toilet, and an information signboard.

DESCRIPTION

The facilities near the trailhead are gorgeous, featuring picnic tables and an all-access trail. Further afield the trails are old ranch roads and nicely graded footpaths; the whole place is thoughtfully designed and well maintained. The ranch is grazed by cattle, and most trails show it—lots of cow plops, mud in winter, and eroded hillsides. If you can look past that, you'll enjoy Fernandez Ranch's easy loops and appreciate the option to stage at the developed trailhead and create longer, more solitary hikes through the adjacent East Bay Municipal Utility District (EBMUD) watershed (permit required).

From the parking lot, walk across the sturdy bridge, then bear left onto Black Phoebe Trail. This level path is all-access for 0.5 mile, as it edges between a fenced pasture and a creek. On my hike I watched a group of turkeys pick their way though the pasture; the cows were nonplussed. At 0.6 mile Black Phoebe Trail ends at a signed junction; bear right onto Whipsnake Trail.

DISTANCE & CONFIGURATION: 3.7-mile loop

DIFFICULTY: Easy

SCENERY: Grassland and woods

EXPOSURE: About equal parts sunny and shaded

TRAIL TRAFFIC: Light

TRAIL SURFACE: Dirt trails and fire roads

HIKING TIME: 2 hours

DRIVING DISTANCE: 20 miles from the Bay Bridge toll plaza

ACCESS: Daily, sunrise–sunset. Spring is the most lovely. No fee.

WHEELCHAIR ACCESS: There are designated

handicapped parking spots, and the first part of the hike is wheelchair accessible.

MAPS: At trailhead's information signboard and tinyurl.com/fernandezranchmap

FACILITIES: Vault toilets but no water; picnic tables

CONTACT: 925-228-5460, jmlt.org/fernandez _ranch.html

LOCATION: 1081 Christie Road, Martinez, CA

COMMENTS: Dogs are welcome and may be off leash in undeveloped areas (unless otherwise posted), provided they are under control. Dog owners must always carry leashes. No drones. Be sure to close cattle gates. You'll need a trail permit to explore EBMUD trails: ebmud.com /recreation/buy-trail-permit.

Whipsnake Trail winds slightly uphill following a small feeder creek. Here I saw a young coyote on the trail. In April buckeyes were days away from flowering; expect clouds of butterflies when these native trees bloom. After a sharp turn left, the trail passes through a cattle gate and veers right. On my April visit, as I ascended easily through California bay and coast live oak woods, froths of yellow buttercup brightened the understory. I got a big shock when I spotted a skunk digging through the leaves a few feet off the trail. Luckily it tottered off when it saw me. There is plenty of poison oak in the understory as well, mixed through other less itchy native shrubs, including wood rose and snowberry. As Whipsnake Trail climbs, the woods gradually thin and yield to big white oaks. There are partial views to the northeast that improve as the trail reaches a viewpoint (and the hike's high point) at 1.4 miles. Here views unfold to the north and stretch across Carquinez Strait to the mountains of Napa County. Just downhill, note the prominent windmill—you'll get a closer look on the return leg of the hike. Whipsnake Trail descends gently through oak-dotted grassland back into the woods and reaches a signed junction on the far side of a bridge at 2.1 miles. Turn left, walk a few feet slightly uphill, and then at a second trail marker, continue left/straight.

Now on Woodrat Trail, you'll climb easily through woods and patches of grassland. Lupines and blue dicks were blooming on my April hike. At 2.8 miles Woodrat Trail ends at a junction and the gated EBMUD boundary. If you have a permit, you can wander around the Pinole Watershed on a segment of the Bay Area Ridge Trail (to the left), or, to extend this hike, pass through the gate, turn right, and walk to a second gate, where you will reenter Fernandez Ranch. From there, explore Franklin Ridge and/or Canyon Loop and Vista Trails, and return to the Windmill Trail via Woodland Trail. For this hike, turn right onto Windmill Trail.

Fernandez Ranch

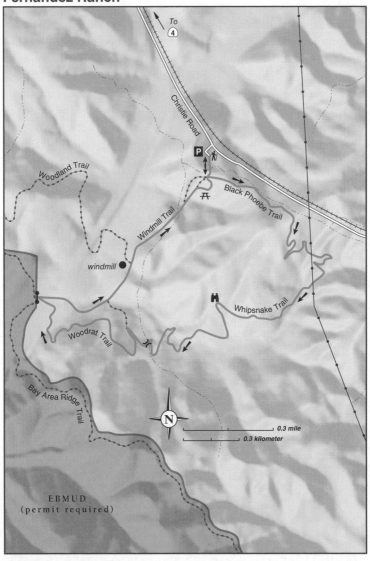

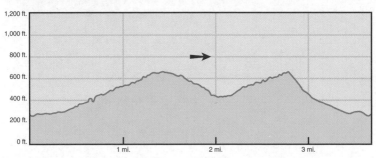

The old ranch road drops sharply out of grassland into a pocket of California bay and buckeye woods where I noticed turkey tracks stamped onto the trail. When the trail returns to grassland at 3 miles, the connector back to Whipsnake breaks off to the right. Continue straight. On an April hike, pipevine swallowtail butterflies fluttered across the hillside on the left. The trail levels out and passes the windmill and a junction with Woodland Trail at 3.2 miles. Continue straight on Windmill Trail.

The last stretch is a gentle meander through grassland. I enjoyed watching swallows near their birdhouse, and a few steps farther startled some quail along the trail. Windmill Trail splits at 3.4 miles—either leg returns to the trailhead, rejoining at the bridge near the trailhead.

• •

GPS TRAILHEAD COORDINATES N37° 59.935' W122° 12.290'

DIRECTIONS From the Bay Bridge toll plaza, drive northeast on I-80 about 16 miles. In Hercules, exit CA 4 E. Drive east 4.4 miles and exit right onto Christie Road (this exit is unmarked—the road looks like a driveway; the exit is just before a railroad trestle crossing over CA 4). Drive south on Christie Road about 0.75 mile to the signed trailhead on the right. *Note:* You must reach this trailhead via eastbound CA 4, and Christie Road dead-ends past the trailhead.

Sweeping through grassland on Whipsnake Trail

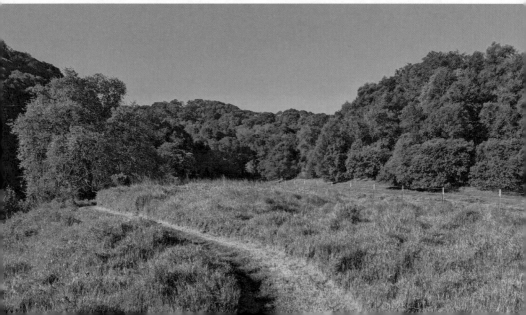

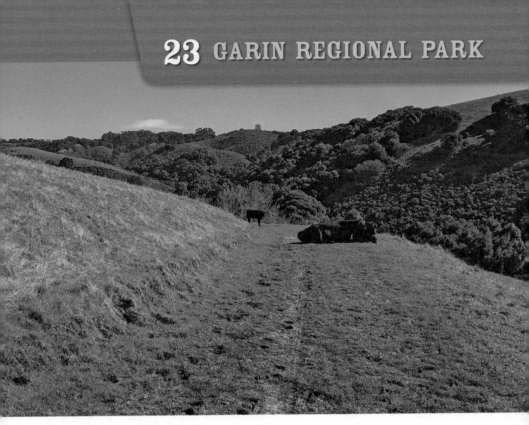

Bovine welcoming committee at Garin Regional Park

LOOP AROUND GRASSY PEAKS perched above Hayward on this 3.3-mile hike that offers spectacular views. On a weekday, you might have the place to yourself. On my latest hike, my son and I saw as many humans as coyotes (two of each!).

DESCRIPTION

Garin and neighboring park Dry Creek Pioneer sprawl across ridges just a mile uphill from busting Mission Boulevard. Trails unfold from the parking lots to the northeast and southwest, like a butterfly drying its wings. Most visitors explore Dry Creek Pioneer Regional Park, which has picnic areas, a visitor center, and a kite field. Folks with small children can loop around Jordan Pond, picnic, and fly a kite. Hikers (or cyclists) up for a challenge should consider combining any of the fire roads that climb to a grassy ridge; loops range from 3 to 6 miles. The Garin parcel is quieter, with only a few trails.

For this hike, begin from the edge of the parking lot on a paved trail, following the sign for Vista Peak Loop. At a level grade, the wide path accompanies lovely little Dry Creek, on the right. Tall sycamores and a few plum trees shade the way. At 0.3 mile, just past two pit toilets, the paved path swings left to Arroyo Flats group camp. Veer right and pass through a cattle gate onto Vista Peak Loop.

DISTANCE & CONFIGURATION: 3.3-mile balloon loop

DIFFICULTY: Easy

SCENERY: Views and grassland

EXPOSURE: Only the first 0.25 mile is shaded.

TRAIL TRAFFIC: Light

TRAIL SURFACE: Dirt fire roads and 1 paved trail

HIKING TIME: 1.5 hours

DRIVING DISTANCE: 34.5 miles from the US 101/I-280 junction in San Francisco

ACCESS: Opens daily at 8 a.m.; closing hours vary by season (check website). $5 entrance fee (when kiosk is staffed).

WHEELCHAIR ACCESS: There are designated handicapped parking spots, and the first 0.25 mile of this hike is wheelchair accessible.

MAPS: At Garin Barn Visitor Center and tinyurl.com/garinparkmap

FACILITIES: Restrooms and drinking water at Garin Barn Visitor Center

CONTACT: 888-327-2757, ebparks.org/parks/garin

LOCATION: 1320 Garin Ave., Hayward, CA

COMMENTS: Dogs welcome ($2 fee)

The wide multiuse trail climbs slightly through grassland. At the first bend, Old Homestead Trail heads off on a dead-end journey. Stay left. Vista Peak Loop ascends at an easy grade, passing a patch of willow on the left. At 0.5 mile the loop splits (you can hike in either direction); turn right.

We came across some cows on this stretch, and in winter the trail may be muddy. On a February hike meadowlarks called sweetly across the grassland, and several western bluebirds perched on dry stalks of fennel along the path, showing off their gorgeous sky-blue feathers. Still climbing easily, you already have great views south to Dry Creek Pioneer Regional Park. The trail curves left and the grade picks up a bit as the path bisects a little grove of coast live oak and California bay trees. Then it's back to sunshine and a sustained climb. When the trail reaches a saddle at 1.2 miles, Bailey Ranch Trail veers off to the right, leading up and over a hill before ending at the edge of a residential neighborhood. Continue left on Vista Peak Loop.

The trail curves left and drops to a signed junction at 1.3 miles. Ziele Creek Trail offers an extension to this loop, although trails along Ziele Creek are prone to mud in wet months: follow Ziele Creek Trail and Garin Woods Trail (the sole hiking-only path at Garin) back to Vista Peak Loop, and rejoin this hike at our next junction. Sticking to our 3.3-mile loop, continue straight on Vista Peak Loop.

A few minutes of uphill climbing leads to the ridgeline, with sweeping views west across the bay. Ignore a side path leading left, and stay right, looping around the top of Garin Peak. As the trail arcs left, the views get even better, stretching north past San Francisco to Marin's Mount Tamalpais, and south beyond San Jose. The trail descends past a huddle of coast live oaks and small boulders on the left. At 2 miles you'll reach a signed junction. There are almost always cows here, munching or reclining in the grassland. Turn left, continuing on Vista Peak Loop.

Descending gently, the trail continues to circuit the peak. My son spotted a young coyote uphill near the rocky knoll on our hike (our second coyote sighting

Garin Regional Park

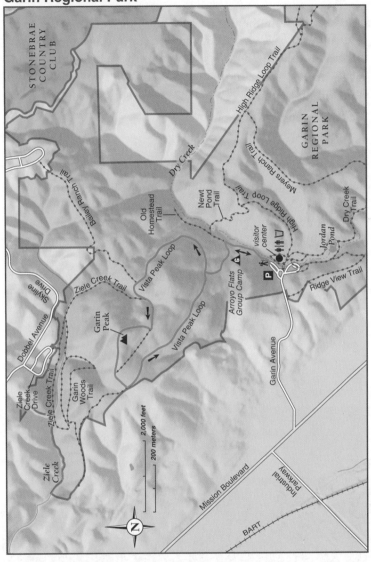

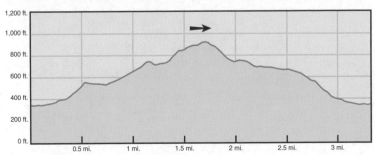

was a short distance from the trailhead on our return leg). To the south, Mission Peak's summit is conspicuous from this angle, as are the low rolling hills of Coyote Hills, on the edge of the bay. By spring, mustard plants splatter the grassland yellow. Across from an old stand of eucalyptus, there's a single swale of chaparral, with sagebrush dominating. Coast live oaks creep up the hillside near a pair of olive trees. At 2.8 miles you'll return to the other end of the loop. Bear right and retrace your steps to the trailhead.

• •

GPS TRAILHEAD COORDINATES N37° 37.786' W122° 01.720'

DIRECTIONS From the US 101/I-280 intersection in San Francisco, drive south on US 101 about 16 miles, then take Exit 414B, CA 92 E/Hayward. Drive east across the San Mateo Bridge, then take Exit 26A/B, I-880. Keep right at the fork and merge onto I-880 S. Drive south about 2 miles, then take Exit 25, Industrial Parkway. Turn left onto Industrial Parkway and drive east 2 miles. Turn right onto Mission Boulevard, and almost immediately get into the left lane to turn left onto Garin Avenue. Drive uphill on Garin 1 mile to the park entrance kiosk.

Pick a clear day and enjoy views galore from Vista Peak Loop Trail.

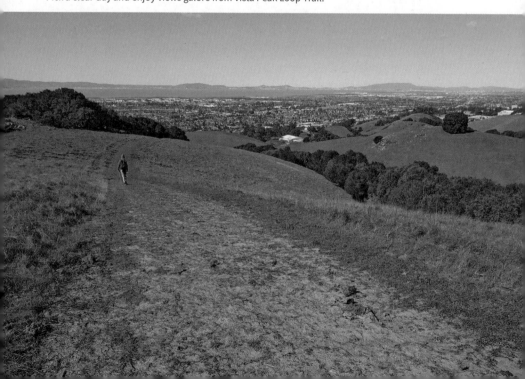

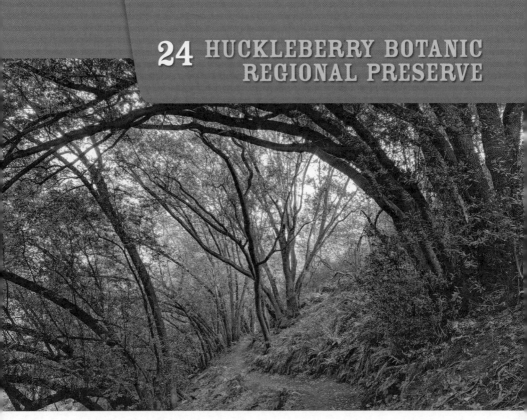

California bays arch over Lower Huckleberry Loop Trail.

THE MOST VISIBLE of the East Bay's open spaces is dominated by rolling grassland, but Huckleberry Botanic Regional Preserve, in the hills above Oakland, offers a tour through a variety of vegetation, including chaparral and woods. Along this short and easy 1.8-mile loop, numbered posts and a free brochure guide hikers through a wide assortment of plants, some of which are uncommon in the area.

DESCRIPTION

This small preserve sits on an unusual deposit of shale and chert—"poor" soil that's well suited to native plants. Although surrounding neighborhoods feature grassland, forests of eucalyptus, and redwood-crammed canyons, Huckleberry is a little oasis of manzanita barrens; scads of huckleberry bushes; and a gorgeous woodland of madrone, California bay, ferns, coast live oak, hazelnut, and currant. This is an arboretum-quality collection with an ever-changing palette of colors, textures, and tastes.

Huckleberry Preserve hosts two segments of long trails: Skyline National Trail and Bay Area Ridge Trail. Skyline National Trail is a 31-mile multiuse path that passes through a string of six big East Bay parks. Bay Area Ridge Trail extends more than 375 miles through nine Bay Area counties.

DISTANCE & CONFIGURATION: 1.8-mile loop

DIFFICULTY: Short but with steep sections

SCENERY: Mixed woodland and chaparral

EXPOSURE: Mostly shaded

TRAIL TRAFFIC: Moderate

TRAIL SURFACE: Narrow dirt trails

HIKING TIME: 1 hour

DRIVING DISTANCE: 11.5 miles from the Bay Bridge toll plaza

ACCESS: Daily, 5 a.m.–sunset. Winter is best for blooming manzanitas, but any time of year is good. No fee.

WHEELCHAIR ACCESS: Not recommended for wheelchairs

MAPS: At trailhead's information signboard and tinyurl.com/huckleberrymap

FACILITIES: Pit toilets at trailhead

CONTACT: 888-327-2757, ebparks.org/parks /huckleberry

LOCATION: On Skyline Boulevard, just south of Elverton Drive, Oakland, CA

COMMENTS: No dogs allowed

From the small staging area, walk a few feet to the information signboard, where you can pick up a brochure and map, then continue on Huckleberry Path. Tangles of blackberry and creambush crowd a hillside on the right, but the trail quickly enters an area well-shaded by coast live oaks and California bays. After 200 feet, where the two legs of the loop split, bear left. A few short zigzags drop the trail into a cool, shaded canyon, where you'll make a slow and steady descent. Look for the first numbered post of the tour on the right, identifying a madrone (the interpretive panels progress counterclockwise, so this post, #21, is the last of the tour—hiking this direction you count down). At 0.4 mile Skyline National Trail, on the left, heads out of the preserve toward Sibley Volcanic Preserve. Veer uphill to the right. California bays arch over the trail as it begins an easy ascent. The tour identifies ferns. A tiny-leaved, sweet-smelling plant called yerba buena hugs the ground in several places. The vegetation shifts subtly to include more coast live oak. In a few exposed areas, sticky monkeyflower and California coffeeberry bask in the sunlight.

At 0.9 mile Skyline Trail continues straight, while Lower Huckleberry Loop Trail bears right. (You can extend this hike by taking Skyline another 0.4 mile and then picking up Upper Pinehurst Trail on the way back to Upper Huckleberry Loop Trail.) Climb right on Connector Trail. A few sets of steep stairs quickly ascend through California bay and coast live oak woods to a junction at 1 mile. Walk a few feet to the right, then turn right, following the sign labeled TO 6. The path ascends easily out of the woods to a sunny manzanita barren. On a clear day, views stretch to include Mount Diablo to the east. If you happen to be visiting during the manzanita bloom (generally December–February), hummingbirds and bees are common, gorging themselves on the sweet nectar from the manzanitas' small white flowers. Return to the previous junction, then turn right.

The preserve's namesake, huckleberry, dominates the trail, which winds through the towering, mazelike hedges of the evergreen shrub. In August, huckleberry plants are crammed with small, dusky, blueberry-like fruit, a favorite of local

Huckleberry Botanic Regional Preserve

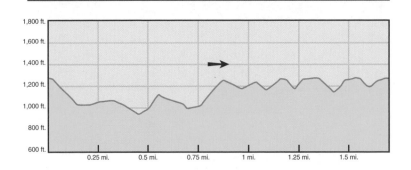

birds and even coyotes, who feed from the lower branches. At 1.3 miles bear right to another manzanita barren, where the brochure assists you in identifying canyon live oak. Retrace your steps back to the main path, then turn right. Chinquapin and silk-tassel accompany manzanita and huckleberry as the trail continues at a nearly level grade. Douglas iris blooms in clusters along the trail in spring.

At 1.7 miles you'll return to the hike's first junction and reach the end of the loop. Continue straight and return to the trailhead, retracing your steps on Huckleberry Path.

NEARBY ACTIVITIES

Learn more about Bay Area plants at the **East Bay Regional Parks Botanic Garden** (510-544-3169, ebparks.org/parks/tilden/botanic_garden.htm), at Wildcat Canyon Road and South Park Drive, in Tilden Park, Berkeley. The garden is open daily except January 1, Thanksgiving, and December 25.

• •

GPS TRAILHEAD COORDINATES N37° 50.560' W122° 11.705'

DIRECTIONS From the Bay Bridge toll plaza, drive about 0.5 mile east and bear right onto I-580 E. Drive 1.5 miles, then take Exit 19B, CA 24. Drive east on CA 24 about 5 miles, and at the far side of the Caldecott Tunnel, take Exit 7A onto Fish Ranch Road, the first post-tunnel exit—stay in the right lane. Drive north on Fish Ranch Road about 1 mile, then turn left onto Grizzly Peak Boulevard. Drive 2.4 miles, then turn left onto Skyline Boulevard. Drive 0.6 mile on Skyline, then turn left into the preserve parking lot.

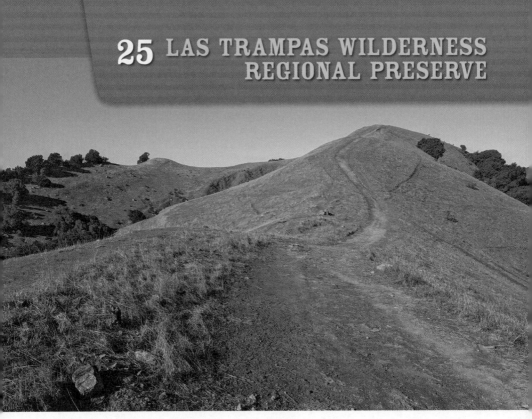

Following the ridgeline at Las Trampas Regional Wilderness

SPANISH FOR "THE TRAPS," Las Trampas is like two parks in one: from the trailhead, at the bottom of a wide canyon, you can hike east to chaparral-coated Las Trampas Ridge or west to grassy Rocky Ridge. Pick this western loop in spring, after the rains have stopped, for a steady climb to Rocky Ridge, where you can enjoy sweeping views and search for wildflowers.

DESCRIPTION

Begin from the parking lot. The paved fire road is the return route—pass through a metal gate and then a cattle gate onto Elderberry Trail, to the left of the vault toilets. At a slight ascent, the wide trail sweeps across the grassy base of Rocky Ridge, dips to cross a seasonal creek, and then runs along a corral on the left. At 0.4 mile you'll reach a junction with a spur leading left to Bollinger Creek Road. Turn right to remain on Elderberry Trail.

After such an easygoing intro, the subsequent climb is a bit of a shock—the trail shoots uphill, initially through a woodland of California bay, coast live oak, and black oak. Even when Elderberry Trail steps out into grassland, there's still no relief from the sharp grade, which feels especially harsh in summer's heat. As you ascend, there are nice views uphill toward the ridgetop and across Bollinger Canyon to Las Trampas Ridge. The grade tapers off, and then the trail begins a campaign of brief rolling

DISTANCE & CONFIGURATION: 4.7-mile loop

DIFFICULTY: Moderate

SCENERY: Grassland, woods, views, and rock formations

EXPOSURE: Nearly equal parts shaded and exposed

TRAIL TRAFFIC: Light–moderate

TRAIL SURFACE: Dirt fire roads, dirt trail, and paved fire road

HIKING TIME: 2.5 hours

DRIVING DISTANCE: 31.8 miles from the Bay Bridge toll plaza

ACCESS: Opens daily at 8 a.m.; closing hours vary by season (check website). Best in spring; muddy in winter; hot in summer. No fee.

WHEELCHAIR ACCESS: Not recommended for wheelchairs

MAPS: At trailhead's information signboard and tinyurl.com/lastrampasmap

FACILITIES: Vault toilets at trailhead

CONTACT: 888-327-2757, ebparks.org/parks/las_trampas

LOCATION: 18012 Bollinger Canyon Road, San Ramon, CA

COMMENTS: Although Las Trampas is designated as a regional wilderness, the western part of the park has some decidedly domestic inhabitants: cattle, which create muddy conditions during the rainy season. If the described trails are muddy—you'll know right away—the park's ungrazed eastern section provides good alternative hiking.

ups and downs. Paintbrush and California poppy are common in spring, blooming in sunny stretches of sagebrush and poison oak. In March, you might catch a few old fruit trees cloaked in a froth of fragrant flowers, gooseberry bushes in bloom, and buds on maple trees unfurling. Look for newts on the trail after heavy rains in winter or early spring.

Leaving the woods behind, Elderberry Trail's last stretch is a moderately steep ascent through grassland to the ridge. In mid-March the slope on the right is a kaleidoscope of flowers, including ivory-colored creamcups, purple filaree, and orange California poppies and fiddlenecks. At 2 miles Elderberry Trail ends at a junction with Rocky Ridge View Trail. The segment to the left ends at the park boundary after less than 0.5 mile. Before turning right, make use of the bench on the left—it's the only one on this loop.

Rocky Ridge View Trail clings to the ridgeline, ascending in fits and starts at a steep grade through grassland. Wonderful views unfold with every step uphill, from Mount Diablo in the east and west all the way to the Golden Gate Bridge on clear days. Cattle seem to love this ridge, and you'll often see lots of cows hanging out up here. On a hike in March one year, I watched an unidentifiable animal running at a fast pace, back and forth on a hillside across the canyon to the left. It was too dark for a coyote and lacked the long tail of a mountain lion but had a longer tail than a bobcat. What was this mysterious creature? I'll never know, as I forgot my binoculars that day.

Be sure to stop and examine the rock formations along the trail—the seashells are easy to pick out in these remnants of the Orinda Formation. It's hard to believe that this ridge, about 30 miles east of the Pacific, originated under the ocean. At 2.4 miles Devil's Hole Trail departs to the left, looping through the remote part of the park where I saw that mysterious animal. Continue straight. On a breezy day the

Las Trampas Wilderness Regional Preserve

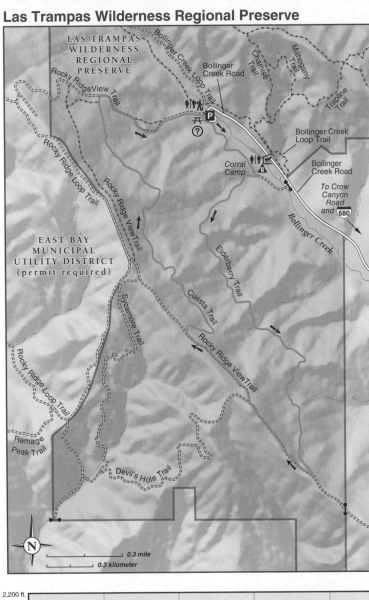

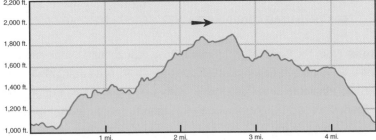

howling wind is absolutely deafening, but on a hot day you might wish for a little airflow. Rocky Ridge View Trail drops a bit off the ridgeline before reaching a junction at 2.8 miles. Turn right onto Cuesta Trail. (*Note:* In winter consider substituting Rocky Ridge View Trail for Cuesta—less mud.)

This little path descends moderately through coyote brush, makes a sharp left, and then levels out a bit while maintaining a general downhill trend. Like Elderberry Trail, Cuesta Trail has a fair amount of elevation wobble, but it's nothing dramatic. Sheltered from the bulk of the ridge, this is an excellent wildflower trail, despite the best efforts of the park's substantial cow population. In late winter, milkmaids, shooting stars, and buttercups are common; in mid-March, mule-ear sunflowers bloom along with California poppies, creamcups, and loads of purple bush lupine, all nicely accented against the green grassland. Some small pockets of California bay nestle in the crooks of the hillsides, but otherwise the descent is under full sun. At 3.6 miles a path heads straight, while the real trail curves right and downhill. This path starts out fine but then deteriorates, so stay right. At the 4.1-mile mark Cuesta Trail ends at a junction with a paved fire road, Rocky Ridge View Trail. Turn right.

The descent, moderately steep and steady, is a popular out-and-back route for locals walking with their dogs. Coast live oaks overtake the grassland as the trail winds downhill. After winter rains, you may hear and see small rivulets draining off the mountain toward Bollinger Creek, downhill to the left. At 4.7 miles Rocky Ridge View Trail ends at a gate back at the parking lot.

NEARBY ACTIVITIES

With herds of cattle and steady equestrian traffic, most of the park feels a bit like a private ranch, but the wilderness designation rings true in the far western section of Las Trampas and the adjacent property, a massive hunk of land managed by the East Bay Municipal Utility District (EBMUD). In the watershed, trails are open to hikers by advance permit only. With a permit, a car shuttle, and plenty of water, you could hike through Las Trampas and EBMUD lands to the Chabot Staging Area, a trek of nearly 11 miles. Get more information at ebmud.com/recreation/east-bay-trails.

• •

GPS TRAILHEAD COORDINATES N37° 48.952' W122° 03.005'

DIRECTIONS From the Bay Bridge toll plaza, drive east about 0.5 mile and bear right onto I-580 E. Drive 1.5 miles, then take Exit 19B onto CA 24. Drive east 12 miles on CA 24, then take Exit 15A south onto I-680. Drive south 10 miles and take Exit 36 onto Crow Canyon Road. Drive west (right) about 1 mile, then turn right (north) onto Bollinger Canyon Road. Continue about 4.5 miles to the trailhead, at the end of the road.

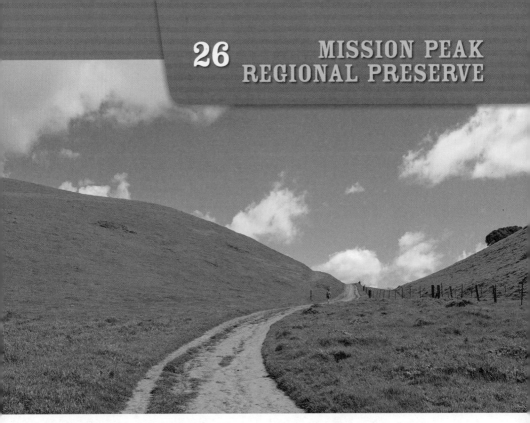

Climbing up Mission Peak from the Ohlone Trailhead is easier and less crowded.

ON THIS MISSION PEAK excursion, you'll begin at the edge of a Fremont residential neighborhood, hike up fire roads, and then take a little trail straight to the summit with 360-degree views—an ascent of more than 2,000 feet.

DESCRIPTION

To get to the Mission Peak trailhead, you turn off a heavily trafficked street, drive 0.5 mile, and boom—you're there, at the base of a mountain. Most mountains require long drives, but heck, you can get to Mission Peak by bus!

Leave from the parking lot on Hidden Valley Trail. The multiuse fire road skirts a short, wide hill. After just 0.1 mile Peak Meadow Trail departs to the right, but stay left on Hidden Valley Trail. The route ahead really stands out in late winter and early spring, when the grass is bright green. After a brief descent, the trail crosses a feeder to Aqua Caliente Creek, bends left, and begins to climb. Ascending at a sharp grade through grassland, you might catch a glimpse of hang gliders drifting downhill from farther up the mountain. Hidden Valley Trail draws near a wooded canyon and creek on the left, and coast live oaks and California bays along the trail offer snatches of shade. You might also notice a few islands of sagebrush, poison oak, and sticky monkeyflower floating in the sea of grassland along the trail.

DISTANCE & CONFIGURATION: 6.1-mile out-and-back

DIFFICULTY: Strenuous

SCENERY: Grassland and views

EXPOSURE: Almost completely exposed

TRAIL TRAFFIC: Heavy

TRAIL SURFACE: Dirt fire roads and trail

HIKING TIME: 3 hours

DRIVING DISTANCE: 45.5 miles from the I-280/US 101 junction in San Francisco

ACCESS: Opens daily at 6:30 a.m.; closing hours vary by season (check website). Spring is pleasant; winter is muddy; avoid during summer heat waves. No fee.

WHEELCHAIR ACCESS: Not recommended for wheelchairs

MAPS: At trailhead's information signboard and tinyurl.com/missionpeakrpmap

FACILITIES: Vault toilets and drinking water at trailhead

CONTACT: 888-327-2757, ebparks.org/parks/mission

LOCATION: Fremont, CA

COMMENTS: Dogs welcome (no fee)

City noises fade markedly as you climb, and as things quiet down, don't be surprised if you hear turkeys gobbling back and forth across the hillsides. Wild-turkey populations are on the rise in the Bay Area, and Mission Peak has its share of them. At 1.5 miles Peak Meadow Trail departs again on the right, dropping back toward the trailhead. Continue uphill on Hidden Valley Trail. Here you'll often come across some of the many cows that graze Mission Peak. Unpleasant cattle-versus-people conflicts do occur in Bay Area parks, and if you think bovines are sweet-tempered creatures, you may change your mind if a herd of them starts galloping toward you. Sometimes the cattle seem to act completely on caprice, but there are ways to minimize conflicts: In general, give cattle plenty of room, and don't get between a mother and her calf. Be sure to close all cattle gates you encounter, and if you're hiking with a dog, either leash it or keep it close and under voice control. Cattle, like people, seem friskiest in spring.

The trail grade slackens a bit, and Mission Peak's summit gets closer with every step. You may notice rocks on the sides of the trail, and their numbers increase until, as you reach a junction at 2.2 miles, the entire steeply sloping hillside leading to the summit is littered with rocks and boulders. At the base of the ridge, Grove Trail starts on the right. Stay left on Hidden Valley Trail. Mission Peak's remaining bulk rises sharply out of a pretty little valley, but the trail ascends a gentler route. Although the slope under the summit is incredibly sharp and rocky, you may see cattle grazing up there. Still ascending at a moderate grade, the trail sweeps through grassland where fiddlenecks bloom in late winter.

At 2.4 miles the last stretch of Hidden Valley Trail meets Peak Trail in the vertex of a big triangle-shaped junction. Stay right, then bear right again onto Peak Trail. Peak Trail pushes uphill through grassland to a signed junction at 2.6 miles. Turn right, remaining on Peak Trail. The path ascends, sweeping right onto the northeastern side of the peak. The trail shrinks from a wide track to a narrow and rocky path; look back over your shoulder from time to time to savor increasingly long views east

Mission Peak Regional Preserve

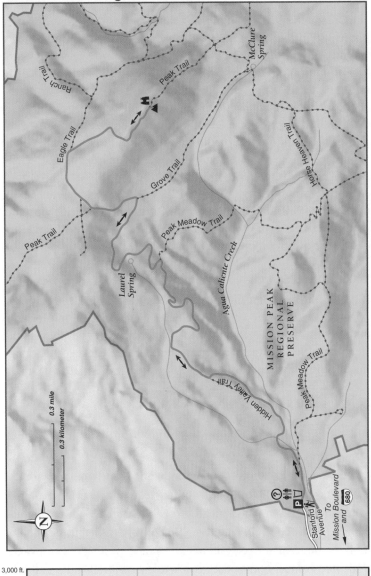

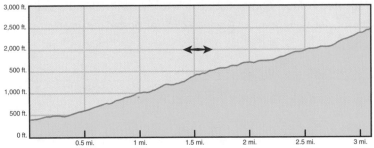

across the Ohlone Regional Wilderness. Peak Trail picks through rock outcrops as it ascends steeply. Finally, at 3.1 miles, you'll reach the top: elevation 2,517 feet.

From the summit, the entire South Bay sits at your feet. A funny little scope points out prominent natural features within visual range, including Mount Diablo to the north. Return to the parking lot the same way you came.

Note: Mission Peak is an exceptionally popular hike departing from an undersize trailhead. The East Bay Regional Park District encourages hikers to begin Mission Peak hikes from Ohlone College (parking fee required). Park at lots E, G, or H or the new parking structure, and start from the side of Pine Street on YSC Trail (signed for Peak Trail access), then take Peak Trail all the way to the top. Another option is to start a hike from Ed Levin County Park and trek to Monument Peak, just a few miles south of Mission Peak. Both peaks share the same ridgeline and fantastic views, but Ed Levin has more parking. Visit sccgov.org/sites/parks/parkfinder/Pages/Ed-Levin.aspx for more info.

NEARBY ACTIVITIES

Mission Peak is the western gateway to the **Ohlone Regional Wilderness** (ebparks.org/parks/ohlone), a 9,737-acre area that requires an advance permit for entry ($2 if purchased in person, $4 if purchased by mail/phone/web). The Ohlone Trail makes a 28-mile journey through the wilderness, and there are backpacking campsites for hikers making the entire trip.

• •

GPS TRAILHEAD COORDINATES N37° 30.263' W121° 54.498'

DIRECTIONS From the I-280/US 101 junction in San Francisco, follow US 101 south 15 miles, then take Exit 414B for CA 92. Keep left, following signs for CA 92 E/Hayward. On the other side of the San Mateo Bridge, take Exit 26A for I-880 toward San Jose. Drive about 14 miles south on I-880, then take Exit 12, Warren Avenue/Mission Boulevard. Drive northeast on Mission Boulevard about 0.6 mile, passing under I-680, and turn right on Stanford Avenue. Drive about 0.5 mile to the trailhead at the end of the street. Park in the lot, not along Stanford Avenue. Follow all posted parking restrictions.

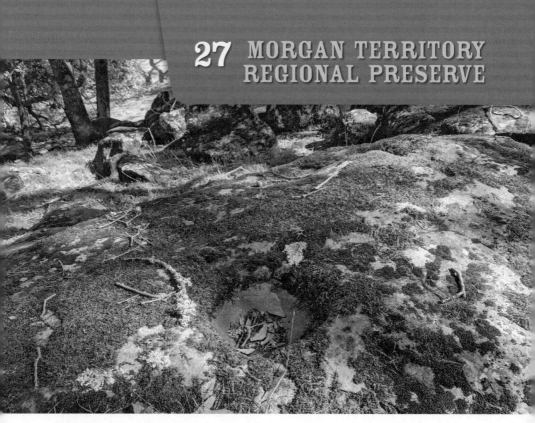

American Indian grinding bowl at Morgan Territory

MORGAN TERRITORY'S NAME whispers of the wilderness, evoking pioneers, wagon trains, and epic journeys. This loop rambles through a lavish landscape of grassland and oaks, with good birding and wildflower-spotting.

DESCRIPTION

Begin near the information signboard on Volvon Trail. After about 150 feet, Coyote Trail begins on the left. Stay right on Volvon. The path crosses through a cattle gate, curves uphill, and meets a fire road entering from the right. Mount Diablo's twin peaks loom in the distance to the north. Sweeping through grassland dotted with oaks, California bay, and buckeye, Volvon rises then begins an easy descent. A fire road doubles back to the right at 0.35 mile; continue left. Volvon Trail meanders through a small, bowl-shaped valley where johnny-tuck, California buttercups, fiddlenecks, and blue dicks bloom in spring. At 0.7 mile Whipsnake Trail heads off to the right; bear left. A few steps later, Volvon Trail veers left; turn right onto Blue Oak Trail.

The fire road winds gently uphill through graceful old oaks. Popcorn flower and filaree, two diminutive spring flowers, sprawl through the grass in early April. There are more sweeping views of Mount Diablo as Blue Oak Trail descends easily, but the surrounding landscape is also a visual delight, with rolling, grassy hills and

DISTANCE & CONFIGURATION: 5.1-mile balloon with 2 out-and-back strings

DIFFICULTY: Easy

SCENERY: Grassland, chaparral, and oaks

EXPOSURE: Partial shade throughout

TRAIL TRAFFIC: Light

TRAIL SURFACE: Dirt fire roads and trails

HIKING TIME: 2.5 hours

DRIVING DISTANCE: 44.7 miles from the Bay Bridge toll plaza

ACCESS: Opens daily at 8 a.m.; closing hours vary by season (check website). Late

winter and spring are best; summer is often very hot. No fee.

WHEELCHAIR ACCESS: Not recommended for wheelchairs

MAPS: At trailhead's information signboard and tinyurl.com/morganterritorymap

FACILITIES: Vault toilets and drinking water at trailhead

CONTACT: 888-327-2757, ebparks.org/parks/morgan

LOCATION: 9401 Morgan Territory Road, Livermore, CA

COMMENTS: Dogs welcome (no fee)

oaks stretching in every direction. On a February hike, snowy Sierra peaks were clearly visible off to the east.

Miwok Trail breaks off to the right at 1.3 miles, descending toward the Los Vaqueros Watershed. Continue left on Blue Oak Trail. In spring, carpets of goldfields appear, as blue and valley oaks begin to leaf out. Hummingbird Trail sets off to the left at 1.4 miles, connecting to Volvon Trail, but stay right on Blue Oak Trail. Here you can get a close look at the blue oaks lining the trail. The Volvon, a local American Indian tribe, would grind oak acorns into an edible mush using mortar rocks, some of which have been discovered inside this preserve. Continue straight on Blue Oak Trail, which gently rises and falls through a more wooded area dominated by oaks and buckeyes, where blue dicks and woodland stars bloom along the trail in spring. Other than bird cries or the soft chattering of squirrels, all is quiet. At 2.1 miles Blue Oak Trail ends at a T-junction. Turn right, back onto Volvon Trail.

At 2.15 miles you'll reach a cattle gate and junction with Valley View Trail; continue straight. The trail ascends to a saddle between hills. Views stretch east across the flatlands of the Central Valley to the Sierra, and north past Mount Diablo to Mount Saint Helena. Here, 2.4 miles into the hike, you could extend your journey on a 1.5-mile loop around Bob Walker Ridge to the right. Retrace your steps back to the junction with Blue Oak Trail, and turn right, continuing on Volvon Trail.

This segment of Volvon Trail rises gently through grassland peppered with oaks and boulders. Land slopes off to the right, revealing views across Morgan Territory Road to a grassy ridge that is also part of this wilderness. A few manzanitas mix into the landscape—in winter, when they are fragrant with white blossoms, bees swarm the shrubs. At 3.3 miles Hummingbird Trail sets off to the left, connecting to Blue Oak Trail. Turn right to remain on Volvon Trail.

Big gnarled oaks line the trail as it rises to a stretch of sunny chaparral. At 3.5 miles turn right from a signed junction onto Prairie Falcon Trail. The narrow

Morgan Territory Regional Preserve

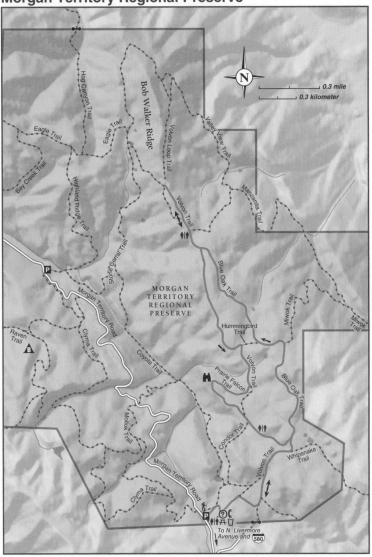

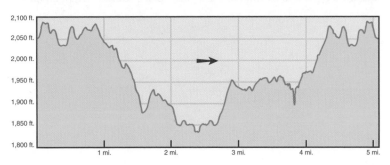

hiking-only path initially winds through grassland, with buckeyes and California bays mixed through oaks, but then dives into chaparral. Some short stretches are rocky. Look for Fremont's star lily, buttercup, and Indian warrior blooming here in late February. Prairie Falcon Trail is squeezed by chaparral shrubs, and you may smell black sage and pitcher sage on your shirt later. The path reaches the top of a rock outcrop with exceptional views and a steep drop-off (use caution). Look north for yet another great Mount Diablo vista. On a February hike I could hear Marsh Creek rushing downhill and see smears of snow on a hillside on the far slope of the canyon— a few days earlier the area had received a rare 6 inches of snow. Prairie Falcon turns away from the viewpoint and continues to poke through chaparral at a slight ascent. A second viewpoint offers one last scenic offering. The path climbs through an open area with a sloping rock floor, weaves though chamise and toyon, and returns to oak grassland and a junction at 4.1 miles. Turn right, back onto Volvon Trail.

A few steps later Condor Trail breaks off on the right, an alternate return path. Continue straight on Volvon Trail. After one last pass through manzanita, the oaks muscle their way back into the scenery. On a muddy hike, I could easily see bobcat, skunk, and mountain lion prints pressed into the trail. At 4.3 miles you'll reach an area I call Squirrel Triangle. A path (not on the map) shortcuts a meadow on the right and squirrel burrows are everywhere. Continue on Volvon to the junction with Blue Oak Trail, then retrace your steps back to the trailhead.

• •

GPS TRAILHEAD COORDINATES N37° 49.118' W121° 47.741'

DIRECTIONS From the Bay Bridge toll plaza, drive east about 0.5 mile and bear right onto I-580 E. Drive about 16 miles south; at the I-238 split, stay left on I-580. Continue east about 18 miles, then take Exit 52 onto North Livermore Avenue. Drive north on North Livermore. After about 3.5 miles, the road makes a sharp left and becomes Manning Road. Shortly after, turn right onto Morgan Territory Road. Drive about 5.5 miles on the narrow, winding, one-lane road to the signed park entrance, on the right.

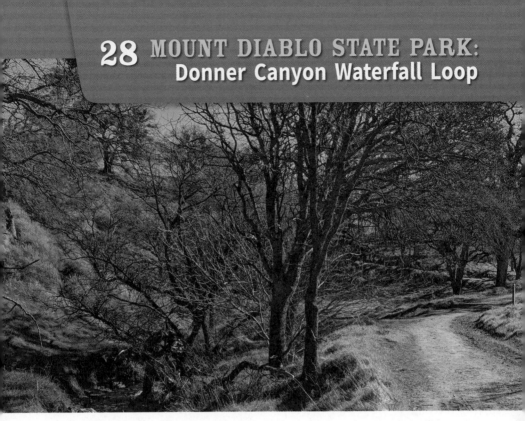

Heading up Donner Creek at Mount Diablo State Park

THIS HIKE ON Mount Diablo's northeastern slopes is the perfect antidote to the winter doldrums. Spring seems to visit Donner Canyon very early, gracing its rugged hillsides with fresh grass and blooming wildflowers and shrubs, even in February. Choose a clear day after a series of storms to see Donner Canyon's waterfalls at their peak.

DESCRIPTION

Rugged Mount Diablo, where temperatures soar to uncomfortable heights in summer, seems an unlikely host to waterfalls. Most of our Bay Area cascades are tucked back in forested canyons, but these falls run out in the open, dropping down rocky, steep hillsides covered with chaparral and pines. Although the falls aren't massive, they are pretty, and you can see them from several perspectives along this loop. If you can arrange it, drop everything and head for this hike when snowfall accumulates on Diablo's peaks. The road to the top of the mountain is usually closed then, but since snow rarely makes a dent on the lower reaches of Mount Diablo, you can enjoy views of dusted peaks without having to trudge through snow.

Depart from the Mitchell Canyon Trailhead, initially on Mitchell Canyon Road. After about 370 feet turn left, at a signed junction, onto Oak Road. The wide fire road climbs at a stiff grade through oak-dotted grassland. At 0.2 mile a fire road

141

DISTANCE & CONFIGURATION: 7.4-mile balloon loop with a long string

DIFFICULTY: Strenuous

SCENERY: Chaparral, grassland, oaks, and waterfalls

EXPOSURE: Mostly exposed

TRAIL TRAFFIC: Moderate–heavy

TRAIL SURFACE: Dirt fire roads and trails

HIKING TIME: 4 hours

DRIVING DISTANCE: 26.5 miles from the Bay Bridge toll plaza

ACCESS: Daily, 8 a.m.–sunset. Best in winter and early spring. $6 day-use fee (cash or check only).

WHEELCHAIR ACCESS: There is designated handicapped parking, and wheelchair access is unobstructed, but this hike's trails are initially very steep and other trails present barriers; thus, wheelchairs are not recommended.

MAPS: Park maps are available when the visitor center is open on weekends and holidays; order a free map published by Save Mount Diablo in advance (savemountdiablo.org/activities /diablo-trail-map), or download at tinyurl.com /mtdiabmap.

FACILITIES: Restrooms and drinking water at trailhead

CONTACT: 925-837-2525, tinyurl.com /mtdiablosp

LOCATION: 96 Mitchell Canyon Road, Clayton, CA

COMMENTS: No dogs allowed

drops off to the left; continue straight and soon you'll reach a second junction at 0.3 mile, with Coulter Pine and Mitchell Rock Trails. Turn left to remain on Oak Road. After a quick descent you'll reach a junction with Murchio Road, at 0.4 mile. Turn right.

The broad multiuse trail sweeps across grassland sprinkled with large oaks. The fire road is often muddy in winter, so look for animal tracks. On a January hike I saw coyote, bobcat, turkey, and horse tracks. At 0.8 mile Murchio Road crosses Bruce Lee Road. Continue straight. There are nice views to Eagle Peak, the bulk of the mountain's peaks, and, to the east, Black Diamond Mines. Murchio Road dips steeply to a seasonal creek, then rises again and meets a junction with Back Creek Trail at 1 mile. Keep going straight on Murchio Road. After a level bit, the fire road drops past a massive old eucalyptus and ends at 1.2 miles. Turn right onto Donner Canyon Road.

As you follow along Donner Creek you'll have good views uphill to Mount Diablo's highest peaks. The wide multiuse fire road weaves gently uphill through oaks, with some buckeyes along the creek. You may see buttercups along the trail in February, as well as fresh leaves on buckeye trees. At 1.9 miles a path breaks off to the left, heading to the Donner Cabin site, and a few steps later there's a junction with a path to Donner Cabin Trail on the right. Ignore both, but just around the corner at 2 miles, Hetherington Loop Trail sets off on the left; bear left.

After a few steps the narrow path crosses Donner Creek. There is no bridge, just a casual rock-hop (if the water level is very high, consider turning back and ascending via Donner Canyon Road). Once across the creek, Bruce Lee Spring Trail starts from a signed junction. Turn left. (Hetherington is an optional route, but you'd need to cross a deeper section of the creek again up the trail.)

Mount Diablo State Park:
Donner Canyon Waterfall Loop

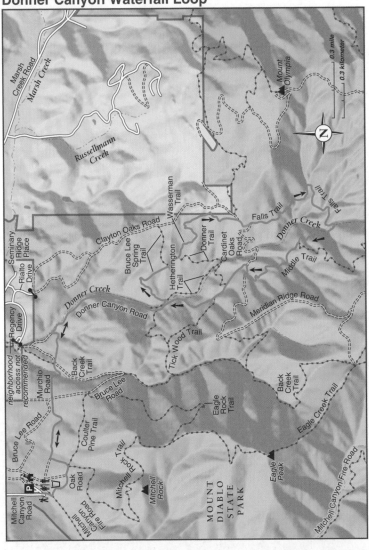

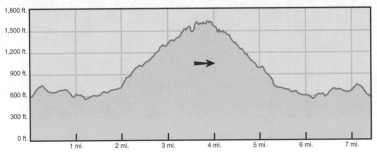

Bruce Lee Spring Trail climbs steeply through an open forest of oak with a grassy understory. At 2.3 miles Bruce Lee Spring Trail swings off to the left, connecting to Clayton Oaks Road. Continue straight, now on Donner Trail. The path keeps climbing, to a junction at 2.5 miles with Wasserman Trail. Turn left. The ascent continues on the narrow path, through oaks and then chaparral. Finally, at 3.1 miles, Wasserman Trail ends at Cardinet Oaks Road. Turn right.

The wide fire road descends slightly, with impressive views north. At 3.2 miles turn left at a signed junction onto Falls Trail. This is where an already scenic hike becomes spectacular. Falls Trail, just a little slip of a path, angles at a slight incline across a hillside of sagebrush, bush lupine, toyon, poison oak, pines, oaks, and grassland. The initial view of the waterfalls, even at a distance, is dramatic; water seems to appear out of thin air and gush out of creases in the hillside across the canyon. As you progress farther along the rocky trail, you'll have nice views uphill of several falls running down the side of steep Wild Oat Canyon. When Falls Trail dips to cross the creek, check out the broad but short waterfall just a few feet upstream. The trail ascends sharply then returns to a more moderate grade. Ceanothus, cercocarpus, and pines are common along the path.

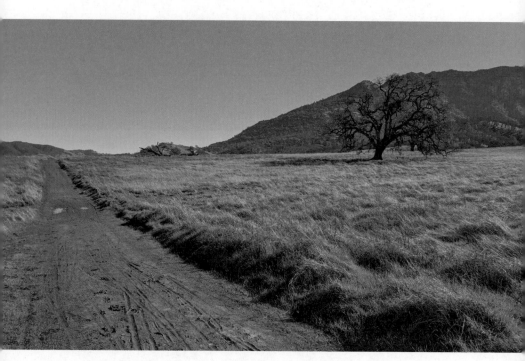

A big oak frames a view of Mount Diablo's peaks from Murchio Road.

Here, at the hike's highest elevation, look north for an ideal overview out of Donner Canyon and beyond. The trail descends to cross another creek, just below a small cascade (the water continues downhill to the last fall, but you have to get past it to see it). Climb uphill on the far side of the creek, then look back for my favorite view of the falls—a sheer, frothy drop that's breathtaking when the water flow is heavy. You'll cross one last creek and ascend a bit to a grassy area where hound's tongue blooms in late winter. At 4.3 miles Falls Trail ends at a signed junction. Middle Trail heads uphill to the left, climbing steeply toward Prospector's Gap. Continue right on Middle Trail toward Meridian Ridge Road.

Middle Trail descends a little, through a thicket of manzanita that fails to obscure views of the opposite side of the canyon and Mount Diablo's summit. You'll pass through an area with more dense vegetation, including toyon, chamise, and California bay, where chaparral currant blooms along the trail in February. After one last sunny stretch, Middle Trail ends at 4.8 miles. Turn right onto Meridian Ridge Road.

Your time on this fire road is brief—less than 0.1 mile down the trail you'll reach Cardinet Junction. Turn left onto Donner Canyon Road. The fire road descends through manzanita, yerba santa, ceanothus, poison oak, and pine. Shooting stars bloom in the understory in winter. At 5 miles Hetherington Loop drops down to the creek on the right. Continue straight. At 5.1 miles Tick Wood Trail sets off to the left, climbing toward Back Creek Trail. Press on downhill on Donner Canyon Road. This next stretch is notorious for sticky mud in winter. Oaks return to dominate the landscape. At 5.4 miles you'll again reach the junction with Hetherington Loop, on the right. Continue straight and retrace your steps back to the trailhead.

• •

GPS TRAILHEAD COORDINATES N37° 55.233' W121° 56.490'

DIRECTIONS From the Bay Bridge toll plaza, drive about 0.5 mile east and bear right onto I-580 E. Drive 1.5 miles, then take Exit 19B onto CA 24. Drive east 13 miles on CA 24 to the I-680 split, then take Exit 15B onto Ygnacio Valley Road. Travel east about 7 miles on Ygnacio Valley, then turn right onto Pine Hollow Road. Drive east about 1.7 miles, then turn right onto Mitchell Canyon Road. Continue about 1.5 miles to the trailhead at the end of the road.

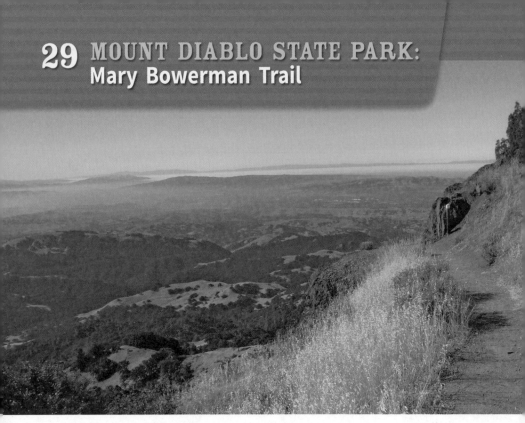

Savor the long view from Mount Diablo's Mary Bowerman Trail.

MARY BOWERMAN TRAIL (formerly known as the Fire Interpretive Trail) offers perspective without perspiration. Less than a mile and gently graded, the trail makes a circuit just beneath Diablo's summit. The first section of the loop is paved and suitable for wheelchairs and strollers, but the remainder of the trail is a standard rocky mountain path.

DESCRIPTION

A drive to the top of Mount Diablo is a classic Bay Area day trip. A twisty, scenic road leads to the mountain's highest peak, which is crowned with a stone observation tower and a little museum. On clear days, Diablo is famous for views that stretch across the San Joaquin Valley to snowcapped Sierra peaks. If you want to supplement a summit trip with a hike but you don't have much time or are hosting out-of-town guests who are active but not really hikers, this loop trail just down the hill from the summit is perfect, featuring awesome views, a self-guided tour of mountain vegetation, and a fraction of the summit crowds.

From the large parking lot, walk uphill toward the summit along the side of the park road; the signed trailhead begins on the left, just past where the park road splits into one-way sections. Mary Bowerman Trail, marked with interpretive posts, begins under the shade of interior live oaks and canyon live oaks. Post 2 juts out

DISTANCE & CONFIGURATION: 0.7-mile loop

DIFFICULTY: Easy

SCENERY: Chaparral, grassland, and views

EXPOSURE: First stretch is shaded; the rest is exposed.

TRAIL TRAFFIC: Light

TRAIL SURFACE: Initial section is paved; the rest is a narrow dirt path.

HIKING TIME: 30 minutes

DRIVING DISTANCE: 36 miles from the Bay Bridge toll plaza

ACCESS: Daily, 8 a.m.–sunset. Any time of year is good, but the park is hot in summer. When snow dusts the mountain, the road to the top is closed. Pay $10 fee at entrance kiosk on the way up the mountain.

WHEELCHAIR ACCESS: There is designated handicapped parking, and the first part of the hike is wheelchair accessible.

MAPS: At entrance station or Summit Museum Visitor Center (open daily, 10 a.m.–4 p.m.), or download at tinyurl.com/mtdiablospmap. An interpretive guide to the trail is available at the trailhead and at tinyurl.com/mbowermanguide.

FACILITIES: Restrooms and water at the summit

CONTACT: 925-837-2525, tinyurl.com /mtdiablosp

LOCATION: Contra Costa County, CA

COMMENTS: No dogs allowed

from a cluster of poison oak. This deciduous plant is astoundingly variable and can grow as a vine, ground cover, or hedge. Here it's a little shrub, naked in winter but clothed again by spring with distinctive "leaves of three." Poison oak's oil, urushiol, is so strong that when any part of the plant comes into contact with clothing, the oil can survive multiple washings, reinfecting the wearer with an itchy rash. (Make sure to wash oil-contaminated clothing separate from other clothing, using the hottest water, largest load size, and longest cycle setting.)

As Mary Bowerman Trail progresses, you'll move out of the trees into a more open area, where greenstone, graywacke, and chert rocks are identified by Posts 3, 4, and 5. Look left for views north past Mitchell Canyon to northern Contra Costa County. At 0.2 mile the pavement ends at a wooden platform. This is a great place to whip out the binoculars. Even if you can't see Mount Lassen, you'll enjoy great close-up views of Diablo's rugged North Peak.

As the trail bends right, you might notice a dramatic change in vegetation. Here chaparral plants, including ceanothus and cercocarpus, dominate with some live oaks and pines mixed through the evergreen shrubs. I've seen mountain lion prints on the trail, but sightings of these shy creatures are not common—cougars prowl mostly at night.

The trail crosses an open, rocky hillside, then approaches Devil's Pulpit on the left. This dusky-red rock formation, composed of chert, has resisted weathering that eroded the surrounding earth. Rough paths scramble downhill to the formation and North Peak Trail, but Mary Bowerman Trail curves right as sparsely vegetated slopes roll downhill to the south. The summit buildings are visible uphill as the trail snakes through yet another plant community.

Mount Diablo State Park: Mary Bowerman Trail

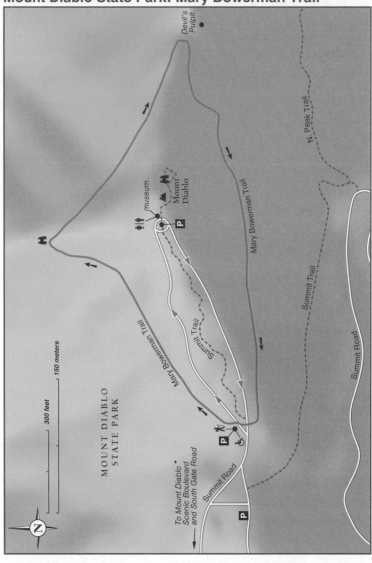

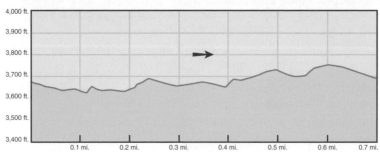

If you're visiting in fall, note that Mount Diablo is tarantula habitat. Tarantulas, which emerge from their burrows to mate in the fall, are autumn regulars on the mountain. These hairy spiders are relatively harmless, their bites about as dangerous as wasp or bee stings. Even if you don't see them on the trails, you may spot a few crossing the park roads. Give them a wide berth and they'll ignore you—they have more important things on their arachnid minds!

The last three posts mark juniper, yerba santa, and chamise, which crowd the trail along with some poison oak. At 0.7 mile the trail ends across the street from the trailhead. Turn left and walk back to the parking lot.

NEARBY ACTIVITIES

The **Summit Museum Visitor Center** (925-837-6119, mdia.org/summit-museum) is located at the actual summit, a short distance from this trailhead. It highlights the cultural and natural history of the park with exhibits on geology, American Indian history, and the park's ecosystems, plus an observation deck with telescopes. Admission to the museum is free.

• •

GPS TRAILHEAD COORDINATES N37° 52.857' W121° 55.025'

DIRECTIONS From the Bay Bridge toll plaza, drive east about 0.5 mile and, bear right onto I-580 E. Drive 1.5 miles, then take Exit 19B onto CA 24. Drive east 13 miles on CA 24, then exit south onto I-680 (Exit 15A). Drive south 7 miles, then take Exit 39, Diablo Road, and turn left. Following the green PARKS signs, drive east on Diablo Road about 1 mile to the junction with El Cerro Boulevard. Turn right and continue about 3 miles on Diablo, then turn left at the stop-signed junction with Blackhawk Road onto Mount Diablo Scenic Boulevard. Drive 3.8 miles carefully uphill to the entrance kiosk, where you'll pay the day-use fee. (As you enter the park, Mount Diablo Scenic Boulevard becomes South Gate Road.) *Note:* This stretch of road is narrow; keep an eye out for bicyclists. Continue uphill on South Gate 3.2 miles to a stop sign and junction, then turn right onto Summit Road. Keep climbing another 4 miles on Summit. Just before the road splits into two one-way segments near the summit, park in a large paved lot on the right (or continue to the summit, then drive back down to this lot).

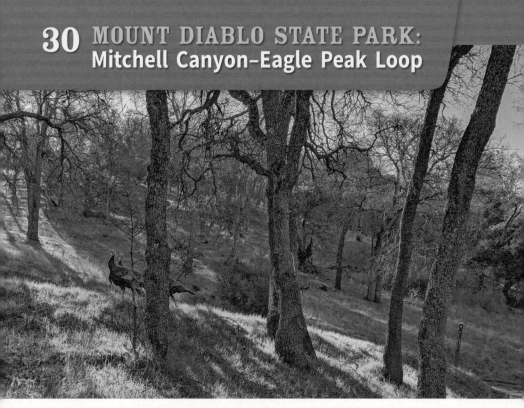

30 MOUNT DIABLO STATE PARK: Mitchell Canyon–Eagle Peak Loop

Wild turkeys on Oak Road at Mount Diablo State Park

THIS CREEK-TO-PEAK Diablo tour begins at Mitchell Canyon and climbs on fire roads, easily then steeply, to Murchio Gap. Here the fun really begins, on a rollicking singletrack excursion over knife-edged Eagle Peak. From the exposed peak top, enjoy views, then continue downhill at an often-steep grade back to the trailhead.

DESCRIPTION

Mitchell Canyon is a popular staging area for long Diablo hikes. From here, you can make an all-day excursion to Diablo's summit, a 14-mile round-trip from 590 to 3,849 feet and back again—one of the Bay Area's toughest day hikes. The trek to Eagle Peak described here doesn't have the same cachet as the bottom-to-top hike, but I prefer the shorter loop. When the long trek to the top of Diablo nears the summit area, you'll commonly cross paths with loads of visitors around Juniper Campground and hear and see cars on a trail paralleling Summit Road—jarring contrasts to the quiet found on most of the mountain. Peaceful and lonely, far from the developed parts of the park, Eagle Peak provides excellent hiking with awesome views.

Begin from the trailhead on the signed Mitchell Canyon Fire Road. As you pass through the gate, pick up the Mitchell Canyon Interpretive Guide, an excellent accompaniment to the first 2 miles of this hike. The broad fire road starts out

DISTANCE & CONFIGURATION: 7.7-mile loop

DIFFICULTY: Strenuous

SCENERY: Chaparral, creek, and views

EXPOSURE: Almost all full sun

TRAIL TRAFFIC: Moderate around the trailhead and on Mitchell Canyon Road; light farther afield

TRAIL SURFACE: Dirt fire roads and rocky trails

HIKING TIME: 4 hours

DRIVING DISTANCE: 26.5 miles from the Bay Bridge toll plaza

ACCESS: Daily, 8 a.m.–sunset. Good any season but summer due to the heat; exceptional wildflowers in spring. Pay $6 fee (self-register; cash or check only) at entrance gate.

WHEELCHAIR ACCESS: There is designated handicapped parking, and wheelchair access is unobstructed, but most of this hike's trails are very steep and present barriers; thus, wheelchairs are not recommended.

MAPS: Obtain the official park map at Mitchell Canyon Interpretive Center (open weekends only), order a free map published by Save Mount Diablo in advance (savemountdiablo.org/activities/diablo-trail-map), or download a map at tinyurl.com/mtdiabmap.

FACILITIES: Restrooms and water at trailhead

CONTACT: 925-837-2525, tinyurl.com/mtdiablosp

LOCATION: 96 Mitchell Canyon Road, Clayton, CA

COMMENTS: A trekking pole is handy for the Eagle Peak traverse. Check for ticks from late spring through autumn, when the grass is high. No dogs allowed.

climbing gently through grassland dotted with blue, coast live, and valley oak. At 370 feet, Oak Trail, the return leg of this loop, begins on the left—continue straight on Mitchell Canyon Fire Road. In spring you may see sticky monkeyflower, Chinese houses, paintbrush, and Ithuriel's spear in bloom along the trail, blended through a mixture of oaks, pines, and chaparral plants, including sagebrush, California coffeeberry, poison oak, and pitcher sage.

At 0.6 mile Black Point Trail departs on the right. Continue on Mitchell Canyon Fire Road, where the trail's namesake creek runs along the left and pockets of riparian trees such as willow and alder are common. Swallowtail butterflies were out in abundance on my May hike, along with variable checkerspots and mylitta crescents, flitting to and fro. In spring look for Mount Diablo fairy lanterns, a yellow globe lily found only on and around Mount Diablo. On other Diablo hikes, I had seen a few of these fairy lanterns, but all along the length of the Mitchell Canyon Trail I saw dozens and dozens of them, as well as staggering amounts of wind poppy, a beautiful, four-petaled orange flower.

On the right, Red Road drops down from Black Point at 1 mile—once again, continue on Mitchell Canyon Fire Road. As the canyon broadens slightly, views begin to unfold uphill to the left of rocky, steep-sided Eagle Peak. The fire road starts to climb with a bit more purpose, somewhat shaded by coast live oaks and a few bigleaf maples, buckeyes, and California bays. At about the 2-mile mark, the grade picks up significantly, and although there are some nearly level stretches, the climb is long and sustained. Stay alert for cyclists descending. On warm days, every bit of shade and cooling breeze is welcome.

Mount Diablo State Park: Mitchell Canyon–Eagle Peak Loop

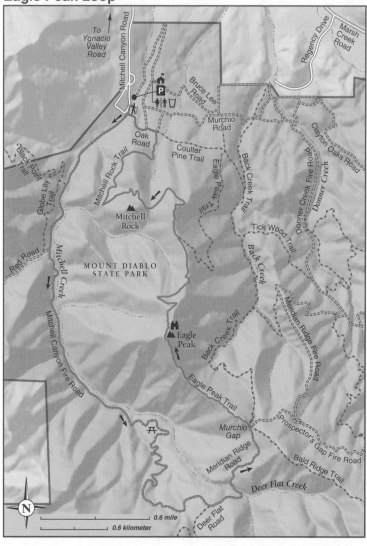

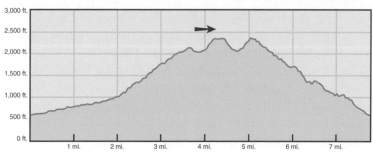

With the creek left behind in the low reaches of the canyon, the surrounding slopes are dry and play host to many chaparral plants, with Coulter pine, sagebrush, ceanothus, goldenbush, cercocarpus, poison oak, toyon, sticky monkeyflower, and black sage prominent. There's plenty to look at along the trail, particularly in spring, when a variety of flowers bloom, including linanthus, paintbrush, lupines, onions, mule-ear sunflower, and clarkia. Views continue to open up to Eagle Peak on the left and out of the park back to the north.

The ascent, following a series of sweeping curves, seems never-ending, but abruptly the grade tapers off slightly, and then the fire road sweeps right and reaches a flat on the right, at 3.4 miles. Two picnic tables provide rest spots. When you're ready, press on uphill at a moderate pace through oaks and pine to the Deer Flat junction at 3.6 miles. Deer Flat Road continues to climb toward the summit on the right, but our route, Meridian Ridge Road, swings left.

The fire road descends through oak, pine, poison oak, and California hop tree, offering a break from all that climbing. The relief is short-lived, though—once the trail crosses Deer Flat Creek, it begins to ascend steeply. Continue on Meridian Ridge Road, ascending past a grassy slope on the right, where California poppies bloom in big patches in April. The trailside vegetation shifts to chaparral, with lots of yerba santa, manzanita, pine, and chaparral pea enjoying the sunny exposure. The climb ends at Murchio Gap at 4.4 miles, where trails depart in every direction: traveling clockwise, Eagle Peak Trail begins; then Back Creek Trail; the continuation of Meridian Ridge Road; and little Bald Ridge Trail, across the road to the right. Turn left onto Eagle Peak Trail.

The slight path skirts a rock outcrop, climbing through ceanothus, chamise, yerba santa, black sage, goldenbush, and hop tree. As Eagle Peak Trail starts to descend, loose rock on the path presents a challenge—if you've brought a trekking pole, you'll definitely be glad. When you reach the saddle, you'll get a brief, level respite as the trail punches through thickets of chamise. Look to the left for a view of Mitchell Canyon Fire Road's snaking uphill route and back to the right for views of Diablo's summit area. As the trail begins to climb again, you'll enter a rocky, grassy area, where juniper and pine are common and, in early May, tons of clarkia, buckwheat, and jeweled onion brighten the grass as it begins to fade to gold. The ascent over these exposed slopes is sharp, with a couple of very rocky sections.

Finally, at 5 miles, you'll arrive at the top (2,369'), unsigned but obvious. There's remarkably little real estate here, and the peak slopes drop sharply off this knife-edged ridge. You'll surely want to pause and enjoy the views, which encompass the entire northern part of the mountain, including the summit and North Peak, as well as rolling ridges on the right and left, and hills well off into the distance. In winter, with strong binoculars, you might be able to see the waterfalls dropping out of Donner Canyon. On a May hike, I observed a horned lizard that scampered a few feet from me, almost perfectly camouflaged in the surrounding tan pebbles. Birders and butterfly enthusiasts could spend some time on this peak, watching hawks and swallowtails soaring or fluttering overhead.

The trail clings to the ridgetop, then drops off to the left, beginning a descent. There are more steep, rocky patches to traverse as Eagle Peak Trail swings through some shaded areas where you might notice chaparral currant blooming in winter. Mostly the hillsides are cloaked in an army-green coat of chamise, black sage, and toyon. Continuing down the sloping ridgeline, a second small peak is crossed, and the trail just keeps dropping. At 5.9 miles Eagle Peak Trail swings sharply right, descending off the east side of the mountain. Continue straight, now on Mitchell Rock Trail.

The narrow path rises, then drops to the side of a red-rock outcrop on the right. Some pines shade the trail as you make a transition into a mixture of grassland and chaparral. Look for a good variety of flowers in spring, including California poppy, coyote mint, mariposa lily, Chinese houses, paintbrush, milkweed, owl's clover, and blue-eyed grass. Although the trend is firmly downhill, there are a few short, easy uphill stretches. The trail veers off the ridgeline into pure grassland and, other than a few forays through chaparral patches, stays that way all the way downhill. You'll pass Mitchell Rock, a pillow-basalt outcrop, on the left. By mid-May, thigh-high grass crowds the trail as it weaves downhill, reaching a junction with Coulter Pine Trail at 7.5 miles. Turn left, now on Oak Road.

Shortly you'll reach a junction with a trail on the right leading downhill toward the water tower. Continue straight on Oak Road, and descend steeply through blue oaks and grassland to a junction with Mitchell Canyon Fire Road at 7.7 miles. Turn right and return to the trailhead.

• •

GPS TRAILHEAD COORDINATES N37° 55.233' W121° 56.490'

DIRECTIONS From the Bay Bridge toll plaza, head east about 0.5 mile and bear right onto I-580 E. Drive 1.5 miles, then take Exit 19B onto CA 24. Drive east about 13 miles on CA 24 to the I-680 split, then take Exit 15B onto Ygnacio Valley Road. Travel east about 6.7 miles on Ygnacio Valley, then turn right onto Pine Hollow Road. Drive east about 1.7 miles, then turn right onto Mitchell Canyon Road. Continue to the trailhead at the end of the road, about 1.5 miles.

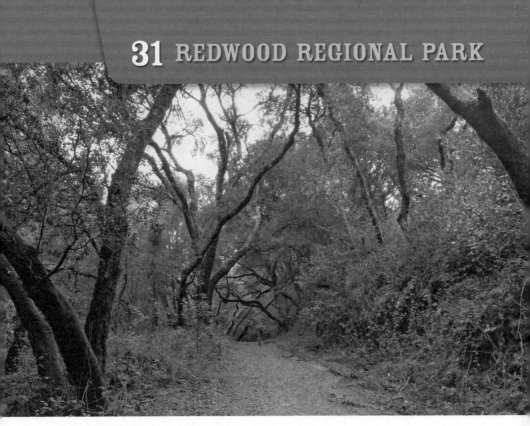

A hiker ascends through the woods on Prince Trail.

THE NEXT TIME you find yourself gazing east from Mount Tamalpais or the Marin Headlands, think of this: towering above the East Bay hills in the 1800s was a row of redwoods so tall that ship captains used them to navigate through the Golden Gate into San Francisco. Although the giant trees were logged by the turn of that century, second-growth redwoods now fill canyons where rainbow trout spawn and ladybugs hibernate in the winter, wildflowers bloom in spring, and other wild creatures scamper through the woods year-round. This easy 4.1-mile loop drops into a redwood canyon and then climbs back to a nearly level trail, which returns to the trailhead.

DESCRIPTION

Redwood Regional Park is mostly just one big canyon, and although it has some neighborhood access points, most people enter from either end of the park. There are many loop options, so hikers can mix and match on canyon and ridge trails. Hikers, equestrians, dog walkers, runners, and cyclists frequent Redwood trails, but it's still easy to find peace and quiet, particularly on the paths closed to cyclists.

Starting from the Skyline Gate Staging Area, begin on West Ridge Trail. At a level grade, the wide fire road sweeps past some eucalyptus into a more natural setting of chaparral currant, California bay, madrone, coast live oak, toyon, hazelnut,

DISTANCE & CONFIGURATION: 4.1-mile loop

DIFFICULTY: Easy

SCENERY: Redwoods and a mixture of grassland and shrubs

EXPOSURE: Shaded in canyon; partial sun on ridges

TRAIL TRAFFIC: Moderate–heavy

TRAIL SURFACE: Dirt fire roads and trails

HIKING TIME: 2 hours

DRIVING DISTANCE: 10.5 miles from the Bay Bridge toll plaza

ACCESS: Daily, 5 a.m.–10 p.m., unless otherwise posted. Nice year-round, although trails are muddy in winter. Free from this trailhead; main park staging area requires a $5 fee.

WHEELCHAIR ACCESS: There are designated handicapped parking spots, and wheelchair access to trails is unobstructed, although not recommended during muddy seasons. Folks in wheelchairs should be able to navigate a short distance on both East and West Ridge Trails.

MAPS: At trailhead and tinyurl.com/redwood regionalparkmap

FACILITIES: Vault toilets at trailhead

CONTACT: 888-327-2757, ebparks.org/parks /redwood

LOCATION: 8490 Skyline Blvd., Oakland, CA

COMMENTS: Dogs welcome ($2 fee)

and creambush. At 0.6 mile French Trail sets off into the canyon on the left, but keep going on West Ridge Trail.

The sea of trees parts occasionally to reveal views southeast out of the canyon. Redwoods creep up from the canyon in places, contrasting with patches of grass and chaparral. When you reach the junction with Tres Sendas Trail at 1.1 miles, turn left and begin to descend.

The narrow trail can get quite muddy in winter when storm runoff filters downhill, plumping a little stream. It doesn't take long to make the transition from ridge to canyon at a moderate grade. In just a few minutes, you'll find yourself in the clutches of a gorge filled with redwoods, California bays, and ferns. French Trail joins Tres Sendas from the right at 1.5 miles, and the two paths run together briefly, until French veers off to the left. Continue right on Tres Sendas as it descends deeper into groves of redwood. Look for trilliums blooming in spring. At 1.8 miles Starflower Trail heads uphill on the right. Stay left on Tres Sendas. The trail crosses Redwood Creek and ends at 1.9 miles. Turn right onto Stream Trail (for a shorter hike, turn left and return to the trailhead—in winter chances are excellent you'll see loads of ladybugs on this stretch of trail).

As Stream Trail follows along Redwood Creek, fences line the trail to protect the fragile riparian environment. Here in the heart of the canyon, it's almost completely shaded all day, and the trailside vegetation is a lush tangle of ferns and blackberry vines. Moss is draped over boulders and swathed around redwood trunks. On one winter hike, I came upon thousands of ladybugs hibernating. The orange beetles looked like a pile of maple leaves from a distance, but up close I marveled at how they huddled together on branches and leaves of the understory vegetation. Observing ladybugs is a highlight of Bay Area winter hikes, and I've since seen them

Redwood Regional Park

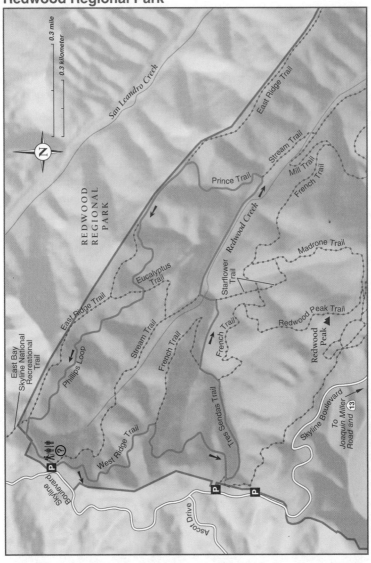

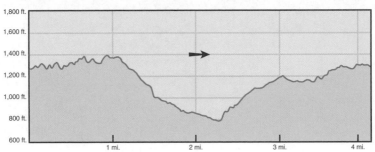

several other times. Stream Trail descends slightly to a junction at 2.3 miles. Turn left onto Prince Trail.

As the broad trail climbs at a moderate grade out of the canyon, redwoods and California bays give way to coast live oaks and madrones; then the trees thin and coyote brush, poison oak, and blackberry dot grassland. Prince Trail ends at 2.7 miles. Turn left onto East Ridge Trail.

The wide fire road follows the park boundary at a nearly level grade. Coyote brush, pine, coast live oak, and madrone seem to stand off from the trail, permitting views back across the canyon to the west ridge. Although dogs are frequent visitors to the park, there's plenty of wildlife here, and you might examine the sandy trail surface for telltale animal signs. Bobcat prints are decidedly feline, though their feet are considerably larger than those of domestic cats. Coyotes leave spadelike prints and are fond of marking their territory at junctions, leaving piles of scat as calling cards for other coyotes where deer trails and paths cross. Deer are the most common hoofed animal in the Bay Area, and their crescent-shaped prints are easy to pick out. In summer months, when the trails are dry, you might see squiggly paths left across trails by traveling snakes. At the 2.9-mile mark, East Ridge Trail continues to the right, while Phillips Trail swings off to the left. Either route is an option, but I prefer Phillips, so bear left.

Many colorful mushrooms brighten the Redwood Regional Park woods in winter. Remember: Look but don't touch!

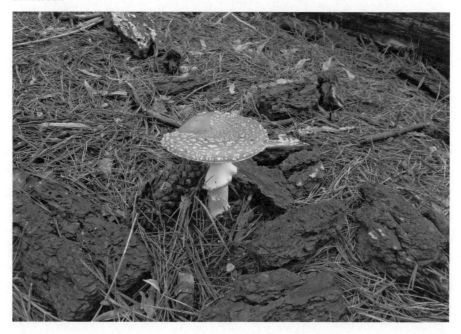

The trail undulates a bit through coyote brush, pine, and madrone. You might hear (and see) hawks perched on tall trees nearby. Eucalyptus Trail crosses Phillips at 3.2 miles; continue straight. Eucalyptus trees, imported in the 1800s from Australia, are a common fixture in East Bay parks. Timbermen hoped the fast-growing trees would provide profitable lumber crops, but their wood turned out to be unsuitable for building purposes. Another exotic plant you might notice along the trail is cotoneaster, a landscaping shrub with glossy leaves and red berries. Unlike that of toyon, a native shrub that also bears red berries, cotoneaster's fruit is poisonous to humans, although birds eat the berries.

Phillips Trail runs downslope from the ridge on the right until the trail merges into East Ridge Trail at 3.9 miles. The trail straight across the junction leaves Redwood Park and heads north into Huckleberry Preserve on the East Bay Skyline National Recreation Trail, a 31-mile path that runs through six East Bay parks. Bear left and follow East Ridge Trail another 0.2 mile back to the trailhead.

NEARBY ACTIVITIES

Sibley Volcanic Regional Preserve (6800 Skyline Blvd., Oakland; 888-327-2757; ebparks .org/parks/sibley), a few miles north of Redwood Regional Park, features a self-guided loop through the remains of a volcano.

• •

GPS TRAILHEAD COORDINATES N37° 49.896' W122° 11.116'

DIRECTIONS From the Bay Bridge toll plaza, drive east about 0.5 mile and bear right onto I-580 E. Drive 1.5 miles, then take Exit 19B onto CA 24. Drive east 3.5 miles on CA 24, then take Exit 5 onto CA 13 S. After about 2.5 miles, take Exit 3, Park Boulevard. At the foot of the exit ramp, make a left onto Park Boulevard, then turn right onto Mountain Boulevard. Drive on Mountain Boulevard 0.3 mile, then make a slight left onto Ascot Drive. Drive uphill on Ascot 1.5 miles, then turn left on Skyline Boulevard. Drive north on Skyline 0.7 mile, and turn right into the Skyline Gate parking lot and staging area.

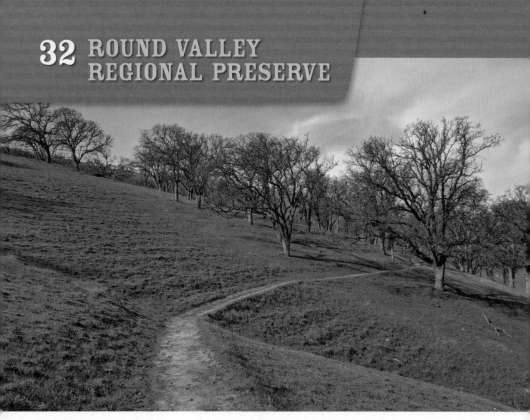

Bare oaks stretch up a hillside on Hardy Canyon Trail.

ROUND VALLEY'S SINGLE trailhead is on a lonely country road that winds through the eastern foothills of Mount Diablo. Hikers can take long out-and-back or shuttle hikes through this preserve and neighboring Los Vaqueros Watershed, but this hike is an easygoing, three-creek, 4.4-mile tour through rolling hills of oak woods and grassland.

DESCRIPTION

Hikes at Round Valley scratch that peace-and-quiet itch. You may hear the occasional plane overhead, but traffic noise fades once you leave the trailhead, and the flanks of Mount Diablo block views of suburban sprawl to the west. This is one of those spots that make Bay Area life delightful for folks who love the outdoors.

Round Valley is part of a little-known greenbelt. The East Bay Regional Parks District–managed Round Valley and Morgan Territory Regional Preserves abut Mount Diablo State Park and Los Vaqueros Watershed (owned and run by the Contra Costa Water District), creating a huge block of protected land. Wildlife-viewing is exceptional through all these parklands; Round Valley is protected habitat for the San Joaquin kit fox, and golden-eagle sightings are frequent.

From the trailhead, follow the obvious route over a bridge to a junction with Hardy Canyon Trail, the return segment of the loop. Pass through the gate to the

DISTANCE & CONFIGURATION: 4.4-mile loop

DIFFICULTY: Moderate

SCENERY: Grassland, oaks, and views

EXPOSURE: Mostly full sun; some partial shade

TRAIL TRAFFIC: Moderate

TRAIL SURFACE: Dirt fire road and trails

HIKING TIME: 2 hours

DRIVING DISTANCE: 57.5 miles from the Bay Bridge toll plaza

ACCESS: Opens daily at 8 a.m.; closing hours vary by season (check website). Summer is often very hot. No fee.

WHEELCHAIR ACCESS: Not recommended for wheelchairs

MAPS: At trailhead's information signboard and tinyurl.com/roundvalleymap

FACILITIES: Vault toilets and drinking water at trailhead

CONTACT: 888-327-2757, ebparks.org/parks /round_valley

LOCATION: 19450 Marsh Creek Road, Brentwood, CA

COMMENTS: No dogs allowed. In summer, temperatures can exceed 100°F. Use sunscreen, and wear a hat and loose-fitting clothing.

right, on Miwok Trail. This fire road begins a moderate climb along the preserve boundary, downslope from an oak-studded hillside. On a winter hike I watched a small flock of white-breasted nuthatches flit from tree to tree.

After a short dip, as the trail rises again, go straight onto an unsigned but well-worn path, which shortcuts a roller-coaster stretch best suited to equestrians. The path descends and feeds back into the fire road, which crosses Round Valley Creek and meets a dead-end trail at 0.5 mile. Stay left on Miwok Trail.

The trail now follows along Round Valley Creek at an easy grade. Hills rise to the right and left, marked with many lovely trees, including blue and coast live oak and buckeye. On one cold February morning, the mud was frozen and grass was frosted with white. There are usually quite a few squirrels scuttling about in the grassy areas off the trail, and you might see hawks sitting in trees near squirrel burrows. I've also seen golden eagles soaring above this part of the preserve in autumn. Miwok Trail ascends a bit and reaches a junction at 1.3 miles. The valley stretches south from here.

Turn left onto Hardy Canyon Trail, a narrow path that ascends through grassland and blue oak. Cattle that graze throughout the preserve seem to prefer the valley basin, but you might meet a few up in these hills as well. During the wettest months of the year, rain cascades downhill in the creases of the hillsides, where buckeyes thrive. Look for coyote and bobcat prints on the trail—dogs are not permitted at Round Valley, so all prints are most likely from wild residents of the area.

Although the grade never increases beyond moderate, you might want to stop occasionally to enjoy the northwest views, which extend beyond the boundaries of the preserve to include Mount Diablo's main and north peaks, an unusual perspective of the East Bay's tallest mountain.

Hardy Canyon Trail sticks to a course downslope from the hilltop, effectively looping around the hill. As you climb, the oaks thin a bit and grassland dominates the landscape. The trail jogs left then right on a little switchback around a long, thin rock

Round Valley Regional Preserve

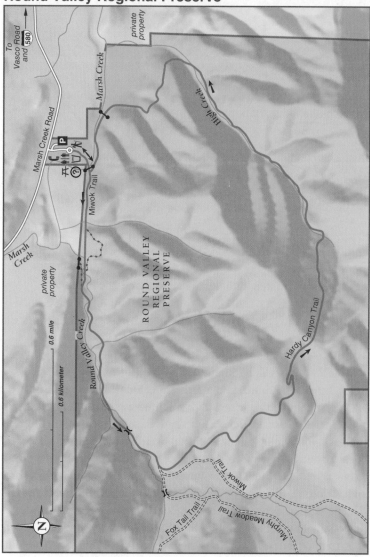

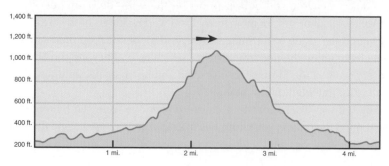

formation that resembles a sloping wall. After one last gentle ascent through grassland, the trail reaches a slight saddle. The trail almost immediately starts downhill to the left. You never reach the hilltop, but then again, with views this nice, you don't need to.

The preserve boundary is a short distance to the right, and the adjacent property is the Los Vaqueros Watershed. The two properties don't connect here, but if they did, it would create a great hiking loop opportunity (you can enter the watershed from a gate on Miwok Trail at the south end of Round Valley). As Hardy Canyon Trail descends to the east, scattered cow paths (one leading to a watering trough) make navigation a bit tricky. Aim for the crease between this hill and another to the right. On a February morning I could see snowy Sierra peaks way off to the east. Gradually you'll enter an area with a high concentration of blue oaks, as the trail adopts a course along the banks of High Creek. Here, as in other parts of the park where water runs in winter and spring, buckeyes grow clustered together. Buttercups are the first flower of the year, setting out yellow flowers in February. Hardy Canyon Trail climbs slightly then descends back toward the creek.

At 3.6 miles you'll reach a crucial (unsigned) junction. Be sure to bear left and cross the creek—the path to the right heads into private property. As you make your way gently uphill through oaks and grassland, an occasional vehicle on Marsh Creek Road may be audible. Hawks are common in this part of the preserve, using the trees to scope out small mammals in the adjacent meadow to the right.

The trail descends into grassland then sweeps left to reach a gate. On the other side you'll follow along yet another waterway, Marsh Creek, where cottonwoods and sycamores share their autumnal-tinted leaves in November. At 4.3 miles the trail rises up to meet Miwok Trail back at the hike's first junction. Turn right and return to the parking lot.

• •

GPS TRAILHEAD COORDINATES N37° 52.108' W121° 45.012'

DIRECTIONS From the Bay Bridge toll plaza, drive east about 0.5 mile and bear right onto I-580 E. Continue on I-580 about 36 miles southeast and take Exit 55 onto Vasco Road in Livermore. Turn left and drive north on Vasco Road about 14 miles to the junction with Camino Diablo. Turn left onto Camino Diablo, drive about 3.5 miles, and continue left onto Marsh Creek Road. Drive west on Marsh Creek Road about 1.5 miles to the preserve entrance on the left.

33 SUNOL REGIONAL WILDERNESS

Hikers on McCorkle Trail, with Flag Hill in the background

SUNOL'S JAGGED PEAKS and grassy ridges are surrounded by open space, cushioning the impact from nearby East Bay towns and highways. There's a lot of real estate here, with natural wonders that include rock formations, creeks, and small waterfalls in winter and spring.

DESCRIPTION

Describing a Bay Area location as Yosemite-esque is bold. California's famous national park is a natural jewel with soaring granite domes, massive waterfalls, and a sense of peace found nowhere else. But attach "little" to Yosemite and apply the term to a spot at Sunol, and it fits. Sunol's Little Yosemite area is remarkably serene and gorgeous, with a boulder-strewn rushing creek, big rock formations, and towering oaks and sycamores. All this beauty is accessed via an easy 2.2-mile out-and-back hike. Put in a little more effort and reach Little Yosemite by climbing up and down through grassland, and be rewarded with sweeping views. Your choice!

Start at the gated Camp Ohlone Road. Right away you'll make friends with Alameda Creek as you cross the waterway on a long, sturdy bridge. Say goodbye to the stream for now—you'll see it again down the trail. At 0.1 mile, turn left onto signed McCorkle Trail. (If you are opting for the easy out-and-back, continue straight.) After squeezing through a very narrow V-stile, the multiuse fire road begins to climb

DISTANCE & CONFIGURATION: 2.7-mile balloon loop, with 2.2-mile out-and-back option

DIFFICULTY: Easy

SCENERY: Grassland, oaks, creek, and rock formations

EXPOSURE: Mostly full sun

TRAIL TRAFFIC: Heavy

TRAIL SURFACE: Dirt trails and fire roads

HIKING TIME: 2 hours

DRIVING DISTANCE: 42 miles from the Bay Bridge toll plaza

ACCESS: Opens daily at 8 a.m.; closing hours vary by season (check website). Late winter and spring are best—not a good summer choice;

exceptional wildflowers in spring. Pay $5 fee at entrance kiosk.

WHEELCHAIR ACCESS: Folks in wheelchairs should be able to navigate the 2.2-mile out-and-back trek to Little Yosemite, on Camp Ohlone Road. Note that there are several cattle grids across the trail that may be difficult to traverse. There is no designated handicapped parking; arrive early to park in this lot.

MAPS: At entrance kiosk and tinyurl.com /sunolmap

FACILITIES: Pit toilets at trailhead

CONTACT: 510-544-3249, ebparks.org/parks /sunol

LOCATION: 1895 Geary Road, Sunol, CA

COMMENTS: Dogs welcome ($2 fee)

though oak-dotted grassland. In winter when the deciduous oaks are leafless, note that they are not exactly empty. Big bunches of parasitic mistletoe are obvious from afar. When you get a closer look at the oaks, you might see galls. Wasps cause these irregular plant growths by laying their eggs on the oaks. Developing larvae introduce chemicals into the trees, triggering the growth. The galls become a nursery for wasp larvae, which then grow to maturity and leave the galls. Although there are many different-colored and -shaped galls, one of the most common is the oak apple gall, which looks to me a bit like an Asian pear.

The grade is moderate, and as you climb, vistas unfold almost immediately. Look north for a view of the rock outcrops at Flag Hill. Yellow buttercups bloom along the path in March. The trail dips and then climbs some more to a signed junction at 0.7 mile. Canyon View Trail drops back down toward park headquarters on the left, and McCorkle Trail continues uphill straight ahead (if you're enjoying the climbing, you can extend this hike by proceeding on McCorkle, then taking Cerro Este Road to Little Yosemite). Turn right onto Canyon View Trail.

This slight hiking-only path slips across a hillside scored with cattle meanders. As Canyon View curves left, oaks fade back and the path ascends easily through grassland. California poppies are common here in spring. The trail descends gently to a muddy spot where a large sycamore stands, off to the left. On my January hike there were lots of cows munching along the path. The trail rises again to a rocky spot, then veers left and clings to the hillside. You'll have nice views here down to the Little Yosemite area and west toward the Calaveras Dam. A spur leads right to a large rock outcrop—if you check it out, be cautious of the drop-off. Sagebrush makes an appearance in the oaky grassland. Canyon View Trail descends easily to a junction with Cerro Este Road at 1.3 miles. Bear right, following the signs toward Little Yosemite.

Sunol Regional Wilderness

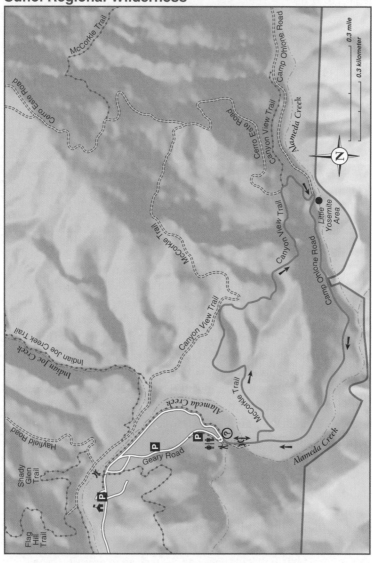

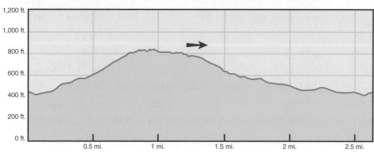

Cerro Este Road weaves through some large coast live oaks and a few California bays, then drops to a junction and the Little Yosemite area at 1.5 miles. A few picnic tables make good lunch spots. Just across from the junction, along Camp Ohlone Road, paths lead down to Alameda Creek, where water rushes around and over giant boulders. Use caution here, as rattlesnakes are sometimes sighted near the water (and there is better creek access down the trail). When ready, turn right (west) onto Camp Ohlone Road.

The wide multiuse trail descends easily along Alameda Creek. Just before a cattle grid, a path on the left leads down to the creek (explore if interested). On the right side of Camp Ohlone Road, the steep, grassy slope is freckled with lupines in spring. A few oaks provide occasional shade. Other than one brief and easy uphill stretch, it's effortless downhill walking, with Alameda Creek occasionally visible. Sprawling buckeyes bask on a grassy shelf on the left. Camp Ohlone Road completely levels out and reaches the junction with McCorkle Trail at 2.5 miles. Continue straight, retracing your steps back to the trailhead.

NEARBY ACTIVITIES

Del Valle Regional Park (7000 Del Valle Road, Livermore; 888-327-2757, ebparks.org /parks/del_valle) offers a similar, slightly tamer terrain of rolling oak savanna, plus a campground and a lake for swimming, boating, and fishing.

• •

GPS TRAILHEAD COORDINATES N37° 30.594' W121° 49.722'

DIRECTIONS From the Bay Bridge toll plaza, drive east about 0.5 mile and bear right onto I-580 E. Continue on I-580 about 25 miles, then take Exit 44B to merge onto I-680 toward San Jose. Drive south 8.3 miles, then take Exit 21A onto CA 84/Calaveras Road. Stay in the left lane of the exit ramp, turn left, drive under the freeway, and then stay in the left lane through a stop sign to remain on Calaveras. Drive south on Calaveras about 4 miles to the junction with Geary Road, and turn left. Continue on Geary almost 2 miles to the park entrance kiosk, then continue past the visitor center to parking lots at the end of the park road.

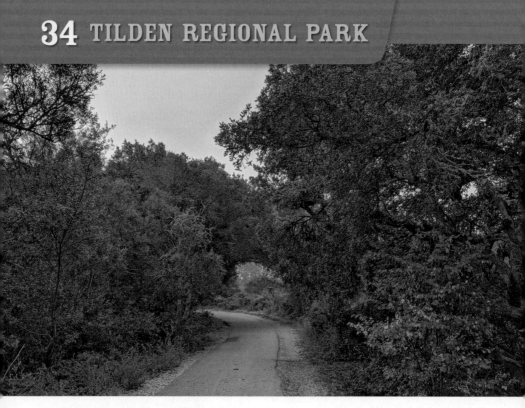

Paved Nimitz Way offers easy walking.

THIS EASY HIKE hosts walkers from the very young to the very old. It's a favorite for anyone looking for easy yet scenic exercise, and dogs are welcome.

DESCRIPTION

Tilden Regional Park is a recreation paradise in the backyard of East Bay communities Berkeley and Kensington. In addition to miles of trails that connect to adjacent parks, enabling long rambles, Tilden provides exceptional opportunities for family fun, with a merry-go-round, a swimming lake, pony rides, steam trains, and picnic areas that can be reserved.

Countless future hikers have been introduced to the great outdoors at Tilden, often on an easy out-and-back excursion on Nimitz Way. With a little one strapped to a parent's chest or snuggled in a stroller, baby's first hike is one that the entire family can enjoy, with excellent facilities, a paved trail with only gentle elevation changes, plenty of benches along the way, and wonderful views of the East Bay and beyond.

Walk west from the parking lot toward the Nimitz Gate. A gated trail on the right leads to East Bay Municipal Utility District (EBMUD) property and is accessible only by advance permit. Once through (or around) Nimitz Gate, begin hiking on paved Nimitz Way. This trail runs north 3.5 miles to a peak in Wildcat Canyon Park, but if you're hiking with a child in a stroller or a dog, you'll likely want to

DISTANCE & CONFIGURATION: 3.9-mile out-and-back

DIFFICULTY: Easy

SCENERY: Views, grassland, and eucalyptus forest

EXPOSURE: Mostly full sun

TRAIL TRAFFIC: Heavy

TRAIL SURFACE: Paved

HIKING TIME: 1.5 hours

DRIVING DISTANCE: 12.6 miles from the Bay Bridge toll plaza

ACCESS: Daily, 5 a.m.–sunset; good year-round. No fee.

WHEELCHAIR ACCESS: There is designated handicapped parking, and this trail is wheelchair accessible, although it is not flat.

MAPS: At trailhead and tinyurl.com/tilden rpmap

FACILITIES: Vault toilets at trailhead

CONTACT: 888-327-2757, ebparks.org/parks /tilden

LOCATION: Wildcat Canyon Road, Berkeley, CA

COMMENTS: Dogs are permitted on this hike but prohibited on some other Tilden trails.

turn back before entering cattle-grazed Wildcat Canyon. The broad multiuse trail enters weedy grassland downslope from the ridgeline to the right. Some pines tower overhead; along the trail you might notice cardoon, a relative of the artichoke with similarly leafy vegetation and big buds that unfold to reveal pretty, thistly flowers. Expect good birding here year-round; the most commonly spotted birds include scrub jays darting from tree to tree, and vultures and red-tailed hawks perched on power lines. To get glimpses of local or migratory songbirds, you'll likely need a good pair of binoculars.

The trail undulates gently past clusters of poison oak and young coast live oak. On the left side of the trail, views unfold across the Berkeley flats to the bay, Mount Tamalpais, and San Francisco. The first of many benches along the route appears. Spring flowers include blue-eyed grass, mule-ear sunflowers, checkerbloom, and yellow bush lupine, but tangles of blackberry, coyote brush, and poison oak choke out most of the grassland (and flowers) in this stretch. High-tension power lines run along the trail for a while. Around the 1-mile mark, the trail descends noticeably, then levels out again. Look for shrubby willows on the right, partly screening a seasonal boggy pond. At 1.3 miles a trail departs on the left, heading downhill toward Tilden Nature Area, where no dogs are allowed. Continue straight on Nimitz Way.

The trail is lined with coyote brush, poison oak, diminutive coast live oak, and California bay. In summer, great clusters of sweet pea and cow parsnip draw bees and butterflies. Nimitz Way enters a eucalyptus grove where on a spring hike I saw several pipevine swallowtail butterflies fluttering through the aromatic woods. At 1.8 miles there's a junction with a trail to Wildcat Peak on the left. This out-and-back path makes a good addition to this hike if you're hiking without a stroller. Continue a bit farther on Nimitz Way, out of the woods to a cattle guard and boundary with Wildcat Canyon Regional Park. Nimitz Way continues north, but this is the

Tilden Regional Park

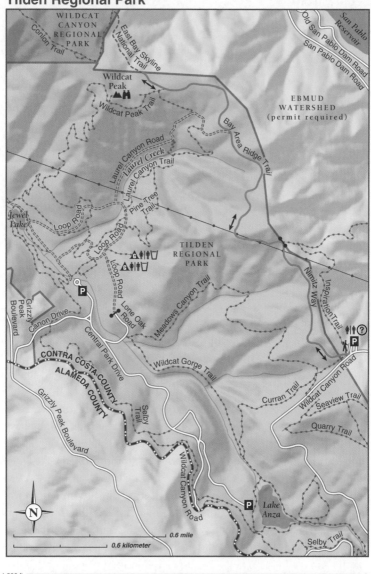

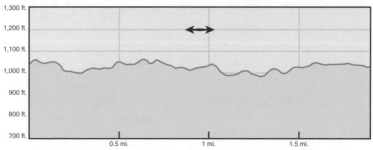

turnaround point for this hike. Enjoy views east, across the hills of Briones Regional Park, all the way to Mount Diablo, then retrace your steps back to the trailhead.

NEARBY ACTIVITIES

Tilden's northern neighbor, **Wildcat Canyon Regional Park** (5755 McBryde Ave., Richmond; 888-327-2757; ebparks.org/parks/wildcat) provides more hiking choices on trails that climb up and down mostly grassy slopes grazed by cattle.

• •

GPS TRAILHEAD COORDINATES N37° 54.303' W122° 14.671'

DIRECTIONS From the Bay Bridge toll plaza, drive east about 0.5 mile and bear right onto I-580 E. Drive 1.5 miles, then take Exit 19B onto CA 24. Drive east about 5 miles on CA 24 and, at the far side of the Caldecott Tunnel, take Exit 7A onto Fish Ranch Road, the first post-tunnel exit—stay in the right lane through the tunnel. Drive north on Fish Ranch Road about 1 mile, then turn right onto Grizzly Peak Boulevard. Drive 1.4 miles, then turn right onto South Park Drive. After 1.5 miles, bear right onto Wildcat Canyon Road. Continue about 1 mile to the Inspiration Point trailhead, on the left.

Note: South Park Drive closes annually November–March to protect migrating newts. If it's closed on your visit, continue on Grizzly Peak to Golf Course Road, turn right, and then turn right again onto Shasta Road. Finally, bear right onto Wildcat Canyon Road and continue to Inspiration Point.

Nimitz Gate at the Inspiration Point Trailhead

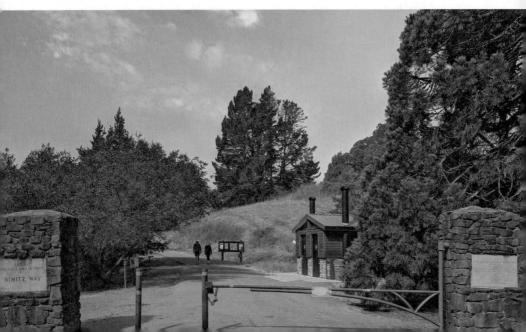

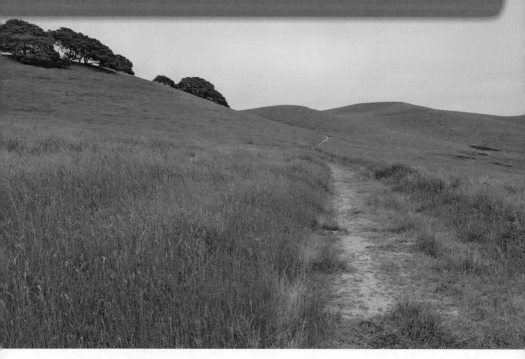

Lonely stretch of trail at Vargas Plateau

"NOBODY GOES THERE anymore. It's too crowded." If you are a dedicated Bay Area hiker, you may identify with this Yogi Berra quote. It's a common complaint—trailheads are overflowing and paths are packed at many parks and preserves. For epic one-of-a-kind places, you may just grin and bear it, but sometimes I crave nearly empty trails, like the ones at Vargas Plateau.

DESCRIPTION

This East Bay preserve east of Fremont is only a few minutes from I-680 and suburbia, but Vargas Plateau is quiet, uncrowded, and peaceful. When I visited in early May, I saw dozens of squirrels, some turkeys, many red-winged blackbirds, cows, and just three other people.

We are lucky to have this oasis. When the property transitioned from land bank to preserve, neighboring landowners brought a lawsuit against the East Bay Regional Park District (EBRPD), forcing a closure. Their concerns were well founded; roads to Vargas Plateau are very narrow and winding. EBRPD worked to improve access and the preserve reopened. Note that the EBRPD strongly discourages access via the Mission Boulevard end of Morrison Canyon Road. Please drive carefully to the trailhead via Vargas and Morrison Canyon Roads, accessed from I-680. Do not park

DISTANCE & CONFIGURATION: 3.8-mile balloon loop

DIFFICULTY: Easy

SCENERY: Grassland and oaks

EXPOSURE: Mostly sunny, some shade

TRAIL TRAFFIC: Light

TRAIL SURFACE: Dirt fire roads and trails

HIKING TIME: 1.5 hours

DRIVING DISTANCE: 41 miles from the Bay Bridge toll plaza

ACCESS: Opens daily at 8 a.m.; closing hours vary by season (check website). Good year-round but best in spring. No fee.

WHEELCHAIR ACCESS: Not recommended for wheelchairs

MAPS: At trailhead's information signboard and tinyurl.com/vargasmap

FACILITIES: Vault toilets at trailhead

CONTACT: 510-544-2268, ebparks.org/parks /vargas

LOCATION: 2536 Morrison Canyon Road, Fremont, CA

COMMENTS: Dogs must be leashed 200 feet from any trail or park entrance; in parking lots, picnic areas, and developed areas; and on some trails. They must be under voice control at all times. Roads to trailhead are very narrow. Drive slowly. No roadside parking.

on the side of the road anywhere on the outskirts of the preserve, and consider carpooling or visiting on a weekday.

I got an immediate feeling for the place from the trailhead. A mountainous black bull sprawled beside a big red barn at the edge of the parking lot. Neither failed to obstruct a sweeping view west. Birds were everywhere—I saw a yellow-billed magpie from my car, and many other birds on my hike.

Start at the signed trailhead near the vault toilet. Once past a stand of eucalyptus, the trail rises gently, passes through a cattle gate, and reaches Golden Eagle Trail. Turn left.

The wide fire road climbs easily through grassland. Great views immediately stretch west. Golden Eagle Trail dips to a creek crossing where two cows stood like statues as I passed them. Then the trail climbs again, at an easygoing grade. Off on a hillside I watched a male turkey tend to his harem, displaying his feathers and gobbling. Above the hillside, a white-tailed kite hunted for breakfast and a vulture hoped for something dead and munchy. Golden Eagle Trail levels out and reaches a junction at 0.6 mile. Trails heading off to the left are dead ends. Turn right.

The wide path drifts gently downhill through grassland infested with squirrels. I saw lots of red-winged blackbirds here. At 0.9 mile the trail forks at a signed junction. The trail doubling back to the right leads to a park residence. Bear left (northwest) on Upper Ranch Trail.

Upper Ranch Trail passes through an area that is soggy in wet months. In this part of the park I really clicked into the "plateau" theme—red-winged blackbirds, a tablelike, damp meadow with gulls flying overhead. It's as if a lower-elevation parcel on the edge of a marsh was plopped on top of a hill. Strange and wonderful! Upper Ranch Trail shrinks, squeezed on both sides by an ocean of gently waving grass. Views begin to unfold to the north, including Pleasanton Ridge. The lumpy

Vargas Plateau Regional Park

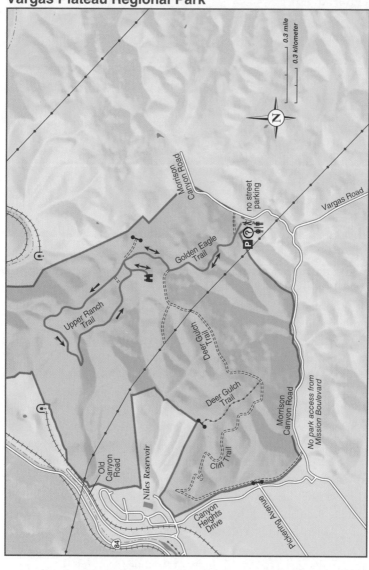

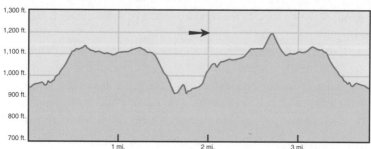

path begins to descend, gently at first, and then with more purpose, reaching a small stock pond and the hike's low point at 1.65 miles. Upper Ranch Trail immediately widens and ascends along the edge of a California bay and coast live oak wood. Poison oak is common in the understory; you might also notice mugwort, sticky monkeyflower, honeysuckle, and creambush. After only a short time in the shade, the trail steps back out into grassland, climbing all the while. On an early May hike, blue-eyed grass and California buttercup were yielding to yarrow. Upper Ranch Trail ascends along the narrow spine of a ridge and the going is steep for a bit—a good reason to stop and soak in the views, which continue to impress. The trail levels out and sweeps past a hill topped with a cluster of coast live oaks. At 2.6 miles you'll reach a junction with a spur to a viewpoint (optional, but nice). Turn right.

The wide, rocky trail ascends to a hilltop with 360-degree views. Look south to admire Mission Peak, southeast to Sunol, north to the hills of Pleasanton Ridge and Garin, and west across the bay to the Santa Cruz Mountains. A bench would be a nice addition here. When ready, retrace your steps back to the previous junction, turn right onto Golden Eagle Trail, and retrace your steps back to the trailhead.

• •

GPS TRAILHEAD COORDINATES N37° 34.481' W121° 55.964'

DIRECTIONS From the Bay Bridge toll plaza, drive east about 0.5 mile and bear right onto I-580 E. Drive south then east on I-580 E about 25 miles, then take Exit 44B onto I-680 S toward San Jose. Follow I-680 south about 12 miles, then take Exit 18 for Vargas Road. At the base of the exit ramp, turn left onto Vargas Road. Drive 1.6 miles north, then turn right onto Morrison Canyon Road. Continue 0.4 mile carefully on the narrow road to the trailhead on the left.

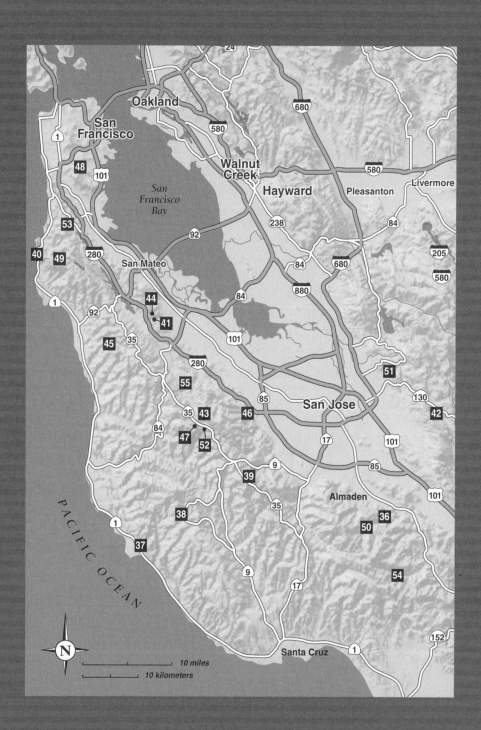

PENINSULA AND SOUTH BAY

(Including San Mateo, Santa Clara, and Santa Cruz Counties)

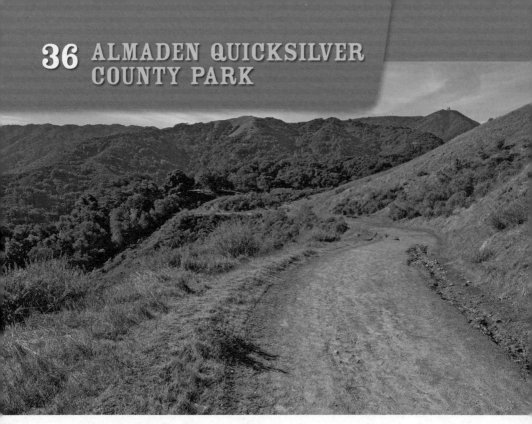

Wood Road Trail with Mount Umunhum in the distance

IF YOU PREFER your history laced with fresh air, Almaden Quicksilver is an ideal hiking destination. This more than 4,000-acre park, a former mercury mine, has over 37 miles of trail that wind past mining artifacts, shuttered shafts, and former settlements. In addition to the mining remnants, there are plenty of natural wonders here: scads of wildflowers, gorgeous oaks scattered in grassland, and a healthy animal population.

DESCRIPTION

On a typical day at Almaden Quicksilver, oak leaves whisper in the breeze, rattlesnakes bask in the sun, wildflowers bloom with abandon, and coyotes scamper across hillsides. It's hard to believe that the park once teemed with human activity as the most productive mine in California history. For decades, the Ohlone tribe used cinnabar, a cinnamon-colored mineral, for pigment, trade, and religious ceremonies. After learning of the cinnabar deposits from the Ohlone in 1845, Mexican mining engineer Andrés Castillero determined that the mineral could be heated to release its stored mercury (quicksilver) and soon applied for and received mineral rights to the land, although he never set up mining operations. A private firm then retained mining rights in 1846. When full-scale operations commenced, settlements, including schools and stores, sprang up on the hillsides. Workers from all over the world

DISTANCE & CONFIGURATION: 8.9-mile balloon loop

DIFFICULTY: Moderate

SCENERY: Grassland, oaks, and chaparral

EXPOSURE: Mostly sunny, some shade

TRAIL TRAFFIC: Light on weekdays; moderate on weekends

TRAIL SURFACE: Dirt fire roads and trails

HIKING TIME: 4 hours

DRIVING DISTANCE: 56 miles from the I-280/CA 1 junction at the San Francisco–Daly City border

ACCESS: Daily, 8 a.m.–sunset. Good year-round but best in spring. No fee.

WHEELCHAIR ACCESS: There is handicapped parking, and wheelchairs may be able to negotiate some trails. However, the entire hike described below is not wheelchair friendly.

MAPS: At trailhead's information signboard and tinyurl.com/almadenquicksilvermap

FACILITIES: None

CONTACT: 408-535-4070, tinyurl.com/almaden countypark

LOCATION: San Jose, CA

COMMENTS: Leashed dogs welcome

mined, crushed, and heated cinnabar to produce mercury, which, although highly toxic, was essential both in the processing of gold and silver and in hat production.

Mine ownership changed throughout the years, and mining ceased in 1927 when the New Almaden Corporation went bankrupt. Piecemeal mining picked up again from 1928 to 1972, but the mines closed for good when mercury use declined and the health risks of the element became known. Santa Clara County bought the land in the early 1970s and, after a thorough cleanup, opened Almaden Quicksilver County Park in 1975. Keep in mind that although the park has been "rehabilitated," some hazards still exist: mice in the park may harbor hantavirus, ramshackle buildings are unstable, and the land surrounding old shafts and mines can still shift. Stick to the trails to stay out of trouble here. This hike climbs on an old mining road to a ridge. From there you'll pass many old mining buildings and remnants on a long loop around the park's tallest hill.

Begin from the trailhead on Wood Road Trail, a dirt fire road that was created in 1876 so workers could transport wood from this oak forest to the furnaces higher uphill. On a cool, peaceful winter morning, it was hard to imagine teamsters hauling wagons of oak on this lovely trail, but it's easy to admire their engineering—the route is scenic and mostly gently graded. It starts out from the trailhead and bends left into coast live oak, madrone, and California bay woods. In February expect the red, white, and blue crew: Indian warrior, milkmaids, and hound's tongue in the understory. A few manzanita shrubs bloom in winter, emitting a sweet aroma. You'll pass under a high-tension power line. Wood Road Trail steps out into a sunny patch of chaparral with a view west to Mount Umunhum. Then it's back into the woods.

The trail continues to rise gently but then exits the woods and drops into grassland. At a flat spot look left for a long view north to San Francisco and Mount Tamalpais. Wood Road Trail starts to climb again, through coyote brush–dotted grassland and pockets of coast live oak. A bench on the right offers a chance to rest and contemplate

Almaden Quicksilver County Park

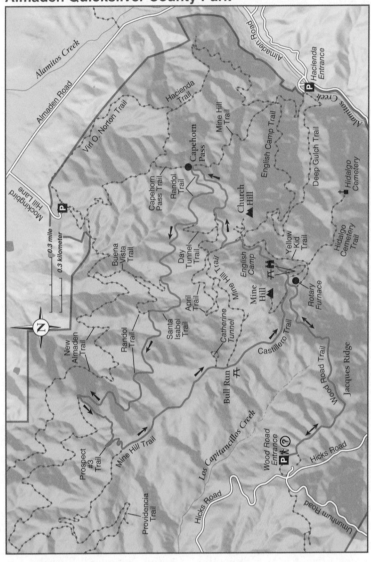

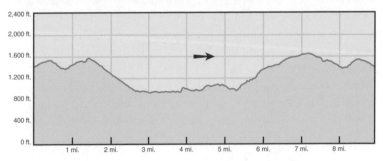

the beautiful Sierra Azul to the west. Although the trail is smooth, winter rains can dislodge small rocks under the sandy surface. Cinnabar, with its deep-red color, stands out. Remember, it's fine to pick them up and take a look, but collecting is forbidden.

The walking remains easy until a junction at 1.35 miles. Yellow Kid Trail heads off to the right. Continue left, then walk to the fenced site of the old rotary furnace, on the right. An interpretive panel shows a photo of the building and explains how the furnace heated crushed ore to release the mercury. A second panel is dedicated to the "Rossi Retort," which permitted quick recovery of the mercury. This panel makes a nice nod to "angle of repose," a term that means "the steepest angle at which a sloping surface formed of a particular loose material is stable." *Angle of Repose* is also the title of a novel by Wallace Steger that partly takes place at what we now call Almaden Quicksilver (it's a great book!).

Once you're done at the rotary furnace site, continue uphill to the left. After a short steep stretch, you'll reach a signed junction at 1.4 miles. Turn right onto Castillero Trail. There's a rest area off to the right, with lovely views south across the South Bay to the Diablo Range, including the telescope dome of Lick Observatory on Mount Hamilton. Just past the picnic tables Castillero Trail meets the trail to Hidalgo Cemetery on the right. Continue straight.

Follow a steady but easy descent through chaparral to a multiple junction at the edge of English Camp, at 1.85 miles. A few buildings still stand where hundreds of miners and their families lived in the late 1800s. Consult the park map and wander around if you wish—there are interpretive signs throughout the area. When ready, continue on Castillero Trail.

Coast live oaks and bigleaf maples shade the nearly level trail. At 2 miles Castillero Trail ends at a signed junction with Mine Hill Trail. Turn right.

The broad fire road descends easily through the woods. At 2.2 miles Day Tunnel Trail breaks off on the left; continue straight on Mine Hill Trail. California bays and coast live oaks thin, often allowing views off to the left; then the trees give way to chamise and sagebrush. At 2.6 miles you'll reach Capehorn Pass. Mine Hill Trail continues downhill to the right. Turn left, then left again, onto Randol Trail.

Angling across the hillside, Randol Trail is nearly level. If you look past the chamise and sagebrush lining the trail, you might begin to notice remnants of mining days. A gigantic pile of tailings on the right marks the spot of Day Tunnel, at 3.1 miles. Interpretive panels feature photos of the area during the mining boom. Day Tunnel Trail heads uphill on the left just past the sealed tunnel site, but stay right on Randol Trail.

Before long, debris piles around Buena Vista Shaft come into view on the right. At 3.7 miles Randol Trail veers right while Santa Isabel continues straight/left. Either trail is an option, but Randol is longer. Bear left onto Santa Isabel Trail.

Spring wildflowers, including shooting stars and baby blue eyes, thrive in the shade of coast live oaks and California bays. Santa Isabel Trail ends at Randol Trail at 4.1 miles. Bear left to once again pick up Randol Trail.

Without major elevation fluctuations, the trail is an easy stroll. You'll pass through cool, shaded canyons and more-exposed areas. Chaparral shrubs including black sage and manzanita occupy a sunny hillside on the left, delighting bees and hummingbirds with their blossoms. Finally the trail reaches grassland and a junction at 5.3 miles. Turn left here onto Prospect #3 Trail.

At a fairly steep grade, the narrow path traverses a sloping meadow dotted with gorgeous mature blue and black oaks. A bountiful display of blossoms spreads through the grass in March—look for linanthus, Johnny-jump-ups, and popcorn flower. Prospect #3 Trail veers into the woods, still climbing but now under the shade of black and coast live oaks. The trail emerges from the woods and ends at a junction at 6 miles. Turn left onto Mine Hill Trail.

If you need an excuse to stop and catch your breath, a pause to admire the views is justifiable. The prominent mountain to the west is Mount Umunhum, the highest peak in the Sierra Azul range. Mine Hill Trail ascends, slightly downslope from the ridgeline, through oaks and grassland. Just past a brief shaded stretch, a trail to Catherine Tunnel branches off to the left at 6.7 miles. Continue straight on Mine Hill Trail, which tapers off to a level grade and reaches, at 6.8 miles, a junction at Bull Run (trail junction 15). A picnic table on the right is a popular rest stop for mountain bikers. Stay right, now back on Castillero Trail.

After a short level segment, the fire road begins a descent. On the exposed sunny hillsides along the trail, you might see California coffeeberry, sagebrush, and poison oak, as well as non-native broom and pampas grass. Keep an eye out for rattlesnakes if the weather is warm. At 7.5 miles you'll return to the junction with Wood Road Trail. Turn right and retrace your steps back to the trailhead.

NEARBY ACTIVITIES

Visit the **Almaden Quicksilver Mining Museum** (21350 Almaden Road, New Almaden; 408-918-7770; tinyurl.com/aqminingmuseum) to learn more about the history of mercury mining here.

• •

GPS TRAILHEAD COORDINATES N37° 10.518' W121° 51.695'

DIRECTIONS From the I-280/CA 1 junction in San Francisco, drive south on I-280 about 37 miles, then take Exit 12B onto CA 85 S. After about 10.5 miles, exit onto Camden Avenue. Drive south on Camden about 2 miles, then turn right onto Hicks Road. Continue on Hicks Road 6.3 miles to the (stop signed) junction with Mount Umunhum Road. Turn left into the signed Wood Road entrance to Almaden Quicksilver, and continue 0.1 mile to the parking lot.

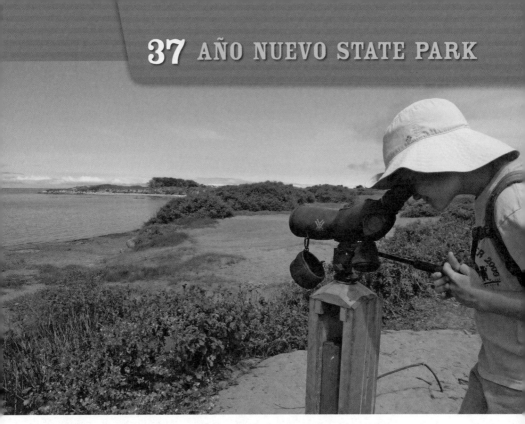

A young visitor uses a spotting scope for a better view of elephant seals lounging on the beach.

ALTHOUGH THIS PARK was created to protect elephant seals and other marine mammals, it is an incredibly restorative destination for humans as well. On this hike you can enjoy fresh sea air, views of the shoreline and mountains, and birdcalls. If you're lucky and the season is right, you might glimpse seals and sea lions basking on the sandy beaches.

DESCRIPTION

Año Nuevo Point was named by Spanish explorer Sebastian Viscaino to commemorate the day he first sailed past the point in 1603, on New Year's Day. At that time, a tribe of Ohlone natives lived in the area, grizzly bears roamed along the coast and through the forested slopes of the Santa Cruz Mountains, and hundreds of thousands of elephant seals swam through the waters off the point. By the late 1800s, the grizzlies were gone and the elephant seals had been hunted nearly to extinction, primarily for their oil-rich blubber. Although their population numbered fewer than 100 when the US and Mexican governments gave northern elephant seals protected status in the 1920s, they slowly began a comeback. Seals were first sighted on Año Nuevo Island in 1955, and in 1961 the first pup was born there. Seals moved onto the mainland to breed. In 1971, the point and island were purchased by the state, and a reserve was established. Since then the elephant seal population has continued to flourish, and sea lions and harbor

DISTANCE & CONFIGURATION: 3.6-mile out-and-back

DIFFICULTY: Easy

SCENERY: Coastal views and elephant seals

EXPOSURE: Full sun

TRAIL TRAFFIC: Moderate

TRAIL SURFACE: Dirt trails; some loose sand

HIKING TIME: 2 hours or more

DRIVING DISTANCE: 48.5 miles from the I-280/CA 1 junction at the San Francisco–Daly City border

ACCESS: Park is open daily, 8:30 a.m.–sunset. Seal-viewing area is open daily, 8:30 a.m.–midafternoon. During seal-breeding season (December 15–March 31), the protection area is accessible only via docent-guided walks (extra fee required), and you must preregister. It can be difficult to secure reservations for the guided walks, so late spring and summer are great times to visit. Pay $10 parking fee at entrance kiosk. April–December 15, obtain a free permit on site to walk through the wilderness area.

WHEELCHAIR ACCESS: There are designated handicapped parking spots, and Año Nuevo Point Trail meets ADA trail standards for 1.3 miles. The ADA trail does not connect with the seal-viewing area, but from mid-December through the end of March, wheelchair users can access the area through a separate reservation. Visit tinyurl.com/equalaccesstours for details.

MAPS: At entrance kiosk and tinyurl.com/ano nuevomap

FACILITIES: Restrooms and water at trailhead

CONTACT: 650-879-2025, tinyurl.com/anonuevosp

LOCATION: Off CA 1, Pescadero, CA (20 miles north of Santa Cruz)

COMMENTS: No food or dogs allowed

seals have found both the mainland and island hospitable for breeding and migratory rest stops. Año Nuevo State Park now hosts the largest mainland breeding colony of northern elephant seals in the world.

Note: The following directions assume you are visiting when reservations are not required, April 1–December 15. If you want to hike from December 15 to March 31, you must have reservations and meet your docent at the Marine Education Center.

Begin at the southwest edge of the parking lot, at the signed trailhead. Walk on the wide, flat path as it bends toward park buildings (the path on the right rejoins the main trail in a bit). Pause at the Marine Education Center for information and/or a visitor permit, then begin hiking on Año Nuevo Point Trail. The wide trail begins a tour through coastal scrub, at a leisurely pace. If you pause to look back to the east, patches of white soil sharply contrast with Chalk Mountain's surrounding dense forest. At 0.2 mile New Years Creek Trail breaks off to the left; continue straight.

Año Nuevo Point Trail sweeps past the edge of a pond where you might notice California aster and swamp knotweed in bloom during late summer. Pelicans are commonly spotted here. On an April hike, I saw dolphins gracefully moving through the ocean just offshore, and a bit farther out, a group of sea otters. At 0.3 mile Cove Beach Trail drops to the sand on the left. Continue on Año Nuevo Point Trail.

The trail slightly ascends through a stand of Monterey pine, then returns to coyote brush–dotted grassland. At 0.8 mile you'll reach a junction and the Natural Preserve Trailhead. Restrooms are a short distance down the path to the right.

In a little exhibit building, interpretive displays describe Steller sea lions, harbor seals, California sea lions, and elephant seals. If you're visiting during the restricted

Año Nuevo State Park

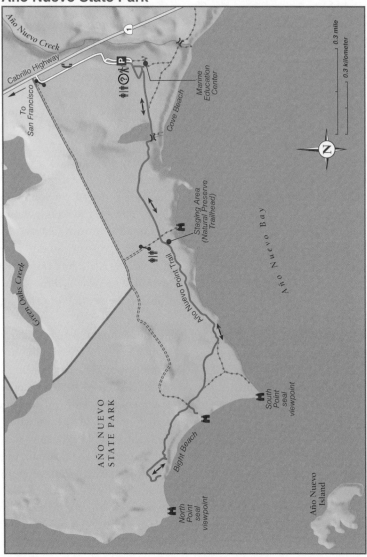

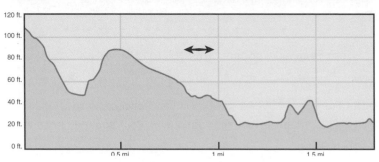

season, this is the turnaround point for your hike; the rest of the year (with your wildlife permit in hand), proceed on Año Nuevo Point Trail.

Gorgeous ocean views unfold as the trail runs along the coast. To the west, the remains of a lighthouse constructed in 1890 are visible on abandoned Año Nuevo Island. Guide wires remind visitors to stay on the trail. As if to emphasize the point, coyote brush, bush lupine, and blackberry form protective thickets, then the shrubs thin and a boardwalk channels visitors over a damp area. Just past an exhibit on a year in the life of elephant seals, the trail shifts to loose sand.

Past this area, the trail network is fluid and may be changed (or closed), with no advance notice, to protect the seals; simply follow the guide wires and signs. The trail climbs a sand dune. At 1.3 miles a path heads left toward the South Point, but stay right, toward the North Point seal overlook. There's a tremendous amount of loose sand to wade through, so if you've ever wanted your own *Lawrence of Arabia* moment, this is your chance. From the top of the dune, the surroundings are scenic and peaceful, with the sounds of the ocean and barking seals, birds swooping over-head, and stunning mountains to the east. The trail descends the dune, flattens, and continues north. You'll pass a second path heading to the South Point viewing area—an optional out-and-back.

Continue on Año Nuevo Point Trail to a signed junction with the boardwalk to the Bight Beach viewpoint. Turn left. A short and beautiful boardwalk leads to the viewing area, where you can often spot seals just offshore. When my son and I visited this viewpoint on an August hike, the docent on duty showed us bits of elephant seal pelt (which, oddly, felt like Astroturf to me) and numerous skulls and bones. Return to the main trail and turn left. Coastal plants such as bush lupine, ragwort, coyote brush, beach primrose, sand verbena, sea rocket, and shrubby willow line the path.

At 1.9 miles turn left at a signed viewpoint junction. The path ends after a few feet, offering sweeping views to Año Nuevo Island and North Point. Return to the trail and turn left. At 2 miles the trail curves sharply left, then ends at a viewpoint above the beach. Docents can answer questions and help you identify whatever mammals are present. When I visited one year in autumn, a few elephant seals were romping in the water. When you're ready, retrace your steps back to the trailhead.

• •

GPS TRAILHEAD COORDINATES N37° 07.184' W122° 18.441'

DIRECTIONS From the I-280/CA 1 junction in San Francisco, drive 1.7 miles south on I-280, then keep right at the fork and continue on CA 1 about 46 miles to the park entrance on the right.

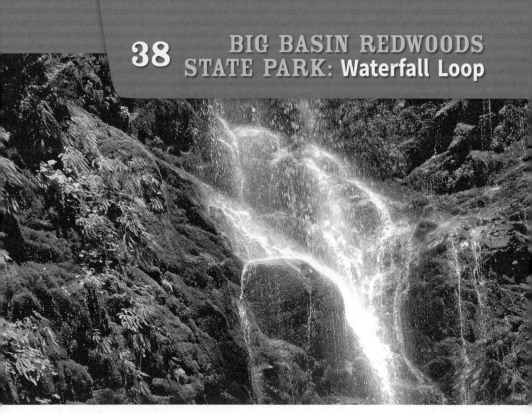

Berry Creek Falls in summer

REDWOODS, CREEKS, AND WATERFALLS—that's what this loop is all about. Nestled in California's oldest state park, this popular hike begins at the Big Basin park headquarters and follows undulating Sunset Trail downhill through forested canyons to a series of three dramatic waterfalls. The return leg, a segment of Skyline to the Sea Trail, rises along murmuring creeks back to the trailhead.

DESCRIPTION

Begin at the edge of the main parking lot on Redwood Trail (look for the massive REDWOOD TRAIL sign). The wide, flat path winds through lovely redwoods. After about 400 feet, you'll reach a junction (bathrooms sit just off the trail to the right). Continue straight on Skyline to the Sea Trail. After crossing Opal Creek on a little bridge, you will reach a T-junction with Skyline to the Sea Trail. Turn right toward Dool and Sunset Trails.

At a level grade, the broad trail runs along Opal Creek, through the outskirts of the park-headquarters area. A trail from a secondary parking lot enters from the right. Noise from vehicles and park visitors fades with each step through redwood, tanoak, and huckleberry woods. After about 0.4 mile Skyline to the Sea continues north on its way to Castle Rock State Park. Turn left onto Dool Trail. The trail rises

DISTANCE & CONFIGURATION: 9.6-mile loop

DIFFICULTY: Strenuous

SCENERY: Redwoods, waterfalls, and creeks

EXPOSURE: Mostly shaded

TRAIL TRAFFIC: Heavy around park headquarters; otherwise moderate

TRAIL SURFACE: Dirt trails, with 1 short, steep downhill scramble over rocks at Silver Falls

HIKING TIME: 6 hours

DRIVING DISTANCE: 62 miles from the I-280/CA 1 junction at the San Francisco–Daly City border

ACCESS: Daily, 6 a.m.–sunset. Good year-round; waterfalls are at their peak in late winter and spring. Pay $10 fee at entrance station or park headquarters.

WHEELCHAIR ACCESS: There is designated handicapped parking, and folks in wheelchairs can explore a grove of tall trees on the 0.6-mile Redwood Loop.

MAPS: At park headquarters and tinyurl.com /bbredwoodsmap

FACILITIES: Restrooms and water at trailhead

CONTACT: 831-338-8860, tinyurl.com /bigbasinsp

LOCATION: 21600 Big Basin Way, Boulder Creek, CA

COMMENTS: Dogs not allowed on trails

easily through the forest, then reaches a junction with Sunset Trail at about 0.4 mile. Turn left.

Sunset Trail begins to climb through tanoaks, Douglas-firs, and redwoods. Many of the trees along the trail have been charred by fire, and some of the huge redwoods have burned-out trunks. Early settlers confined poultry in these hollowed-out trees, which became known as goose pens. At 0.9 mile Sunset Trail crests at the junction with Middle Ridge Road. Continue across the fire road on Sunset Trail, which begins an easy descent. Winding down into a redwood canyon, you might see milkwort and California harebell in summer, and in a short grassy stretch, lingering blossoms of Ithuriel's spear and vetch.

At 1.1 miles a connector to Skyline to the Sea departs on the left, but continue straight on Sunset Trail. A few coast live oaks give way to a forest dominated by redwood and tanoak. The trail ascends gently, crosses a knoll, and drops through woods where trilliums, redwood violets, western heart's ease, and fairy lanterns bloom in spring. At West Waddell Creek, a pretty stream graced with a few bigleaf maples, the trail rises again. Timms Creek Trail begins at 3.2 miles, heading off to the left as Sunset Trail makes a sharp right. Timms Creek Trail, which leads to Skyline to the Sea Trail, is the bail-out route for hikers who are ready to return to the trailhead.

Continue on Sunset Trail, climbing steadily. Sunset Trail crests near a huge fallen redwood, then begins to descend through quiet woods. After crossing Berry Creek, the path ascends again and soon steps out of the woods to bisect a swale of chaparral. Manzanita covers the chalky white hillsides to the left and right, and these low-slung shrubs, mixed through a few knobcone pines, permit views south to the forested canyon surrounding the waterfalls. Bush poppy's cheerful yellow flowers stand out in a sea of green in early summer, preceding the bloom of chamise and fruit on huckleberry shrubs.

Big Basin Redwoods State Park: Waterfall Loop

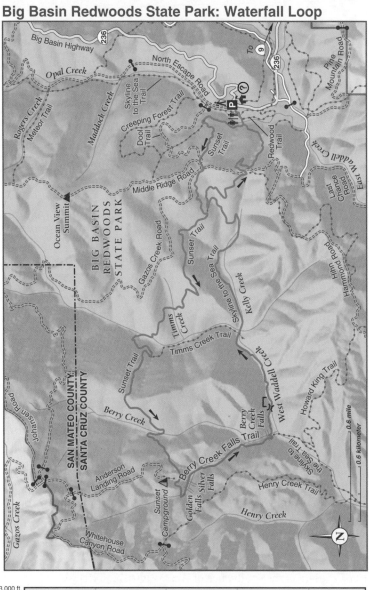

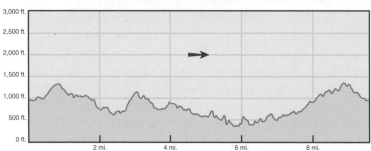

As Sunset Trail leaves the chaparral, live oak, California nutmeg, and Douglas-fir bridge a transition back into redwood and tanoak. At 4.8 miles the trail to Sunset Camp breaks off to the right; continue straight, now on Berry Creek Falls Trail. The sound of rushing water increases as the trail descends. Then, on the right, Golden Falls comes into view. A short switchback drops the trail to the side of the fall, where water slides down a sloping wall of tawny sandstone. The water rushes to a second, short drop, then pools at the top of Silver Falls. As the water shoots straight down 50 feet in a single gasp, the trail clings to the side of the cliff, descending rock stairs. The guide wire on the right is essential: take special care when the water flow is heavy because the steps will be slippery.

Berry Creek Falls Trail reaches the base of Silver Falls, then levels out and follows the creek. When the creek is low, you can jump across to the right and walk a few feet to get a close look at the falls. This interlude between waterfalls is my favorite spot on the hike—West Berry Creek burbles along the trail and sunlight filters through the redwoods to an understory of ferns, where starflower, trilliums, and redwood sorrel brighten the forest floor in spring and butterflies float through the air in summer.

Just past the confluence of West Berry and Berry Creeks, the trail crosses the stream and rises to overlook the top of Berry Creek Falls, a 60-foot drop distinguished by gorgeous ferns and moss covering the rocks around the water flow. There are wonderful views to the falls as the trail descends to a viewing platform near the base of the falls; if it's not crowded, this is an ideal location for lunch. Past the platform, the trail descends to a junction at 5.8 miles. Turn left onto Skyline to the Sea Trail.

A bridge crosses the confluence of Berry and West Waddell Creeks, and then Skyline to the Sea Trail climbs somewhat sharply to a bench where you have one last view to Berry Creek Falls. I lunched here on one hike and enjoyed not only the waterfall view but also the entertainment provided by a band of marauding Steller's jays perched on a nearby fence, hoping for bread crumbs. Past the bench, Skyline to the Sea Trail begins a rollicking course of short ups and downs along West Waddell Creek. Azaleas and bigleaf maples line the stream as the trail crosses the water for the south bank, where you may notice salal and wild rose in the understory of tanoak and redwood. Past some big boulders sitting in the creekbed at 6.7 miles, Timms Creek Trail crosses the creek on the left, at the confluence of West Waddell and Kelly Creeks.

Continue straight on Skyline to the Sea Trail, still climbing, here at a more straightforward uphill pace. The trail wanders through a beautiful redwood forest where clintonia, a lily with magenta flowers, blooms in late spring. Later, in summer, orchids unfurl, including the native reddish-striped and -spotted coralroot and purple-green helleborine, a Eurasian floral import. Skyline to the Sea Trail forks, with the left leg crossing the creek—either path is an option, as they reconnect shortly.

Past the rejoining, Skyline to the Sea Trail crosses Kelly Creek, then begins to climb out of the canyon, away from the creek. The forest remains quiet and shaded, and you might see banana slugs along the trail, particularly in cool, damp weather. At 8.3 miles the connector to Sunset Trail heads uphill to the left; continue straight on Skyline to the Sea Trail. The ascent mellows as you reach the hike's highest elevation, slightly over 1,300 feet.

Skyline to the Sea Trail crosses Middle Ridge Fire Road at 8.8 miles, then descends through redwoods scarred by fire. In spring, starflower and trilliums bloom along the path. At the 9.4-mile mark, bear left at a fork toward park headquarters. At 9.5 miles you'll return to the hike's first junction. Turn right, cross Opal Creek, and return to the trailhead.

NEARBY ACTIVITIES

This is the most popular Big Basin hike (the short Redwood Trail loop is really just a walk), although there are scores of other possibilities. One of my favorite hikes is the out-and-back trek to **Buzzard's Roost,** a sandstone outcrop with incredible views of the park.

• •

GPS TRAILHEAD COORDINATES N37° 10.319' W122° 13.340'

DIRECTIONS From the I-280/CA 1 junction in San Francisco, drive south on I-280 about 36 miles, then take the Foothill Expressway exit. Turn right and drive south on Foothill (which morphs into Stevens Canyon Road after 3 miles). Continue on Stevens Canyon Road 3 miles, then turn left onto Redwood Gulch Road. Continue uphill another 1.4 miles to the junction with CA 9. Turn right onto CA 9 and drive 9.1 miles, then turn right onto CA 236. Proceed on this narrow, winding road 8.2 miles to the park headquarters (left) and parking lots (right).

Weaving through a redwood forest at Big Basin Redwoods State Park

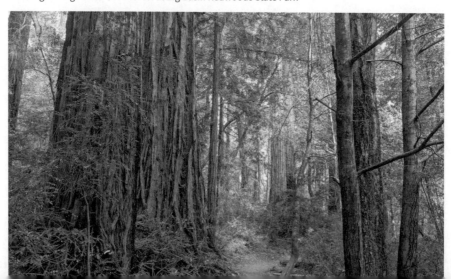

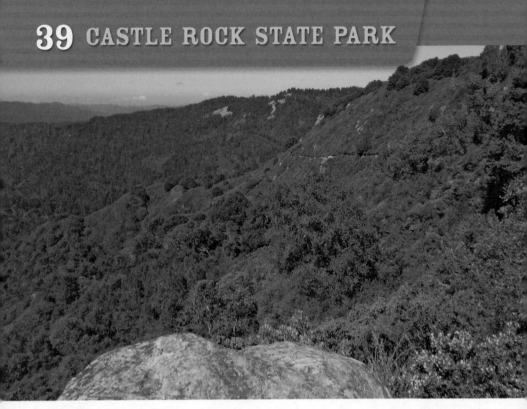

A gorgeous view from (and to!) Saratoga Gap Trail

CASTLE ROCK IS an appropriate and majestic name for a park with so much natural beauty. Starting at the crest of the Santa Cruz Mountains, this hike descends into an evergreen forest; winds through chaparral and oak woods; passes massive boulders and smaller sandstone formations; offers fabulous, sweeping views west; and stops at a waterfall before returning uphill toward the trailhead. On the return leg, a detour visits the park's name-sake rock formation.

DESCRIPTION

Hikers love Castle Rock, and for good reason. It's beautiful year-round and has a few little extras that elevate it to the top tier of Bay Area parks and preserves. One is a variety of vegetation—woods, chaparral, and oak savanna. A second is Castle Rock Falls, less than 1 mile from the parking lot. This 70-foot waterfall nearly disappears in the driest months of the year, but winter storms send water rushing down in a single fall. The third and perhaps most unusual Castle Rock attribute is the tafoni-sandstone formations. Although a few other locations in the area have these formations, Castle Rock's are the biggest and best, with interesting clusters on the trail around the park's namesake, Castle Rock, and along Saratoga Gap and Ridge Trails. The park permits low-impact climbing, so you may see climbers on the largest rock formations.

DISTANCE & CONFIGURATION: 5.3-mile figure eight

DIFFICULTY: Moderate

SCENERY: Chaparral, waterfall, woods, sandstone formations, and views

EXPOSURE: Nearly equal parts shade and sun

TRAIL TRAFFIC: Moderate

TRAIL SURFACE: Dirt trails, with quite a few short scrambles over sandstone rocks

HIKING TIME: 3 hours

DRIVING DISTANCE: 50 miles from the I-280/CA 1 junction at the San Francisco–Daly City border

ACCESS: Daily, sunrise–sunset. Good year-round. Pay $10 fee at pay station in parking lot.

WHEELCHAIR ACCESS: There are designated handicapped parking spots, and the developed part of the trailhead is wheelchair accessible. The hike itself is not wheelchair friendly (one section is impossible to navigate in a wheelchair).

MAPS: Available at tinyurl.com/crspmap

FACILITIES: Restrooms and water at trailhead

CONTACT: 408-867-2952, tinyurl.com/castlerocksp

LOCATION: 15000 Skyline Blvd., Los Gatos, CA

COMMENTS: No dogs allowed

Start at the new Kirkwood Entrance trailhead, on Waterfall Trail. Under deep shade, the narrow trail descends through woods of tanoak, California bay, and Douglas-fir. Old madrones tower above Kings Creek near the junction with Saratoga Gap Trail at 0.3 mile. Turn right onto Saratoga Gap Trail. The trail loses elevation steadily but moderately, following a creekbed. When you arrive at the junction with Ridge Trail at 0.4 mile, cross the creek on a tiny footbridge. Note the giant Douglas-fir in the crook between the trails—easily the size of a mature redwood. Stay right, on Ridge Trail.

The narrow path winds a bit uphill, passing a massive white boulder. Moss-covered live oaks give way to sunny chaparral composed of ceanothus, manzanita, yerba santa, chamise, pitcher sage, toyon, and sticky monkeyflower. Deciding where to cast your gaze is tough, with sweeping views west, rocks and roots underfoot, and weird rock outcrops uphill on the right. These pockmarked boulders are some of the most visible tafoni formations, the sandstone slowly shaped by the elements. Winter rains seep into the rocks, dissolving calcium carbonate; then summer's low humidity draws out moisture containing the mineral. Over time, the rocks develop weak spots and break from the inside out, creating dimples, holes, and small caves.

You encounter the first of the hike's two rock scrambles here, where the trail is very rocky and the route seems to disappear. At the first, the trail climbs before dropping to the left. At the second, ascend to the right, picking your way uphill until the rocks give way to tamer terrain. The trail bends right under a buckeye at the base of Goat Rock, and steps bring the trail to the upper reaches of the rock formation and a junction at 0.8 mile. The path heading right leads to an interpretive shelter. Bear left and, after a few feet, follow the trail left to Goat Rock overlook. This path passes through oak grassland, then ends at a viewpoint. Two interpretive signs help you identify landforms in the distance, including Monterey Bay, the Butano Range, and Big Basin's Eagle Rock. Return to the previous junction and bear left, following the sign for Ridge Trail and Castle Rock Trail Camp.

Castle Rock State Park

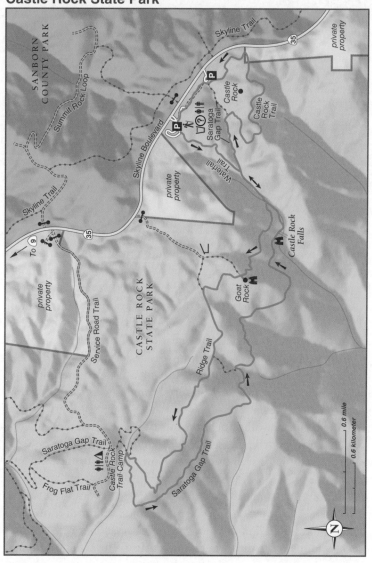

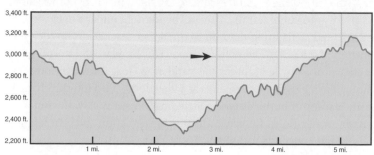

I've seen the sides of the trail, beneath madrones, California bays, and black oaks, torn up—a telltale sign that wild pigs have passed through. The pigs are troublesome residents of the Bay Area, and in this part of the Santa Cruz Mountains you don't have to look far to see the evidence of them. Descended from escaped domestic swine and boars imported for hunting, they dig through topsoil searching for roots and acorns. Mountain lions and coyotes kill some piglets, but adults can weigh more than 300 pounds and have no predators (except cars). Some parks have begun a campaign of trapping and euthanasia, but the problem is nonetheless spreading. The path winds slightly uphill through grassland and trees, where baby blue eyes bloom in April. At 1 mile you'll reach a T-junction. Turn left onto Ridge Trail.

Madrones, black and live oaks, and Douglas-firs form a sparse forest along the trail as it descends easily. A short path veers left, leading to a bird-observation lookout (there are better views to come, however). At 1.3 miles a shortcut to Saratoga Gap Trail heads left. Continue straight on Ridge Trail.

As the trail descends downslope from Varian Peak, stands of madrone, tanoak, and live oak close off views. Just past a spot with a rock formation and some manzanita, Ridge Trail passes beneath some towering knobcone pines. The ridgeline thins, and the trail makes a transition from a course downslope of the ridge to the top of the ridge. Woods prevail until a sudden break in the tree cover, where you'll step out to a cliff edge. Views unfold to the west, across miles of forested ridges. The trail heads back into a forest now dominated by madrone, descending to a junction at 2.1 miles. Castle Rock Trail Camp is to the right. Turn left onto Saratoga Gap Trail.

At a mostly level grade, the trail winds through a forest where, after heavy rains, you may hear water tumbling down Craig Springs Creek on the right. Saratoga Gap Trail bends left and changes its character completely. Under the dappled shade of live oaks, the trail passes beneath a rock outcrop, then descends a short segment of steep steps cut into a boulder. A metal guide wire is helpful—there's a drop-off on the right. Saratoga Gap Trail ascends slightly through chaparral. As it weaves through (and sometimes over) sandstone outcrops, the views west are outstanding. Manzanita and two varieties of ceanothus (wartleaf and buckbrush) bloom in late winter and early spring, while yellow bush lupine, paintbrush, and lizardtail flower in early summer. A few California bays and live oaks shade the trail every once in a while. Watch out for poison oak. As the trail skirts Varian Peak, vegetation shifts to grassland and black oaks. The connector leading back uphill to Ridge Trail starts at 3 miles. Continue straight on Saratoga Gap Trail.

Once past a little bunch of buckeyes in a gully on the right, you'll climb back into chaparral and get a good look ahead to steep, rock-studded hillsides near Goat Rock. But there's a little surprise in a damp crease along the trail: a grove of California bays and a pocket of redwoods. The tour through this cool oasis is short-lived, and Saratoga Gap Trail rises back into chaparral. Keep your eyes open for tafoni with visible caves on the left. There seems to be a "wow" with every step—hawks soaring overhead, flowers blooming at your feet, and, always, the view. The trail squeezes between two boulders, marking a transition to a woodland of California bays, tan and live oaks, and Douglas-firs. You must pick through a pile of little boulders similar to the rock piles on the way to Goat Rock. Waterfall lovers may quicken their step when they begin to hear the sound of rushing water. Hop onto an observation platform on the right for a look down to Castle Rock Falls. The route continues uphill, following the creek. At 4 miles, you'll return to the junction of Saratoga Gap and Ridge Trails. Turn right and head back uphill.

Pass the junction with Waterfall Trail on the left and continue uphill to a signed junction with Castle Rock Trail at 4.3 miles; turn right. The trail ascends gently through a forest of tanoak, madrone, and Douglas-fir to Castle Rock. Unlike the largest tafoni formations toured so far on this hike, Castle Rock is not perched out in the open but nestled among the trees. Does it resemble a castle? It's surely big enough to house a family of lilliputian elves, and it doesn't take too much imagination to see jutting pieces of rock as gargoyles eroded into waves and cascades. The trail opens to fire-road width and passes another large rock formation on the right. Soon after, bear left, following the sign toward the parking lot. After an easy descent the trail ends at the "old" Castle Rock parking lot. Look for the trail at the northwest edge of the lot, the flat return route to the trailhead.

NEARBY ACTIVITIES

Two other parks in the Santa Cruz Mountains feature sandstone formations. **Sanborn County Park** (16055 Sanborn Road, Saratoga, CA; 408-867-9959; sccgov.org) sits on the east side of CA 35/Skyline Boulevard, across from Castle Rock, and **El Corte de Madera Creek Open Space Preserve** (Skyline Boulevard, Redwood City, CA; 650-691-1200; openspace.org) is on the west side of CA 35, about 20 miles north of this Castle Rock trailhead.

• •

GPS TRAILHEAD COORDINATES N37° 13.915' W122° 05.948'

DIRECTIONS From the I-280/CA 1 junction in San Francisco, drive south on I-280 about 37 miles, then exit Foothill Boulevard. Drive south on Foothill about 1.5 miles, then continue on Stevens Canyon Road. After 3 miles, continue right at the junction with Mount Eden Road. Drive about 1.7 miles, then turn left onto Redwood Gulch Road. Continue 1.4 miles, then turn right onto CA 9. After 3 more miles, you'll reach Saratoga Gap (the junction of CA 9 and CA 35). Turn left onto CA 35, and drive south about 2.4 miles to the Kirkwood Entrance, on the right.

The multiuse Devil's Slide Trail squeezes between rock formations.

THE INFAMOUS DEVIL'S SLIDE (the road) is now the incredible Devil's Slide (the trail), a must-hike coastal experience.

DESCRIPTION

This 1.3-mile stretch of pavement vexed drivers and Caltrans for many years. It edges along a narrow shelf above the ocean, with steep cliffs ascending and descending on both sides. The cliffs are composed of two types of soil—granite and shale/sandstone. This unstable mix is a poor foundation for a road, and during winter, landslides were common. In 1995 the stretch was closed for five months, inconveniencing and isolating the towns of Pacifica and Montara. When the road was open, accidents regularly sent cars and trucks tumbling down the cliff. After years of debate, a bypass tunnel was built through Montara Mountain, and Devil's Slide, the roadway, was closed to vehicles. In 2014, it reopened as a multiuse trail and was an immediate hit. There are two trailheads, one on the south side of the Lantos Tunnel and one on the north. Both offer pit toilets, water, and parking. I prefer to start from the south.

Once out of the parking lot, begin walking on the multiuse trail (bikes use the right side; walkers, the left). Immediately I was stunned by the narrow trail width. We used to drive here? Yow. Examine the cliff face to the right (watch for bikes)—the sparkly stuff is granite. The trail ascends just slightly, squeezing through the cliffs.

DISTANCE & CONFIGURATION: 2-mile out-and-back

DIFFICULTY: Easy

SCENERY: Coastline and views

EXPOSURE: Full sun

TRAIL TRAFFIC: Heavy

TRAIL SURFACE: Pavement

HIKING TIME: 2 hours or less

DRIVING DISTANCE: 11 miles from the I-280/CA 1 junction at the San Francisco–Daly City border

ACCESS: Opens daily at 8 a.m.; closing time varies by season and is posted at trailhead. No fee.

WHEELCHAIR ACCESS: There is designated handicapped parking, and the trail is well suited for wheelchairs, although it is not flat.

MAPS: At trailhead's information signboard and tinyurl.com/devilsslidemap

FACILITIES: Vault toilets and drinking water at trailhead

CONTACT: 650-355-8289, parks.smcgov.org /devils-slide-trail

LOCATION: Off CA 1, between Pacifica and Montara

COMMENTS: Leashed dogs welcome

Interpretive panels offer a wealth of information regarding wildlife, history, and more. On my visit, birders had just seen a peregrine falcon on the cliff to the left.

The trail sweeps right and continues to climb, still at a gentle grade. The old structure on the hilltop here to the left was a base-end station, part of a coastal defense network. Every time I drove south, I wanted to stop at just this spot, and surely you will savor the spectacular views. The three rocks jutting up out of the water just off the coast are collectively called Egg Rock. If you've brought binoculars, see if you can spot cormorants or common murres on the rocks. Lucky searchers may get glimpses of whales or seals in the ocean. On clear days, views stretch north past the Pedro Point Headlands all the way to Mount Tamalpais and Point Reyes in Marin County. The cliffs on the right are nearly vertical and mostly bare, but patches of native vegetation thrive amongst non-native interlopers, mostly pampas grass and sweet alyssum. In winter after heavy rains, small waterfalls drop down off the cliff, and near those damp areas look for coyote brush, sagebrush, and ceanothus. In spring when ceanothus is blooming, the heavenly scent mixes delightfully with the fresh ocean air.

The grade picks up a bit, but at the 1-mile mark Devil's Slide Trail crests. Enjoy lovely views from the Northern Overlook. If you want to continue exploring the remaining 0.3 mile of trail, follow the path down to the northern trailhead (trailside vegetation is more diverse and lush along this stretch). Otherwise, you may opt to make the overlook the turnaround point. When ready, retrace your steps back to the trailhead.

• •

GPS TRAILHEAD COORDINATES N37° 34.348' W122° 30.988'

DIRECTIONS From the I-280/CA 1 junction in San Francisco, drive south 1.8 miles and exit onto CA 1 S/Pacifica. Continue on CA 1 for 9.2 miles, then turn right into the parking lot (just past the Lantos Tunnel).

Devil's Slide Trail

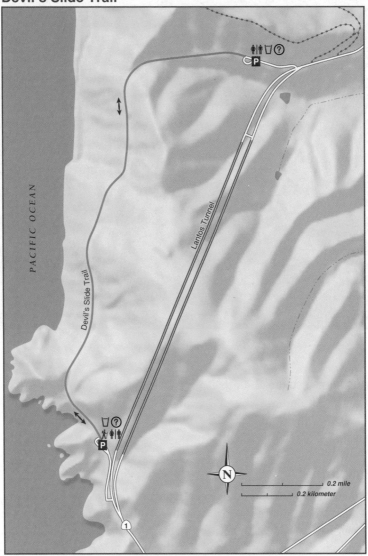

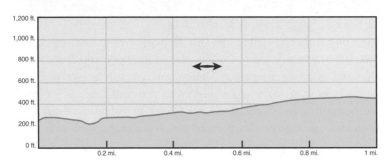

Wildflowers bloom everywhere at Edgewood, sometimes even on rocks.

THIS HIKE ASCENDS gently through coast live oak and California bay woodlands then traverses grassland where hikers here in spring may see drifts of flowers. On the return leg of the loop, a tiny waterfall in a wooded canyon charms visitors after heavy rainstorms.

DESCRIPTION

Edgewood County Park is a little jewel of a park surrounded by a bustling highway, a busy county road, and residential neighborhoods. Thousands of commuters zip past it every day on I-280, and between the traffic noise and the hum of suburban living, there's no confusing Edgewood with the wilderness. However, the park hosts an incredible wildflower display in spring and shelters a community of animals, including hawks, coyotes, deer, and jackrabbits.

Edgewood's chaparral-coated hillsides, serpentine grassland, and oak-forested canyon were nearly lost in a series of threatened developments from the 1960s to 1993, when the parcel became a San Mateo County nature preserve and park. An Edgewood advocacy group works tirelessly to preserve habitats for endangered plants and butterflies, and docent-led hikes offered by volunteers during the park's high season are a great way to learn about the creatures that thrive throughout the 467 acres. Because bicycles and dogs are prohibited in the park and horse traffic is

DISTANCE & CONFIGURATION: 3.5-mile balloon loop

DIFFICULTY: Easy

SCENERY: Mixed woodland, serpentine grassland, and wildflowers

EXPOSURE: Mixture of shaded woods and exposed grassland

TRAIL TRAFFIC: Moderate year-round; heavy during spring peak

TRAIL SURFACE: Well-maintained dirt paths

HIKING TIME: 1.5 hours, plus more time to search for wildflowers

DRIVING DISTANCE: 21.7 miles from the I-280/ CA 1 junction at the San Francisco–Daly City border

ACCESS: Opens daily at 8 a.m.; closing hours vary (check website). Good year-round but exceptional March–May. No fee.

WHEELCHAIR ACCESS: Not recommended for wheelchairs

MAPS: At trailhead's information signboard and tinyurl.com/edgewoodmap

FACILITIES: Restrooms, water, and picnic area near trailhead

CONTACT: 650-368-6283, parks.smcgov.org /edgewood-park-natural-preserve

LOCATION: 10 Old Stagecoach Road, Redwood City, CA

COMMENTS: No dogs allowed

limited to a few trails, Edgewood is very hiker-friendly and is a good destination for a family hike with small kids.

Begin at the edge of the parking lot, following the signs for Sylvan Trail. The path runs along a road heading toward houses, then veers right and reaches a junction with a path leading right to the restrooms. Turn left, following the signs for Sylvan Trail. Along this nearly flat path, which runs parallel to the park boundary, a few plum trees grow, flowering in late winter and fruiting in early summer. A few other "exotic" plants, including acacia and a palm tree, are mixed with native buckeye, California bay, and coast live oak.

After about 0.2 mile you'll reach a signed junction. Bear right onto Baywood Glen Trail and climb up the canyon's shoulder on a series of switchbacks, mostly shaded by mature coast live oaks and California bays. Shooting stars and hound's tongue bloom in the understory in early spring, and in winter you may see birds picking berries off toyon shrubs. Poison oak is abundant, but from autumn to spring when it loses its leaves, it blends in with other benign plants, so beware of bare-branched shrubs. At 0.8 mile the trail crests, emerges from the woods, and reaches a junction with Franciscan Trail; turn left.

Under partial cover of coast live oak and California bay, the trail skirts a hilltop on the right. From a bench crowded by sun-drenched sagebrush, views stretch across the canyon to the southeast. A few steps later you'll cut across the edge of a grassy plateau then reach a junction with Serpentine Trail at 1.1 miles. Continue straight (southeast) on Franciscan Trail. Climb a bit to a junction at 1.4 miles, and turn left onto Live Oak Trail.

Traffic noise from nearby I-280 is steady, but tree cover blocks vehicular views as the trail climbs. When you step out into chaparral, a break in the vegetation permits

Edgewood County Park and Natural Preserve

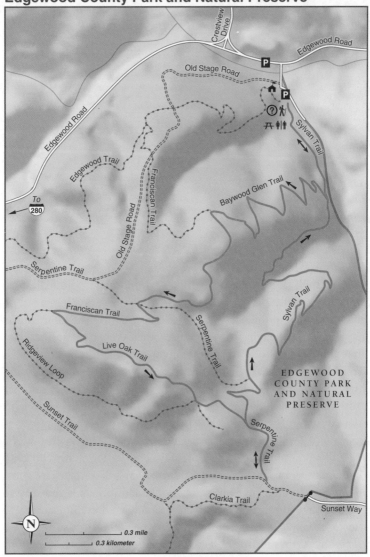

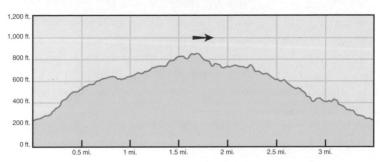

a peek at the Santa Cruz Mountains to the west. A thicket of chamise lines the trail near Edgewood's highest point, but soon you'll descend through some pretty coast live oaks to a junction at 1.8 miles. Continue left on Live Oak Trail.

After a brief descent, turn right onto Serpentine Trail, 2 miles into the hike. Fences protect habitat as the trail enters serpentine grassland, where incredible displays of wildflowers carpet the sides of the trail in spring. Serpentine Trail reaches a junction at 2.1 miles. This is the turnaround point for the hike, but in wildflower season you might explore more in the area. Whatever you choose, retrace your steps back to the junction with Live Oak Trail.

Instead of returning uphill on Live Oak, continue straight on Serpentine Trail. A few zigzags take the trail down a hillside to a junction at 2.4 miles. Keep going straight (north), now on Sylvan Trail.

Initially this part of Sylvan Trail winds downhill through an open forest of oaks, madrone, and patches of grass, but after passing through some chaparral, the path again settles into coast live oak and California bay woods. At about 3 miles a wee waterfall appears on the left after rainstorms. There's one last sunny section before Sylvan Trail reenters woods then returns to the junction with Baywood Glen Trail, on the left, at 3.3 miles. Continue straight on Sylvan Trail and retrace your steps back to the parking lot.

• •

GPS TRAILHEAD COORDINATES N37° 28.387' W122° 16.690'

DIRECTIONS From the I-280/CA 1 junction, drive south on I-280 about 20 miles, and take Exit 29 onto Edgewood Road. Turn left and drive east on Edgewood Road about 1 mile, and turn right into the park. There's overflow parking in a paved lot off Edgewood Road, plus a smaller parking lot inside the park gates.

JOSEPH D. GRANT COUNTY PARK

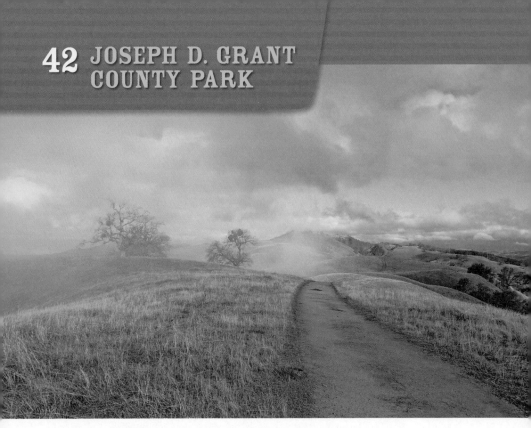

One dreamy morning on Cañada de Pala Trail, I got caught in the clouds.

ON THE HIGH SLOPES of Mount Hamilton, Joseph D. Grant County Park sprawls over 10,000 acres of oak-dotted grassland, less than 15 miles from downtown San Jose. Even though the park is bisected by Mount Hamilton Road, it has an isolated feel to it—I've hiked for hours here and seen only birds, cows, and wild pigs. This hike begins near an old ranch compound, skirts Grant Lake, and then climbs through an oak savanna to the ridgeline. After a sustained jaunt along the grassy ridge, you'll drop through grassland peppered with oaks then retrace your steps back to the parking lot.

DESCRIPTION

Begin on the signed Hotel Trail at the edge of the parking lot. The first steps are paved, but when the pavement swings right, continue straight, passing the pretty old ranch buildings on the left. After 0.1 mile you'll reach a T-junction. Turn left, following the sign toward Mount Hamilton Road.

A few steps down the trail, a hard-to-spot path, Loop Trail, departs on the right. Continue on Hotel Trail, here a wide dirt path. Ascending easily, the trail is lined with young coast live oak and coyote brush, and in spring the sloping grassy hillside on the right hosts big patches of rose clover, along with smatterings of blue-eyed grass, vetch, fiddlenecks, and California poppy. A few cottonwoods and alders thrive

DISTANCE & CONFIGURATION: 7.6-mile balloon loop

DIFFICULTY: Moderate

SCENERY: Grassland and views

EXPOSURE: Almost entirely exposed

TRAIL TRAFFIC: Light

TRAIL SURFACE: Dirt fire roads and trails

HIKING TIME: 4 hours

DRIVING DISTANCE: 62 miles from the US 101/ I-280 junction in San Francisco

ACCESS: Daily, 8 a.m.–sunset. Best in spring— not a summer destination unless you favor dehydration. Trails are often muddy, but this is an awesome winter hike. Pay $6 fee at park entrance (self-register if kiosk is unattended).

WHEELCHAIR ACCESS: Park in the Grant Lake lot; you should be able to navigate about 0.3 mile along Grant Lake.

MAPS: At park entrance, information signboard at trailhead, and tinyurl.com/grantcountyparkmap.

FACILITIES: Restrooms and water at trailhead

CONTACT: 408-274-6121, tinyurl.com /grantcountypark

LOCATION: 18405 Mount Hamilton Road, San Jose, CA

COMMENTS: Leashed dogs welcome. Watch out for wild pigs throughout the park.

on the left on the edge of a damp creek basin where I've seen some of the park's marauding wild-pig population. At 0.5 mile the trail approaches Mount Hamilton Road. Carefully cross the street, then turn left onto Yerba Buena Trail.

The trail approaches then swings to the right of the Grant Lake staging area and reaches a junction at 0.6 mile. Turn right toward Halls Valley Trail. Lakeview Trail breaks off to the right, looping back to Yerba Buena Trail; continue straight. Coyote brush forms thickets on the right, and just off the left side of the trail, ducks, herons, egrets, and cormorants may be seen on Grant Lake. From a junction at 0.9 mile, turn right onto Halls Valley Trail.

The fire road dips to cross a creek, then rises again through coast live oak, valley oak, eucalyptus, and coyote brush. On one hike, I heard the distinctive *whoof* grunts of wild pigs, which were concealed from view in a dense clump of coyote brush just off-trail to the right. I didn't linger because these wild pigs (descendants of game animals and escaped domesticated pigs) can run faster than I can, and some of them wield tusks. Should you come across pigs, be sure to give them a wide berth. Their eyesight and hearing are poor, so they might not see you—give them a good holler and raise up your arms to look big, and they should be on their way.

McCreery Lake Trail begins on the right at 1 mile—another blink-and-you'll-miss-it trail. Continue straight on Halls Valley Trail 0.1 mile, then stay left at a junction with Los Huecos Trail. At an easy grade, Halls Valley Trail begins to ascend through coyote brush; California coffeeberry; poison oak; and black, valley, and coast live oaks. Look for yarrow, Ithuriel's spear, and checkerbloom along the trail in late April, when I once saw a long, dense swath of orange scarlet pimpernel at the edge of the trail. As the grade picks up slightly, you may notice California bay and a few bigleaf maples; their shade fosters a pretty display of shooting stars, blue larkspur, buttercups, and woodland star in spring. Halls Valley Trail passes through

Joseph D. Grant County Park

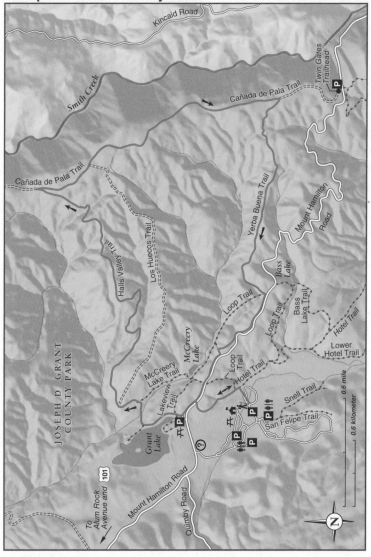

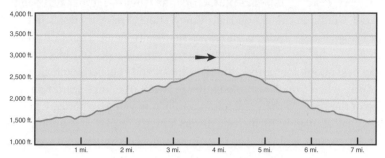

a gate, crosses a creek, and then begins to climb at a steady, moderate grade. On the right in early May, California gilia blooms in a cluster of sagebrush and sticky monkeyflower. The landscape shifts to oak savanna, with lovely blue and valley oaks standing in grassland along the trail, many of them dangling massive clumps of mistletoe, a poisonous, parasitic plant.

Weaving through a landscape of oaks and grassland, the trail permits views north to the highest hills of the park, near Antler Point. In autumn, when the grass is sun-baked blonde, your gaze may be drawn to bright-red patches of poison oak on distant hillsides. On a hot day, every little bit of shade along the trail provides a brief but welcome respite from the sun. With the ridgeline in sight, Halls Valley Trail begins a drop to another creek. Buckeyes blend through California bays on the left—look for fairy lanterns on the right slope in April. The trail makes one last push uphill to the ridge, reaching a junction with Cañada de Pala Trail at 3.2 miles. If you'd like to add 4.5 miles to this hike, you can turn left here and loop to Antler Point; at just under 3,000 feet elevation, it's the highest point in the park. Turn right on Cañada de Pala Trail.

At the peak of wildflower season, the slopes are filled with a variety of common flowers: look for blue-eyed grass, popcorn flower, Johnny-jump-ups, fiddlenecks, California poppy, checkerbloom, blue and white lupine, and blue dicks. On an early-May hike, I enjoyed one of the best wildflower displays I've ever witnessed in the Bay Area, with heavily concentrated blooms all around. It's a far different scene in summer and autumn, when only oaks interrupt the one-dimensional expanse of golden grassland.

Cañada de Pala, the name of this rancho's original grant, rises gently, then reaches a junction with Los Huecos Trail at 3.6 miles. Continue straight. Across a valley to the east, the domes of Lick Observatory are visible, near the highest elevation on Mount Hamilton, 4,373-foot Copernicus Peak. Cañada de Pala Trail crosses through a gate into cattle range, where cows are present in spring and summer. In April and May the transition is abrupt—say goodbye to wildflowers and hello to trim, bare grassland and big sections of muddy trail.

As you follow an easy, rolling course, look for a bench on the right, a good spot from which to gaze at the long views extending downhill to Grant Lake and beyond to downtown San Jose on clear days. The fire road drops away from this hike's highest elevation, about 2,700 feet, and you should be able to see past the rolling hills along the trail to the ridge forming Grant's southwestern boundary. At 4.9 miles Yerba Buena Trail begins on the right. If you'd like to stretch this hike to 9.5 miles, you can continue on Cañada de Pala Trail here and cross Mount Hamilton Road at the Twin Gates Trailhead to Hotel Trail, which returns to the trailhead through the southern part of Halls Valley. To stick to this 7.6-mile hike, turn right onto Yerba Buena Trail.

The trail begins a moderate descent through cattle range. Even when the cows are in the area, some wildflowers escape them, including owl's clover, woodland star, and blue and white lupine. Poison oak is common, growing here in shrub form. Valley oaks keep a distance from the trail, so there is little shade. Bass Lake is briefly visible downhill to the left. One short uphill precedes a steady descent past a few black oaks on the right, through grassland where mule-ear sunflowers, goldfields, johnny-tuck, blue-eyed grass, Ithuriel's spear, California poppy, and buttercups bloom in spring.

At 6.3 miles Yerba Buena Trail nears Mount Hamilton Road—the gate to the road is locked, but there's a step-over bench. A path to Bass Lake sets off directly across the street, but as of this writing Bass Lake Trail is closed. To the right Loop Trail sets off, offering an optional route downhill. Continue on Yerba Buena Trail, which runs along Mount Hamilton Road, finally leaving the cattle range at a gate. The trail here shrinks to a narrower path and keeps to an easy, mostly downhill grade. Look for a big gooseberry bush growing around a rock formation on the left. A connector to Loop Trail begins on the right at 6.6 miles. Continue straight on Yerba Buena Trail.

A trail to McCreery Lake departs on the right at 7 miles. Continue on Yerba Buena Tail to the next junction at 7.1 miles. Turn left, cross the road, and retrace your steps back to the trailhead.

NEARBY ACTIVITIES

This large park offers many hiking possibilities. For mellow, easy loops, pick trails through Halls Valley, such as Lower Hotel and San Felipe.

• •

GPS TRAILHEAD COORDINATES N37° 20.204' W121° 42.890'

DIRECTIONS From the I-280/CA 1 junction in San Francisco, drive south on I-280 about 49 miles, then continue east on I-680 for 1.7 miles. Exit onto Alum Rock Avenue and drive east about 2 miles, then turn right onto Mt. Hamilton Road. Drive about 7.5 miles southeast on this narrow, winding road to the park entrance on the right. Once past the entry kiosk, go straight past the first parking area on the left, then turn left where the road splits and park near the gated entrance to the Hotel Trail.

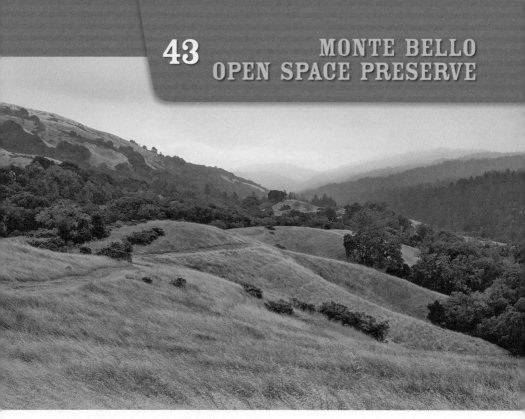

Summer landscape at Monte Bello Open Space Preserve

AT 2,800 FEET ELEVATION, Black Mountain boasts outstanding 360-degree views. Want to look down at the Santa Clara Valley? You got it. Prefer views of the forested Santa Cruz Mountains? No problem—just turn around! This hike descends to cool, quiet Stevens Creek, then ascends out of a canyon to Black Mountain's summit. The return route is all downhill, through grasslands where flowers riot in spring.

DESCRIPTION

Oddly enough, in a preserve where everything seems supersized, I find myself particularly drawn to Monte Bello's most subtle charms. In this open-space preserve, the trails, views, and hikes are long, but I get lost in the little things: new oak leaves unfolding, hillsides covered with miniature flowers, and water trickling down a tiny waterfall. It's the perfect place for a solo hike-as-meditation.

From the parking lot, walk to the signed trailhead, then turn right onto White Oak Trail. The narrow trail follows the edge of grassland along the shoulder of a wooded canyon. Initially there are views south to Black Mountain, but trees soon shade the path and block vistas. At a signed junction at 0.6 mile, stay left on White Oak Trail, which begins to descend.

DISTANCE & CONFIGURATION: 6.9-mile loop with a short out-and-back stretch

DIFFICULTY: Moderate

SCENERY: Grassland, woods, creek, and views

EXPOSURE: Mixed

TRAIL TRAFFIC: Light–moderate

TRAIL SURFACE: Dirt fire roads and trails

HIKING TIME: 3.5 hours

DRIVING DISTANCE: 37.2 miles from the I-280/CA 1 junction at the San Francisco–Daly City border

ACCESS: Daily, 30 minutes before official sunrise–30 minutes after official sunset.

Summer is often very hot; late winter and spring are best. No fee.

WHEELCHAIR ACCESS: There is designated handicapped parking. One short trail segment is wheelchair accessible—from the parking lot south to the viewpoint.

MAPS: At trailhead's information signboard and tinyurl.com/montebellomap

FACILITIES: Vault toilets at trailhead

CONTACT: 650-691-1200, openspace.org /preserves/monte-bello

LOCATION: Page Mill Road, 7 miles west of CA 280 and 1.5 miles east of Skyline Boulevard

COMMENTS: No dogs allowed

The trail passes through madrone and oak woods, then emerges into grassland peppered with huge, old white oaks. Valley and Oregon oak are both classified as white oaks, but Oregon oaks are an unusual find on the peninsula. Some of these gorgeous oaks on the sides of the trail are Oregon oaks, but it takes a practiced eye to tell them apart—oak leaves can vary from tree to tree, and the most distinguishing feature, the acorn, is around for perusal only in autumn (valley oak acorns are slender and long, while those of Oregon oaks are short and fat). Even though it's tough to identify them, it's easy to admire these venerable oaks.

White Oak Trail continues to descend, then adopts a series of switchbacks. The landscape begins to shift as the trail makes its way into a canyon; in the transition, mule-ear sunflowers bloom along the trail in spring, in the last patches of grassland. As the tree cover thickens, you might notice two oaks of the evergreen variety, coast live and canyon live. Other common plants include California bay, bigleaf maple, gooseberry, Douglas-fir, tanoak, wild rose, ferns, and creambush. The springtime flowers, including western heart's ease, trillium, coltsfoot, and pink-flowering currant, are typical to moist, dark woods and creekbeds. In the dead of winter, the trail is often completely covered with fallen leaves. White Oak Trail rises to a junction at 1.8 miles. Skid Road Trail climbs to the right on the way to Skyline Ridge Open Space Preserve. Continue left, following the sign toward Stevens Creek Nature Trail.

This wide trail descends through a forest of Douglas-fir, tanoak, and California bay. At 2.1 miles Stevens Creek Nature Trail heads back toward the trailhead on the left. Continue right, toward Canyon Trail. The trail crosses then follows Stevens Creek. At a second bridge, a tributary drops into the creek from the left, creating a small cascade in the wettest months. Thimbleberry, blackberry, and blue elderberry thrive in the damp canyon beneath Douglas-fir and California bay, and honeysuckle vines drip from live oaks. Fairy lanterns bloom here in spring. The trail begins to

Monte Bello Open Space Preserve

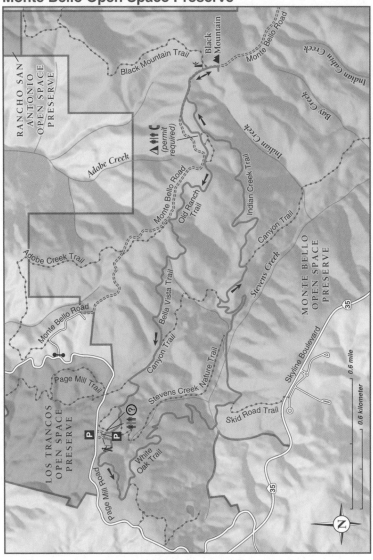

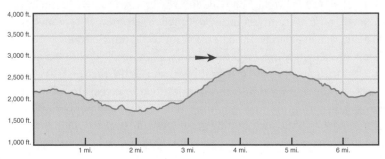

ascend then makes a sharp left, away from the creek. At 2.6 miles the trail ends at a junction with Canyon Trail. Turn right.

Baby blue eyes freckle a small, grassy meadow in spring. The fire road sweeps uphill through a pocket of woods, then reemerges into grassland and descends to a junction at 2.9 miles. Turn left onto Indian Creek Trail.

The wide fire road begins to ascend at a sustained, moderate grade. On one August hike, I caught a glimpse of a young coyote sitting in a patch of sloping grassland near the edge of the woods on the right. Gradually the accompanying vegetation shifts from madrone, oaks, and California bay to a chaparral blend of poison oak, sticky monkeyflower, chamise, toyon, California coffeeberry, ceanothus, and yerba santa. You may also notice clematis, a vine with pretty white flowers in spring and puffy seed clusters in autumn.

As the trail ascends, grassland begins to dominate, and graceful displays of popcorn flower, Johnny-jump-up, chia, owl's clover, fiddleneck, blue dicks, and California poppy appear in spring. At 3.9 miles a path veers off to the left. Continue straight, following the sign toward Black Mountain. The climb continues until Indian Creek Trail ends at a T-junction at 4.1 miles. Turn right onto Monte Bello Road.

As if to compensate for the climb, the last stretch to the summit, on a broad fire road, is easy. A tangle of California coffeeberry, live oaks, ceanothus, madrone, and pitcher sage blocks views to the east, but just past some communication structures, where a trail begins on the left and descends at an extremely steep grade into Rancho San Antonio Open Space Preserve, the trees and shrubs yield to grassland. Continue a little farther on Monte Bello Road to the top of Black Mountain at 2,800 feet—more of a plateau than an apex. Here, savor views east and south, including Mission Peak and Mount Hamilton. Look for a small boulder field on the right, and follow the unsigned but obvious path into this area. The treeless summit offers exceptional views, particularly of Mount Umunhum to the south and a forested ridge running west, much of which is preserved open space. This is a wonderfully scenic spot for a lunch break. When you're ready, return to the junction with Indian Creek Trail, then continue straight on Monte Bello Road.

The fire road descends easily, bordered by woods where you might see mournful duskywing butterflies in summer. When the road forks, stay left, following the BACK-PACK CAMP sign. On the right, the wide fire road passes Black Mountain Backpack Camp, a small, no-frills camp requiring advance reservations. Continue through the camp to a junction at 5.0 miles, and bear left onto Old Ranch Trail.

Almost immediately head right on a slight path, marked with NO BIKES, NOT A THROUGH TRAIL signs. The path climbs through grassland, then ends at a hilltop with the preserve's best views north, extending past San Francisco to Mount Tamalpais on clear days. In spring, Johnny-jump-ups, fiddlenecks, and popcorn flower bloom with abandon through the surrounding grass. Descend back to Old Ranch Trail, then turn right.

The trail descends downslope from the ridgeline, through grassland dotted with coyote brush. The high reaches of a wooded ravine on the left are packed with poison oak, but thankfully Old Ranch Trail keeps its distance. You might see buttercups, owl's clover, California poppy, and blue and white lupine peeking out from spring's lush green grass. Russian Ridge is visible to the northwest, and in the foreground Bella Vista Trail is conspicuous. At 5.5 miles you'll reach a junction with two paths on the right leading to Monte Bello Road. Stay left, now on Bella Vista Trail.

Beautiful views? Yes, indeed, particularly to the north and west. Bella Vista initially sticks to grassland, but as it descends, trailside vegetation becomes more varied and includes small clusters of creambush, California bay, buckeye, live oak, and bigleaf maple nestled in creases of the hillside. Painted lady butterflies are commonly glimpsed along the trail in summer. After a steady, moderate descent, Bella Vista Trail ends at 6.3 miles. Turn right, onto Canyon Trail.

Coyote brush, buckeye, willow, and toyon mix it up along the trail. Activity along the San Andreas Fault, which runs parallel to the fire road, created the little sag pond on the right. Canyon Trail, keeping to a mostly level grade, passes a spur path on the left, then reaches a junction at 6.5 miles. Turn left, following the sign to the Monte Bello parking lot.

The little trail weaves through an old walnut orchard, then sweeps right and ascends slightly. On these grassy slopes high above Stevens Creek, grassland fosters good wildflower displays in spring; on one late-April visit, an entire hillside on the left was covered with pink owl's clover. At 6.8 miles Stevens Creek Nature Trail enters from the left near a rustic stone bench. Before continuing on the trail heading right, take a moment to gaze south, enjoying one last look at Black Mountain and Mount Umunhum. The final stretch to the parking lot is short and level.

NEARBY ACTIVITIES

Los Trancos Open Space Preserve, (650-691-1200, openspace.org/preserves/los-trancos) just across Page Mill Road from the Monte Bello parking lot, offers a self-guided nature tour with an emphasis on earthquakes and geology—the San Andreas Fault runs through both preserves.

• •

GPS TRAILHEAD COORDINATES N37° 19.544' W122° 10.743'

DIRECTIONS From the I-280/CA 1 junction in San Francisco, drive south on I-280 about 29 miles, then take Exit 20 onto Page Mill Road. Drive west on Page Mill Road about 8 miles, and turn left into the preserve parking lot.

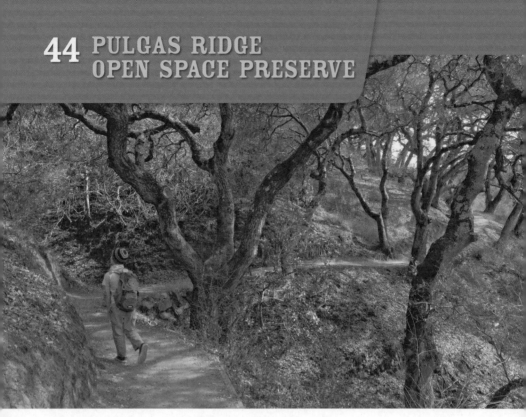

Looking for woodrat nests at Pulgas Ridge Open Space Preserve

THIS HIKE IS an easy loop through woods and chaparral at a preserve for dogs and the hikers who love them (or at least don't mind them).

DESCRIPTION

Pulgas Ridge is a small preserve on the outskirts of San Carlos and Redwood City, just across a canyon from Edgewood County Park and Natural Preserve (see Hike 40, page 197). Both parks share a similar landscape of mixed woods, grassland, and chaparral. Both are right off I-280—a mixed blessing/curse of fast access and highway noise. The biggest difference between the two parks has four legs and a wagging tail: dogs are prohibited at Edgewood but welcome at Pulgas.

From 1926 to 1972, Pulgas Ridge housed a City of San Francisco tuberculosis sanatorium. After the hospital closed, the property was purchased by the Midpeninsula Regional Open Space District (MROSD), and the buildings were torn down in the 1980s. When I first hiked here in 2000, a motley collection of plants growing along the old paved roads was the last relic of the sanatorium era. District staff and volunteers removed cacti, oleander, rockrose, broom, and other non-native specimens, replanting oaks in their stead. Only the crumbling old roads remain.

In 2006, MROSD added a parking lot and two new trails at Pulgas Ridge, greatly increasing loop possibilities. The off-leash dog area is still the preserve's hot spot for

DISTANCE & CONFIGURATION: 2.6-mile loop

DIFFICULTY: Easy

SCENERY: Woods and chaparral

EXPOSURE: Mostly shaded

TRAIL TRAFFIC: Moderate–heavy

TRAIL SURFACE: Dirt trails

HIKING TIME: 1 hour

DRIVING DISTANCE: 21.8 miles from the I-280/CA 1 junction at the San Francisco–Daly City border

ACCESS: Good year-round. No fee.

WHEELCHAIR ACCESS: There is designated handicapped parking, and the first 0.4 mile of trail is wheelchair accessible.

MAPS: At trailhead and tinyurl.com/pulgasmap

FACILITIES: Vault toilet at trailhead

CONTACT: 650-691-1200, openspace.org /preserves/pulgas-ridge

LOCATION: 167 Edmonds Road, Redwood City, CA

COMMENTS: Dogs are permitted on leash on trails and off leash in a designated area.

hikers with canine companions—Dick Bishop (formerly Sagebrush) Trail allows hikers to skip this area altogether. Dusky-Footed Woodrat Trail combined with Hassler and Polly Geraci Trails is another loop option. Regardless of your hiking proximity to the off-leash area, come prepared to cross paths with dogs at Pulgas.

Start from the information signboard at the parking lot, and follow the trail signed TO CORDILLERAS TRAIL. The path accompanies a string of power lines to the left as it traverses a gently sloping hillside. Coast live oaks, California bays, and buckeyes provide shade. The property on the right is private—stay on the trail here and keep it quiet. After some easy undulating, the trail bends right, passes through a narrow, tree-dotted meadow; crosses a road; and meets Cordilleras Trail at a T-junction. Turn left. Now parallel to the road, the trail borders water-district lands; stay on the trail (don't walk on the road). There's not too much to look at along the flat trail—mostly poison oak shrubs, some coast live oaks, and acacias. You might see a few Ithuriel's spear and blue-eyed grass in spring. At 0.4 mile the paved road (here named Hassler Trail) sweeps left and continues uphill. A gated trail heads under the trees to the right. Turn right, enter the preserve, and, after a few feet, turn left onto Polly Geraci Trail.

The narrow path crosses a creek and begins an easy ascent through buckeye, madrone, coast live oak, and California bay woods. At 0.5 mile Dusky-Footed Woodrat Trail breaks off to the right (this is a great option for a longer hike with more substantial elevation change). Continue straight.

The wildflower display begins here in February, with red Indian warrior, blue hound's tongue, white milkmaids, and big displays of fetid adder's-tongue. This plant is easy to miss until you see one, and then you'll likely see it everywhere you look—the smooth green leaves are mottled with brown spots, and the flowers are streaky brown and white. Polly Geraci Trail is a reliable location for this member of the lily family.

The trail switchbacks uphill, climbing out of the shaded canyon to a sun-drenched, sandy chaparral plateau. Chamise and manzanitas dominate this landscape, where

Pulgas Ridge Open Space Preserve

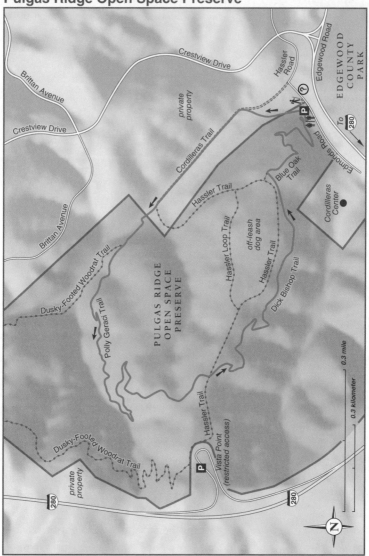

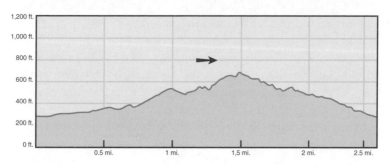

you might also notice sticky monkeyflower, blue elderberry, yerba santa, ceanothus, pitcher sage, and toyon. At 1.5 miles Polly Geraci Trail ends at a signed junction with Hassler Trail. To the right, Hassler runs uphill along the ridgeline, connecting to the Dusky-Footed Woodrat Trail near a Caltrans vista point. To the left, it leads downhill to the off-leash dog area. Continue straight, now on Dick Bishop Trail.

As the trail begins an easy descent, there are sweeping views south to the forested slopes of the Santa Cruz Mountains and, even closer, of Edgewood County Park and Natural Preserve. Sagebrush and coyote brush line the trail initially, but after a while pockets of coast live oaks provide occasional shade. At 2.1 miles Dick Bishop Trail ends at Blue Oak Trail. Turn right.

Under a mix of blue and coast live oak, madrone, and California bay, the narrow trail winds downhill. This is another good stretch for wildflower hunting in spring, with delicate, ivory-hued fairy lanterns appearing in May and golden brodiaea blooming reliably every June. Blue oaks are uncommon on the peninsula—these deciduous native oaks are more at home in southern Santa Clara, Contra Costa, Marin, and Sonoma Counties. Edgewood County Park, less than 0.25 mile south, has plenty of oaks but no blues. Blue Oak Trail ends at st above the trailhead and Edmonds Road. Bear left to the parking lot.

NEARBY ACTIVITIES

If you and your dogs prefer a sunnier Peninsula destination, check out **Pearson-Arastradero Preserve** (1530 Arastradero Road, Palo Alto, CA; 650-329-2423; tinyurl .com/arastradero), about 10 miles south of Pulgas Ridge between Page Mill and Alpine Roads. Arastradero's trails roam gently rolling, grassy hills, and leashed dogs are welcome.

• •

GPS TRAILHEAD COORDINATES N37° 28.504' W122° 16.969'

DIRECTIONS From the CA 1/I-280 junction in San Francisco, drive south on I-280 about 20 miles, and take Exit 29 onto Edgewood Road. Turn left and drive east on Edgewood about 1 mile, then turn left onto Crestview Drive. Almost immediately, turn left onto Edmonds Road. Continue about 0.2 mile to the signed preserve parking lot, on the right.

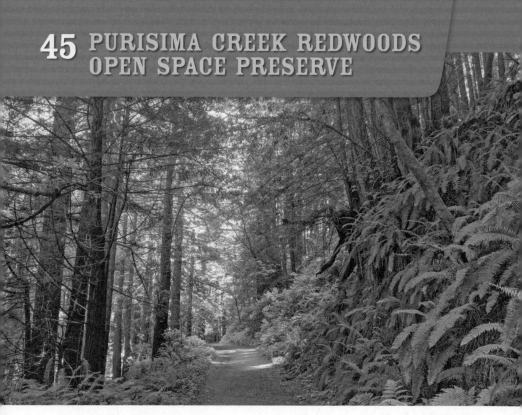

Lush canyon along Purisima Creek Trail

THIS LOOP FOLLOWS Purisima Creek upstream into a canyon, then breaks off through wooded Soda Gulch. You'll wind uphill through chaparral, then descend rapidly on a moderately steep fire road.

DESCRIPTION

Logging was commonplace in the Santa Cruz Mountains, with redwood lumber widely used as building material for San Francisco structures. By the early 1900s most of the redwood giants had been cut and hauled out. Although some small virgin groves of redwoods still stand throughout the Santa Cruz Mountains, usually tucked in hard-to-reach canyons, most of the redwood forests are second-growth woods. Purisima Creek Redwoods is no exception, although when wooded canyons are this gorgeous, I find myself transfixed by the trees rather than by the stumps.

Life along Purisima Creek and the surrounding canyons changes with the seasons. In early winter, redwood needles pad the trails, and after rainstorms, newts can be spotted making their way to the creek to breed. Late winter and spring bring wildflowers to brighten the floors of the darkest canyons. Summer's abundant daylight encourages daylong hikes through chaparral spiced with the aroma of blooming native shrubs.

As you make your way from the parking lot into the preserve, almost immediately you can feel and see the cooling influence of Purisima Creek and the redwoods.

DISTANCE & CONFIGURATION: 6.9-mile loop with a very short out-and-back segment

DIFFICULTY: Moderate

SCENERY: Redwoods, creek, and chaparral

EXPOSURE: Nearly equal parts shade and sun

TRAIL TRAFFIC: Moderate on weekends; light on weekdays

TRAIL SURFACE: Dirt fire roads and trails

HIKING TIME: 3.5 hours

DRIVING DISTANCE: 29 miles from the I-280/CA 1 junction at the San Francisco–Daly City border

ACCESS: Good year-round; cool in summer if you get an early start. No fee.

WHEELCHAIR ACCESS: There is designated handicapped parking, and wheelchair users should be able to roll about a mile along Purisima Creek.

MAPS: At information kiosk a short distance from parking lot and tinyurl.com/purisimamap

FACILITIES: Pit toilets near trailhead

CONTACT: 650-691-1200, openspace.org /preserves/purisima-creek-redwoods

LOCATION: Half Moon Bay, CA

COMMENTS: No dogs allowed

The canyon wall on the right is a tangle of moisture-loving thimbleberry, alder, red elderberry, and ferns. Near the pit toilets and information signboard, Harkins Ridge Trail (your return route) and Whittemore Gulch Trail depart to the left. Continue straight (southeast) on Purisima Creek Trail. Running above the banks of Purisima Creek, the broad trail is nearly flat and almost completely shaded by redwoods. Banana slugs are often sighted curled up on logs and plants. These mollusks are important composters, chewing fallen leaves, needles, and mushrooms and expelling fresh fertile soil.

After 1 mile of easy walking, you'll reach a junction with Borden Hatch Mill Trail. Continue straight on Purisima Creek Trail. The grade picks up a bit but remains easy. Huckleberry makes an appearance in an understory where trillium, starflower, and California larkspur bloom in June. The trail meets Grabtown Gulch Trail at 1.2 miles; continue on Purisima Creek Trail, and press on uphill, delving farther into the redwood canyon. A little bridge marks the confluence of Soda Gulch and Purisima Creek. After one more bridge routing you back across to the south side of the creek, the trail begins to climb with more purpose. At a sharp bend left, you'll leave Purisima Creek behind and, after one last hill, reach a junction at 2.4 miles.

Purisima Creek Trail continues uphill toward Skyline Boulevard. Turn left onto Craig Britton Trail (formerly Soda Gulch Trail). Continuing the journey through the darkest part of the canyon, this Bay Area Ridge Trail segment is a stunner. The narrow path winds through redwoods, angling across steep hillsides. Ferns sprawl through the understory and nestle on the shores of a little creek crossed by a wooden bridge. Winter storms uproot trees, forcing temporary reroutes or scrambles over or around the fallen giants. There's a "wow" around nearly every corner, including a surprising grassy spot where a few coast live oaks and ceanothus shrubs permit views west.

Craig Britton Trail crosses Soda Gulch on another pretty little bridge. The sound of water is supremely refreshing on a hot summer day. Finally, as the trail begins to

Purisma Creek Redwoods Open Space Preserve

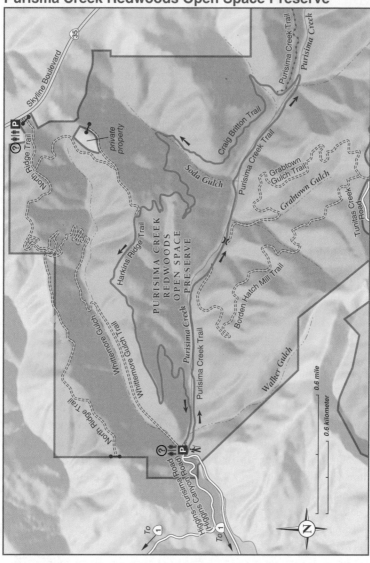

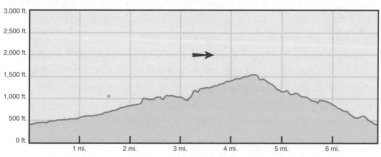

climb, you'll slalom through a very dark patch of redwoods and then emerge on the sun-drenched slopes of the mountain, blinking in the sudden sunlight. Views here stretch to the ocean.

Switchbacks route the trail through ceanothus, coyote brush, toyon, coffeeberry, and lizardtail. Paintbrush, sticky monkeyflower, and cow parsnip are just a few of the wildflowers that linger into summer, thriving under a coastal influence that keeps the hillsides green when inland parks' wildflowers are already dry and brown. A few madrones and coast live oaks shade the trail occasionally, which you'll likely appreciate around noon on a sunny day. At 4.8 miles, where Craig Britton Trail ends at a junction with Harkins Ridge Trail, turn left.

The contrast between Harkins Ridge Trail, a wide, steep fire road, and the intimacy of hiking-only Craig Britton Trail is illuminated immediately. Harkins Ridge sets off downhill like it means business, through towering Douglas-fir and an understory of creambush, hazelnut, huckleberry, yellow bush lupine, and coyote brush. There are a few short uphill bits for variety. Watch out for cyclists zipping down the steepest sections, where the sharp grade might give hikers with unstable knees a pause. Because views have been mostly obscured by the redwoods until this part of the hike, the trail compensates for the steep descent with lots of stunning vistas. To the right you can see North Ridge and the high eastern flanks of Montara Mountain. Dead ahead to the west, hills undulate all the way to the ocean.

The trail soon veers left and begins a series of broad switchbacks, heading down into the canyon. As redwoods exert their influence, look also for hazelnut and currant. Harkins Ridge Trail ends at a junction with Whittemore Gulch Trail at 6.9 miles. Turn left, cross Purisima Creek for the last time, and then turn right toward the parking lot.

NEARBY ACTIVITIES

You can also begin a Purisima hike from the preserve's main trailhead on CA 35, 4 miles south of CA 92.

• •

GPS TRAILHEAD COORDINATES N37° 26.253' W122° 22.237'

DIRECTIONS From the CA 1/I-280 junction in San Francisco, drive 14 miles south on I-280, then take Exit 34 for CA 92 W. Turn left onto Skyline Boulevard and drive 1 mile to the junction with CA 92. Turn right and drive 7 miles to the junction with CA 1. Turn south (left) onto CA 1 and drive about 1.3 miles; turn left onto Higgins–Purisima Road (aka Higgins Canyon Road). Drive on this narrow, winding road about 4.5 miles to the trailhead, on the left just past the tiny white bridge.

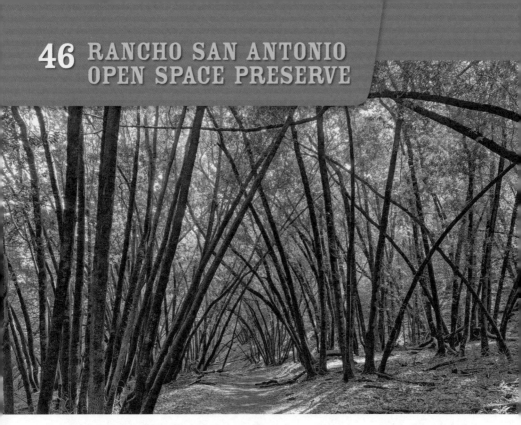

Shaded California bay woods on Upper Wildcat Canyon Trail

AFTER A MILE of gentle strolling, you'll leave the crowds behind and climb through oaks and grassland to a vista point. Press on uphill, through chaparral where coyotes have been spotted, then descend to a shaded canyon and follow a creek back toward the farm. A bypass route skirts the farm area and returns to the trailhead through woods and grassland.

DESCRIPTION

Once you've nailed down a parking space, you'll start this hike with the masses, walking to Deer Hollow Farm. Begin from the parking lot near the restrooms and cross Permanente Creek on a footbridge (not the sturdy vehicular bridge on the other end of the parking lot). On the far side of the bridge, turn right onto Permanente Creek Trail, following the sign toward Deer Hollow Farm. This broad dirt trail runs along the creek through a flat grassy area.

Once past a massive California bay, the trail ends at a multiple junction. Turn left, cross a paved path and the road, and you'll arrive at the boundary with the open-space preserve. Pick up a map from the signboard and continue on Lower Meadow Trail, a wide dirt path through a pretty swatch of grass dotted with coast live oaks and California bays. Orange fiddlenecks bloom along the trail here in late winter, preceding yellow mule-ear sunflowers.

DISTANCE & CONFIGURATION: 6.3-mile figure eight

DIFFICULTY: Moderate

SCENERY: Grassland, woods, chaparral, and creek

EXPOSURE: Nearly equal parts shaded and exposed

TRAIL TRAFFIC: Busy, busy, busy—365 days a year

TRAIL SURFACE: Dirt fire roads and trails

HIKING TIME: 2.5 hours

DRIVING DISTANCE: 38.3 miles from the I-280/CA 1 junction at the San Francisco–Daly City border

ACCESS: Daily, 30 minutes before sunrise–30 minutes after sunset. Good anytime. No fee.

WHEELCHAIR ACCESS: There is designated handicapped parking, and this hike is wheelchair accessible for the first mile.

MAPS: At information signboard 0.3 mile inside park and at tinyurl.com/rsamap

FACILITIES: Restrooms and water at trailhead

CONTACT: 650-691-1200, openspace.org /preserves/rancho-san-antonio

LOCATION: Just east of the I-280/CA 85 junction, near Cupertino, CA

COMMENTS: No dogs allowed. Arrive early on weekends for parking.

When Lower Meadow Trail meets the paved road, cross the street and skirt a permit parking area, then pick up a continuation of the trail. You'll cross a creek then walk on a level grade parallel to the park road. At 0.8 mile a multiple junction sends trails scattering in every direction. Across the paved road to the left, Farm Bypass Trail loops around Deer Hollow Farm. The other two routes (the paved road and a dirt footpath) continue straight, proceeding to the farm. Mora Trail, to the right, avoids the area altogether, climbing up to a grassy ridge. Continue straight on the dirt footpath (Lower Meadow Trail).

This little path rolls gently up and down on the edge of grassland. At 0.9 mile the trail feeds into the paved road. Turn right. The buzz of activity surrounding Deer Hollow Farm includes excited kids, vocalizing animals, and the hum of farm equipment. Along with farm buildings that date back to the 1850s, mature persimmon, pomegranate, and other fruit trees create an old-time, bucolic atmosphere. Although the farm is not open to the public every day, you can still enjoy watching goats and cows from the trail side of the fence and peer into a pretty garden of flowers and vegetables. Wild animals seem ridiculously comfortable near the farm, and you might see deer, turkey, or quail only a few feet off the trail. Just past a barn that wears a historical patina, Rogue Valley Trail heads off to the right at 1.1 miles. Stay left, heading toward Upper Wildcat Canyon Trail.

A few steps past some vault toilets, you'll pass Farm Bypass Trail, which enters from the left. Continue straight through a damp area where willow, bigleaf maple, buckeye, ninebark, and blackberry brambles form a dense wall of vegetation. At 1.2 miles Wildcat Loop Trail continues straight, while a path to Coyote Trail sets off to the left. Turn right onto High Meadow Trail.

An assortment of native plants lines this broad trail, including silktassel, sagebrush, sticky monkeyflower, poison oak, pitcher sage, coast live oak, buckeye, and

Rancho San Antonio Open Space Preserve

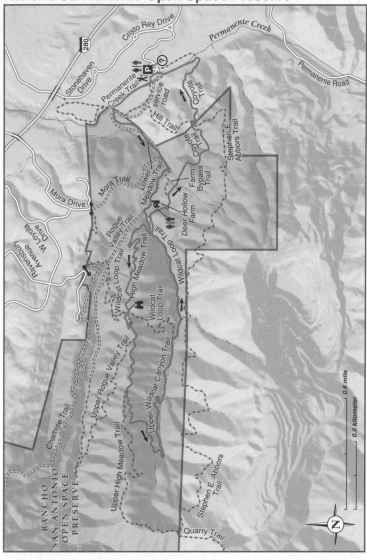

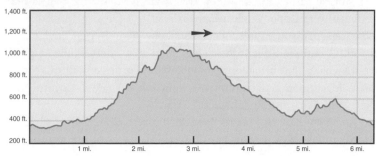

toyon. High Meadow Trail curves uphill at a moderate grade, then turns left and begins a series of long switchbacks, which softens the ascent. As the trail meets the lower reaches of a sloping, grassy meadow, blue oaks and coast live oaks appear. Coast live oaks are evergreen and enjoy each other's company, while deciduous blue oaks stand in more-solitary formations. Blue oaks are easy to pick out in autumn, when their leaves are at their bluest, and in late winter, when they leaf out. Mule-ear sunflowers bloom along the trail in abundance as early as March, and if you visit in late May or early June, you might see a few mariposa lilies.

The trail continues uphill on the edge of the sloping grassy hillside, passing coast live oak, toyon, and a few cercocarpus. Look for several venerable valley oaks that grace the grassland to your left.

At 2.1 miles, moving clockwise at a multiple junction, the first path to the left heads to a vista point, Wildcat Loop Trail descends to Upper Wildcat Canyon Trail, High Meadow Trail keeps climbing, and the other segment of Wildcat Loop Trail drops toward Rogue Valley Trail on the right. Turn left for a short out-and-back on the path to the vista point.

The trail ascends quickly then ends at a belvedere. Straight ahead, the sloping, grassy meadow peppered with oaks descends to the south, framing a view across Silicon Valley to peaks of the Mount Hamilton range. Return downhill to the previous junction, then resume uphill (left) on High Meadow Trail.

After a few steps, the trails split. Either route is an option, but the path on the right is less steep than the fire road, so bear right.

Angling across the hillside, the trail enters a shaded area where California bays mix with coast live oak, sticky monkeyflower, poison oak, and toyon. After a switchback, the path meets and crosses the steep fire road. The difference between the two sides of the hill is remarkable. On these sunny slopes, chamise basks in the sun along with sagebrush and toyon. There are good views to the northwest of Black Mountain, which tops out at 2,800 feet. At 2.4 miles the two legs of High Meadow Trail rejoin for good at a junction where Upper Rogue Valley Trail drops off the ridge on the right. Continue left on High Meadow Trail.

The trail ascends slightly through chaparral and then reaches a junction at 2.7 miles. Upper High Meadow Trail continues uphill straight ahead, presenting a good option for extending this hike 2 miles, on a loop through one of the most remote parts of the preserve. For today's hike bear left onto Upper Wildcat Canyon Trail.

Descending, Upper Wildcat Canyon Trail winds through madrone, toyon, silk-tassel, chamise, California coffeeberry, pitcher sage, and coast live oak. As the trail drops into Wildcat Canyon, a forest of California bays overtakes the landscape; then the trail bends left and runs along a creek. It's hard to believe that this quiet section of the park is less than 2 miles from the farm area. With steep hills rising up to the right and left, this trail really captures the essence of a canyon, and in the heat of summer, the sound of water and the total shade are welcome. In October and November, bigleaf maples create a gorgeous autumnal tableau, releasing their colorful leaves to drift down to the trail and creek. The trail descends gently to a junction with Wildcat Loop Trail at 4.1 miles. Continue right, now on Wildcat Loop Trail.

Creambush, coast live oak, California bay, and blackberries tangle along the trail, accompanying a large colony of western leatherwood. Early wildflowers include trillium, hound's tongue, and milkmaids. A connector to Stephen E. Abbors Trail departs to the right at 4.2 miles, but continue left on Wildcat Loop Trail.

As you make your way out of the heart of the canyon, the trail crosses the creek on tiny bridges under gracefully arching California bays. At 4.7 miles you'll reach a familiar junction with High Meadow Trail. Continue straight a few feet, then bear right toward Farm Bypass Trail.

Buckeyes dominate the landscape as the narrow trail ascends easily. You might notice California bay, poison oak, and pitcher sage, as well as trilliums in late winter. Farm Bypass Trail breaks off to the left at 5 miles, but continue right on Coyote Trail.

Runners favor this trail for its easy grade and abundant shade. In this fairly open woodland, the limited understory vegetation makes it easy to find wildflowers such as woodland star and mission bells. When the trail enters a sunny area, look for clematis, a trailing vine, draped over shrubs. Gooseberry, ceanothus, sagebrush, poison oak, and sticky monkeyflower are common here. Just past some blue oaks, the trail ends at 5.6 miles. Stephen E. Abbors Trail doubles back to the right, and Hill Trail descends on the left, past a water tank. Make a soft right to stay on Coyote Trail, following the sign reading TO COUNTY PARK.

Vetch covers much of the hillside on the right, and coast live oak, California bay, buckeye, and blue oak are scattered about. Where the trail descends to a junction near the equestrian parking lot at 6.0 miles, turn left. The perfectly flat path accompanies Permanente Creek, on the right, screened by willows. At 6.3 miles, you'll reach a junction with a paved bike path and the park road. Turn right and cross the bridge to return to the parking lot.

• •

GPS TRAILHEAD COORDINATES N37° 19.973' W122° 05.271'

DIRECTIONS From the CA 1/I-280 junction in San Francisco, drive south on I-280 about 36 miles, then take Exit 13 at Foothill Expressway. Turn right, drive south on Foothill Boulevard, and take the first right onto Cristo Rey Drive. Drive about 1 mile and turn left into the park.

RUSSIAN RIDGE
OPEN SPACE PRESERVE

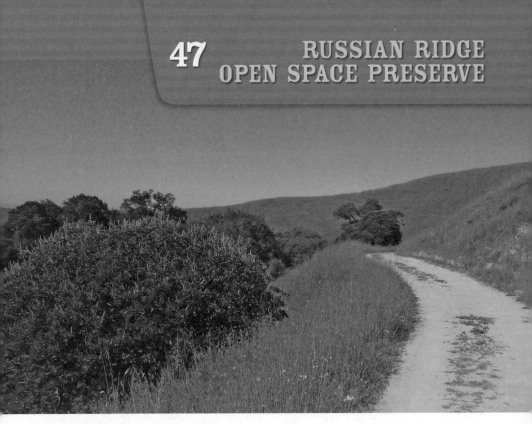

Beautiful spring scenery at Russian Ridge

WHEN SPRING IN ALL ITS GLORY graces the Bay Area, Russian Ridge is one of the top destinations to enjoy swaths of green grass, gentle breezes, and wildflowers. This loop showcases the best of the preserve on an easy circuit through grassland and clusters of venerable live oaks.

DESCRIPTION

Russian Ridge Open Space Preserve sprawls over one of the Santa Cruz Mountains' rare publicly accessible treeless ridges, so the views are incredible. And because the trailhead is right off CA 35, Russian Ridge is easy to get to and easy to hike—it takes just 10 minutes of walking to reach the ridgeline.

If you're on a wildflower mission, you might go no farther than an out-and-back jaunt along the ridge. Usually peaking in early May, a dramatic blossom extravaganza unfolds, with massive carpets of purple lupines and liberal, multihued sprinklings of tidy tips, owl's clover, California poppy, creamcups, and Johnny-jump-ups. Although Russian Ridge is renowned as a wildflower destination, the preserve offers good hike possibilities year-round.

From the trailhead, begin walking uphill on Ridge Trail. The first stretch runs parallel to CA 35, but soon the trail passes a cluster of buckeye and jogs left, cushioning the noise from the road. The trail turns again and now begins to follow the

DISTANCE & CONFIGURATION: 3.7-mile balloon loop

DIFFICULTY: Easy

SCENERY: Grassland, oaks, and wildflowers

EXPOSURE: Mostly unshaded

TRAIL TRAFFIC: Moderate on weekends; light on weekdays; heavy during wildflower peak

TRAIL SURFACE: Dirt trails and fire roads

HIKING TIME: 2 hours

DRIVING DISTANCE: 39 miles from the I-280/CA 1 junction at the San Francisco–Daly City border

ACCESS: Daily, 30 minutes before sunrise–30 minutes after sunset. Good anytime; amazing in spring. No fee.

WHEELCHAIR ACCESS: There are designated handicapped spots. Wheelchair users should depart the Russian Ridge parking lot and wheel along Ipiwa Trail to and around Alpine Pond in adjacent Skyline Ridge Open Space Preserve.

MAPS: At information signboard in parking lot and openspace.org/sites/default/files /map_RR.pdf

FACILITIES: Vault toilets at trailhead

CONTACT: 650-691-1200, openspace.org /preserves/russian-ridge

LOCATION: CA 35 (Skyline Boulevard), about 7 miles south of the CA 35/CA 84 junction, San Mateo County, CA

COMMENTS: No dogs allowed

ridgeline, gaining elevation at an easy pace. Grassland sprawls on both sides of the trail, and as you head northwest, the trail stretches out straight ahead into an inviting ribbon. At 0.6 mile bear left, following the sign marked TO ANCIENT OAKS TRAIL.

Sweeping south downslope from the ridge, the trail passes through some pockets of California bays and oaks. You'll likely hear vehicles on Alpine Road, partly visible in some places on the left. At 0.9 mile ignore a spur trail that heads straight and ends shortly at the road, and turn right from a signed junction onto Ancient Oaks Trail.

Pass buckeyes cuddled up in the creases of the hillside on the left, as the narrow trail crosses through grassland and descends slightly. On clear days, there are long views west to the ocean as well as to Mindego Ridge. California poppy and blue and white lupine dot the grassland through here in spring. You might see gopher snakes sunning themselves on the trail. Where the trail steps into the woods and reaches a junction at 1.2 miles, continue left, on Ancient Oaks Trail.

Although gorgeous live oaks play a starring role along the trail, you might also see madrone and Douglas-fir. In the shaded understory, look for hound's tongue in spring. The trail winds downhill, taking a brief foray through grassland before returning to woods again. Creambush and hazelnut mingle with ferns to create a lush atmosphere, particularly in winter after a rainstorm, when you might catch newts crossing the trail. At 1.6 miles Ancient Oaks Trail ends. Turn right onto Charquin Trail and begin to climb out of the woods, skirting the base of the grassy ridge. In summer, look for painted lady and red admiral butterflies near a wet seep on the right. You'll reach a three-way junction at 1.9 miles—you have an opportunity to extend this hike an additional 1.3 miles, via Alder Spring and Hawk Trails to the left. Bear right, though, on Charquin Trail, toward the vista-point parking.

Ascend easily through quiet grassland. Follow the trail to a crest and junction at 2.2 miles. Continuing straight, the trail ends at Skyline Boulevard, across from a

Russian Ridge Open Space Preserve

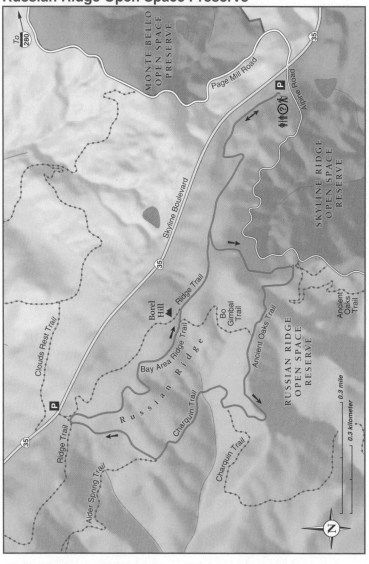

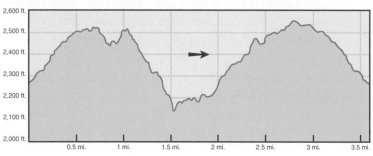

small vista-point parking area. Ridge Trail extends to the left and right. Turn right onto Ridge Trail; after a few steps, the path splits (both trails reconnect after about 0.5 mile)—stay to the right.

Small rock outcrops sit off the sides of the trail, which ascends slightly through grassland just off the ridgeline. This is spot to look for coyotes, active residents of the preserve. Views west are outstanding. Flowers are sprinkled through the grass in spring, a visual snack before the main course still to come. At 2.8 miles Bo Gimbal Trail, connecting to Ancient Oaks Trail, departs on the right, but continue straight on Ridge Trail. A few feet farther uphill, the other leg of Ridge Trail feeds in from the left. Stay to the right.

Now hugging the spine of the ridge, the trail enters an area legendary among Bay Area wildflower enthusiasts. During the peak of the season, usually early May, flowers pop (literally and figuratively) out of the lush green grass along the trail. These are "common" wildflowers, including Johnny-jump-ups, owl's clover, blue and white lupine, California poppy, tidytips, creamcups, clarkia, and blue-eyed grass, but what knocks your socks off is the display's frequency and urgency. Marvel at your leisure, but take care to stay on the trail and, of course, don't pick the flowers! If you follow the change of seasons at Russian Ridge, you'll note that while in spring the grass is short and verdant, by midsummer the hillsides are cloaked in thigh-high grass, and the only flowers still in bloom are usually a few tired-looking tidytips and mule-ear sunflowers.

Continuing, Ridge Trail descends gradually, offering views south to the hills of Monte Bello Open Space Preserve, topped by 2,800-foot Black Mountain. When you reach the junction with the path to Ancient Oaks Trail again at 3.1 miles, continue straight and retrace your steps back to the parking lot.

• •

GPS TRAILHEAD COORDINATES N37° 18.926' W122° 11.316'

DIRECTIONS From the CA 1/I-280 junction in San Francisco, drive south on I-280 about 29 miles, then take Exit 20 onto Page Mill Road. Drive west on Page Mill Road about 9 miles to the junction with CA 35/Skyline Boulevard. Cross Skyline and continue straight onto Alpine Road; then, almost immediately, take the first right into the preserve parking lot.

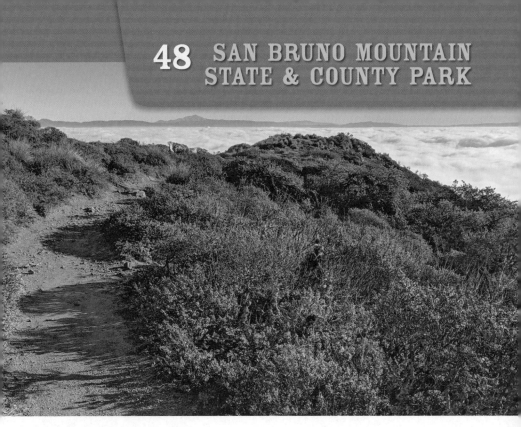

Above the fog at San Bruno Mountain

SPRAWLING JUST SOUTH of San Francisco, San Bruno Mountain is the perfect park for a quick get-out-of-town hike. This 3.6-mile loop climbs through coastal scrub to a ridge where views include the mountains of Marin and San Mateo Counties. After cresting near the mountain's summit, the hike descends back to the trailhead, offering views of San Francisco and Mount Diablo all the way downhill.

DESCRIPTION

One of the Bay Area's most important urban-fringe open spaces, San Bruno Mountain has evaded development plans since the 1960s. One group wanted to shave land off the top of the mountain to fill the bay near San Francisco Airport, and many developers eyed the land for housing tracts. Development plans were firmly squelched in 1976, when the rare mission blue butterfly, which lives only on San Bruno Mountain and San Francisco's Twin Peaks, was placed on the U.S. Fish & Wildlife Service's endangered-species list. Although houses have crept up the sides of the mountain and communications equipment protrudes from the summit area, more than 2,000 acres of San Bruno Mountain are protected, and the mountain, surrounded by densely populated neighborhoods, feels like an island.

DISTANCE & CONFIGURATION: 3.6-mile loop

DIFFICULTY: Easy

SCENERY: Coastal scrub and views

EXPOSURE: Nearly all full sun

TRAIL TRAFFIC: Moderate; the loop is popular in spring.

TRAIL SURFACE: Dirt trails

HIKING TIME: 2 hours

DRIVING DISTANCE: 5.5 miles from the US 101/I-280 junction in San Francisco

ACCESS: Opens daily at 8 a.m.; closing times vary by time of year (check website). Perfect in spring, but bring a jacket in case it's windy. Pay $6 day-use fee at entrance kiosk.

WHEELCHAIR ACCESS: There are designated handicapped parking spots. Wheelchair users should park in the first lot past the entrance kiosk and wheel on paved Old Guadalupe Trail.

MAPS: At entrance kiosk, trailhead, and tinyurl .com/sanbrunoparkmap

FACILITIES: Restrooms and water

CONTACT: 650-589-5708, parks.smcgov.org /san-bruno-mountain-state-county-park

LOCATION: 555 Guadalupe Canyon Pkwy., Brisbane, CA

COMMENTS: No dogs allowed

Removal of invasive vegetation has been a long-term volunteer project for San Bruno Mountain advocacy groups. Eucalyptus, cotoneaster, ivy, gorse, and broom thrive in some areas. Even with so much non-native vegetation, a hiker might see plenty of native plants on just one San Bruno Mountain visit. There is an abundance of common flora, but you'll see lots of unusual and some endangered plants as well, including wallflower, owl's clover, and a few varieties of manzanita. April and May are the peak times for wildflowers.

The San Bruno Mountain loop begins at Radio Road Trailhead. Follow the arrow pointing right (west) to Summit Loop Trail, and wind through the native plant garden to reach signed junction 14, with Eucalyptus Loop Trail. Bear right onto Summit Loop Trail and then, after a few steps, cross the road.

Summit Loop Trail begins a slight descent through an area where eucalyptus, ivy, and Monterey cypress thrive near a creek. On the right, a damp, bowl-shaped meadow fosters willows. Scorpionweed, blue-eyed grass, checkerbloom, fringe cup, and cow parsnip bloom in spring, tangled through coyote brush, coffeeberry, and lizardtail. Guadalupe Canyon Parkway is visible and audible to the north, but the trail soon bends left, crosses April Brook, and then starts climbing south on a few switchbacks.

As you reach a ridgeline, the grade tapers off, and plants along the trail seem to hunker down, keeping a low profile against winds that regularly whip across the mountain. Oregon grape nestles in rock outcrops, and annual wildflowers, here sprinkled through sagebrush, include paintbrush, Johnny-jump-ups, and varieties of owl's clover.

On clear days, views extend north to the Point Reyes Peninsula and Mount Tamalpais. Summit Loop Trail veers left off the ridgeline and runs downslope. Cottontails can be glimpsed at the edge of the trail, but on approach they dive into thickets of coastal scrub composed of California coffeeberry, coyote brush, lizardtail, sticky monkeyflower, twinberry, and poison oak. A cluster of hummingbird sage near a kink in the trail puts forth bold, bright-pink flowers in spring.

San Bruno Mountain State & County Park

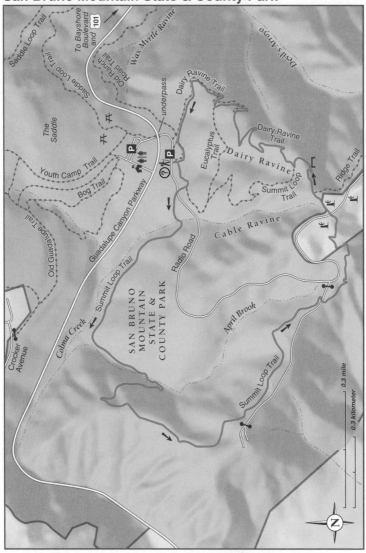

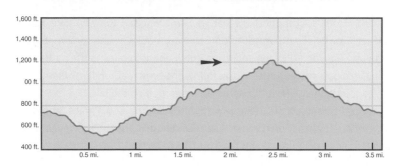

On the final push toward the summit, the trail crosses a paved service road then snakes uphill not far from Radio Road. Nearly every year here in January, I see San Francisco wallflower blooming. In spring, stands of iris burst out of a community of stunted-looking sagebrush, coyote brush, and lizardtail. Tiny-leaved yerba buena trails along the ground, within sight of downtown San Francisco. This plant lent its name to the village that became the city of San Francisco in 1847.

Some shortcuts and one unsigned spur off to the right make the trail a little hard to follow, but just keep heading uphill toward the communications towers. Looking west, the Farallon Islands are often visible if it's not too foggy. At 2.4 miles Summit Loop Trail crosses a paved road. You'll likely want to hurry through this area, which is marred with ugly communications buildings, dishes, and towers (but I did experience my first-ever Bay Area coyote sighting near this junction). After a few steps, a gorgeous blend of coastal scrub signals a return to a more natural setting.

Just as the trail begins to descend, Ridge Trail departs on the right. Continue straight on Summit Loop Trail. At an easy pace, the trail drifts downhill toward a bench off to the right where hikers can gaze north to San Francisco or across the bay to Mount Diablo. In spring, goldfields occupy grassy patches off the trail like an invading army. At 2.7 miles you'll reach a signed junction. Turn right onto Dairy Ravine Trail, which descends on long, fluid switchbacks through coastal scrub. I've seen wildflowers blooming along the trail here as early as mid-January, and during the peak season you'll likely see plenty of scorpionweed, blue-eyed grass, blue dicks, seaside daisy, California poppy, and paintbrush. Soon, Dairy Ravine Trail reaches a signed junction at 3.1 miles. Again, although either trail is an option, bear right to continue on Dairy Ravine Trail.

Winding downhill, the path features views to the remote southern canyons and slopes of the mountain. A signed trail breaks off on the right at 3.5 miles. This is Old Ranch Road Trail, which runs along Guadalupe Canyon Parkway and then ends. Continue straight on Dairy Ravine Trail. One final split offers two options; both return to the trailhead.

• •

GPS TRAILHEAD COORDINATES N37° 41.710' W122° 26.061'

DIRECTIONS From southbound US 101 in San Francisco County, take Exit 429B at Third Street/Cow Palace. Drive south on Bayshore Boulevard about 2 miles, turn right on Guadalupe Canyon Parkway, and drive uphill about 2 miles to the park entrance on the right. Once past the entrance kiosk, follow the park road under Guadalupe Canyon Parkway to the trailhead, near the native-plant garden on the left.

From northbound US 101, take Exit 426A toward the Cow Palace, and drive north on Bayshore Boulevard; then turn left onto Guadalupe Canyon Parkway and follow the directions to the park entrance and trailhead listed above.

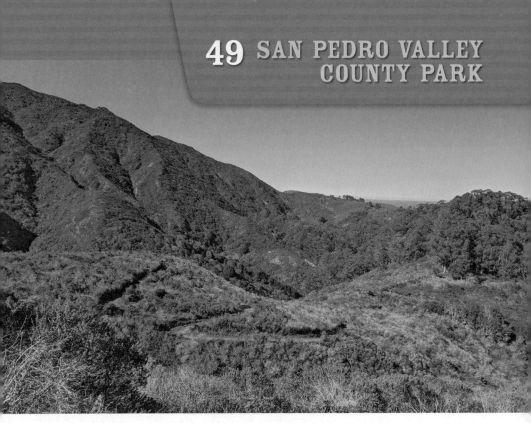

Zigzagging through coastal scrub at San Pedro Valley County Park

AT 3.7 MILES, Hazelnut Trail is the longest path in San Pedro Valley County Park. Designed with plenty of switchbacks, the aptly named trail climbs through coastal scrub and permits sweeping views of the park, Sweeney Ridge, the ocean, and Montara Mountain. The hiking trail makes a sweet loop when combined with Weiler Ranch Road and Plaskon Nature Trail.

DESCRIPTION

Start at the information signboard near the start of Plaskon Nature Trail. Cross the bridge and walk about 90 feet on Plaskon Nature Trail, then turn right at the signed junction with Hazelnut Trail. The hiking and equestrian trail begins under cover of a particularly large and lovely coast live oak. In spring, you may see trillium and forget-me-nots. Hazelnut Trail soon leaves the woods and begins an ascent through grassy chaparral. Poison oak is everywhere and is particularly obvious in autumn and early spring, when its leaves are red-tinged. A few madrones and coast live oaks persist, but gradually the trail transitions into more-shrubby vegetation. Cream-bush, coyote brush, huckleberry, hazelnut, ceanothus, chinquapin, toyon, California coffeeberry, elderberry, and manzanita line the narrow path. You might see vetch and hound's tongue in early spring.

DISTANCE & CONFIGURATION: 4.7-mile loop

DIFFICULTY: Moderate

SCENERY: Coastal scrub and views

EXPOSURE: A few pockets of shade; otherwise exposed

TRAIL TRAFFIC: Light–moderate

TRAIL SURFACE: Dirt fire road and dirt trail

HIKING TIME: 2 hours

DRIVING DISTANCE: 11 miles from the I-280/CA 1 junction at the San Francisco–Daly City border

ACCESS: Opens daily at 8 a.m.; closing times vary by time of year (check website). Good year-round. $6 day-use fee.

WHEELCHAIR ACCESS: There is designated handicapped parking, and folks in wheelchairs can access Plaskon Nature Trail.

MAPS: At entrance kiosk and tinyurl.com /sanpedrovalleyparkmap

FACILITIES: Restrooms and water at trailhead; visitor center at park entrance (open weekends and holidays 10 a.m.–4 p.m.)

CONTACT: 650-355-8289, parks.smcgov.org /san-pedro-valley-park

LOCATION: 600 Oddstad Blvd., Pacifica, CA

COMMENTS: No dogs allowed. Picking or removing wildflowers or other natural material is prohibited.

As you climb you'll initially have views of Weiler Ranch Trail and the valley, followed by glimpses of Sweeney Ridge and Montara Mountain. Cow parsnip crowds the trail in spring, and hedge nettle, hound's tongue, starflower, iris, feathery false lily of the valley, and trillium bloom in the shady spots. Bluewitch nightshade, thimbleberry, currant, yerba santa, and pitcher sage also make occasional appearances.

Hazelnut Trail passes through a eucalyptus grove, resumes a climb through coastal scrub, bisects a second eucalyptus patch, and again emerges in scrub. You might see mission bells in early spring, in bloom along with thimbleberry, and ceanothus. Manzanitas, which start flowering at San Pedro around Christmas, will already have berries developing by winter's end. A series of switchbacks lead to a bench with a view back down Hazelnut Trail and up to Montara Mountain. Thick hedges of huckleberry tower over the trail on the right, where you might see the last blossoms on currant bushes in early spring. As Hazelnut Trail heads east, Sweeney Ridge is visible on a clear day. The trail starts to descend on switchbacks, with the same familiar coastal scrub plants lining the trail. Poison oak, which had abated for a while, returns with a vengeance. Hazelnut shrubs are common, although you might not notice them in the winter when they ditch their leaves. Weiler Ranch Trail comes back into view. On a hot day, a bench under some chinquapin is a perfectly shaded rest spot. You may see milkmaids, paintbrush, and manroot blooming in spring. At 3.7 miles Hazelnut Trail ends at Weiler Ranch Trail. Turn left.

Flat Weiler Ranch Trail, open to hikers, equestrians, and cyclists, runs along the Middle Fork of San Pedro Creek. This wide trail is popular with parents pushing strollers and kids learning to ride bicycles. Dogwood thrives near the waterway. After crossing a bridge, Weiler Ranch Trail follows the contour of the valley floor, where deer are commonly spotted. At 4 miles, Weiler Ranch Trail meets Valley View Trail at a signed junction. Continue straight on Weiler Ranch Trail.

San Pedro Valley County Park

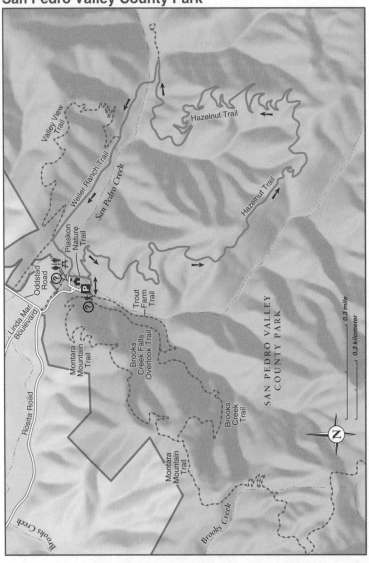

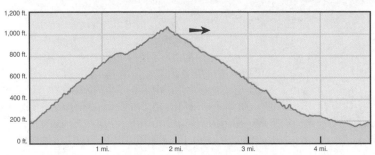

As you near the park's border, Weiler Ranch Trail splits. Either leg is an option, but I prefer to take the path to the left (if you stay to the right, you'll pass the other end of Valley View Trail; turn left and head roughly west). After crossing the creek again, you'll pass two reservable group picnic areas and some restrooms. Weiler Ranch Trail ends at the edge of the parking lot, at 4.5 miles. Turn left and walk on the sidewalk for a few feet, then turn left on Plaskon Nature Trail.

A bridge crosses the South Fork of San Pedro Creek, where you may spot salmon spawning after heavy winter rains. Willow and dogwood, as well as coast live oak, shade the path. At 4.6 miles you'll reach a previously encountered junction with Hazelnut Trail. Continue right on Plaskon Nature Trail to the trailhead.

• •

GPS TRAILHEAD COORDINATES N37° 34.678' W122° 28.523'

DIRECTIONS From the CA 1/I-280 junction in San Francisco, drive south on I-280 for 1.8 miles, then keep right at the fork and follow signs for CA 1 S. Continue on CA 1 for 6 miles, to the junction with Linda Mar Boulevard. Turn left and drive 1.9 miles to the junction with Oddstad Boulevard. Turn right and almost immediately turn left onto the signed park road.

Look for fetid adder's tongue along Hazelnut Trail in winter.

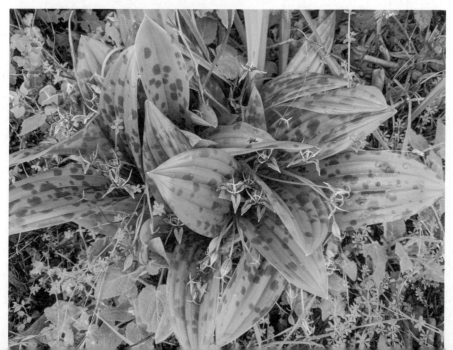

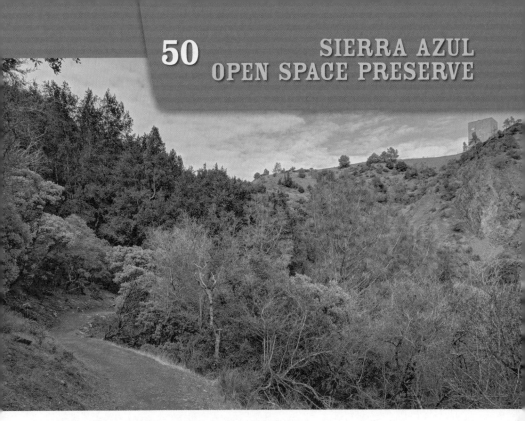

Heading toward the sugar cube on Mount Umunhum Trail

SIERRA AZUL MAY be the biggest Bay Area preserve you've never heard of. With more than 18,000 acres, the massive preserve sprawls over the flanks of Mount Umunhum, in the Sierra Azul range just south of San Jose.

DESCRIPTION

Sierra Azul Open Space Preserve has a long and colorful history. The preserve's highest point, Mount Umunhum, was a sacred spot for American Indians, who graced the rugged peak with its melodious name, which translates as "the resting place of the hummingbird." In the late 1950s, the U.S. Air Force built a radar station at the top of Umunhum, and until 1980, the facility scanned the coast for potential Cold War threats. When the station closed, the Air Force left behind crumbling buildings; contaminated property; and, at the top of the mountain, a prominent six-story radar tower, which still stands today.

The Midpeninsula Regional Open Space District began purchasing Sierra Azul property in the 1980s. Like a jigsaw puzzle in progress, a series of relatively small additions has resulted in one huge but somewhat fragmented preserve. Some areas are still off-limits to the public, while others are surrounded by private inholdings.

Most of the preserve trails are long fire roads that shoot up and down the hillsides at steep grades, making Sierra Azul a favorite with experienced mountain

DISTANCE & CONFIGURATION: 7.8-mile out-and-back

DIFFICULTY: Moderate

SCENERY: Chaparral, woods, and views

EXPOSURE: Mostly shaded, with some full sun

TRAIL TRAFFIC: Heavy

TRAIL SURFACE: Dirt trail, paved sidewalk

HIKING TIME: 3.5 hours

DRIVING DISTANCE: 58 miles from the I-280/CA 1 junction at the San Francisco–Daly City border

ACCESS: Daily, 7 a.m.–30 minutes after sunset. Good anytime but very hot in summer. No fee.

WHEELCHAIR ACCESS: There is designated handicapped parking at the summit. Folks in wheelchairs can navigate the summit area but not Mount Umunhum Trail.

MAPS: At trailhead and openspace.org/sites /default/files/map_SA.pdf

FACILITIES: Vault toilets at trailhead. No water.

CONTACT: 650-691-1200, openspace.org /preserves/sierra-azul

LOCATION: (Bald Mountain Trailhead) Mount Umunhum Road, approximately 1.7 miles from the Hicks Road intersection

COMMENTS: Dogs are permitted on some pre-serve trails, but not on Mount Umunhum Trail or the summit-area paths.

bikers and equestrians. Hikers can make all-day treks along rolling ridgelines, such as the 11-mile (one-way) trip from Lexington Reservoir to the Jacques Ridge trailhead. Sierra Azul rivals some of the largest state parks in the Bay Area for sheer size and diversity, encompassing chaparral, redwood groves, mixed woodlands, headwaters, and grassy slopes, all just a short drive from San Jose. The Summit Area opened to the public in 2017, to great fanfare and excitement. Now all can enjoy the incredible views from the mountaintop.

Start from the parking lot at the Bald Mountain Trailhead. Carefully cross Mount Umunhum Road and walk on the path along the road to the trailhead and an information signboard. Mount Umunhum Trail departs into madrone and California bay woods. The wide multiuse path ascends at a barely perceptible grade, a trend that continues for the entire length of the trail, with an average 6% grade. Running downslope but out of sight of Mount Umunhum Road, the trail passes through a sunny spot with a view uphill to the summit, the turnaround spot for this hike. At 0.3 mile Mount Umunhum Trail reaches a signed junction with Barlow Road. Continue uphill on Mount Umunhum Trail.

Swinging away from the road, the trail weaves through shaded woods and some exposed stretches of chaparral where views stretch to San Jose and beyond. In early February the first blooming wildflower, Fremont's star lily, is common in shaded spots. Foothill pines, with pineapple-size cones, soar above ceanothus, cercocarpus, chamise, and manzanita in the sunny sections. At 1 mile Mount Umunhum Trail crosses a creek on a sturdy bridge—dogwood thrives here. The next segment, climbing through chaparral, pine, and woods, is one of my favorites, especially when the manzanitas are blooming. Two pines stand on either side of the trail like a mystic gate. Back in the woods look for California nutmeg, a conifer with sharp-tipped needles and (in late spring) green, olive-shaped seeds. At 1.35 miles you'll reach the

Sierra Azul Open Space Preserve

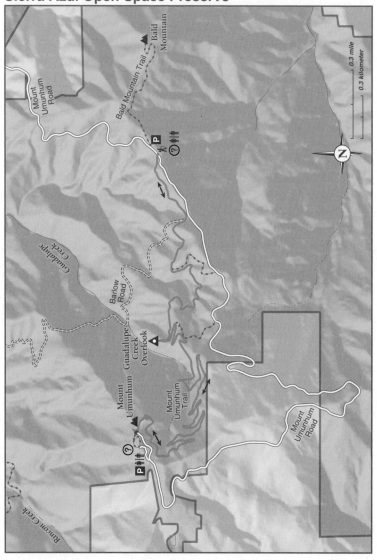

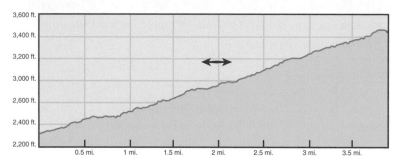

perfect rest spot, the Guadalupe Creek Overlook, on the right. Just a few steps from the main trail, this little spur loop ends at a fenced drop-off. Views of the creek canyon are spectacular and extend far to the east, including Mount Hamilton and Mount Diablo. The sugar cube at the summit area seems within reach! When ready, return to Mount Umunhum Trail and continue uphill.

Another stretch of gorgeous woods yields to another sunny area with chaparral and pine. Switchbacks begin, keeping the climb easy. A second bridge crosses Guadalupe Creek. The next batch of chaparral boasts a little bit of grassland—a good home for spring wildflowers. Just before the third bridge, there's an interpretive panel near the remains of an old cabin. After passing through a dense grove of pine, Mount Umunhum Trail returns to the familiar mix of madrone and California bay. The switchbacks keep coming. Some very tall manzanitas tower over the path; when they bloom in winter, they leave puddles of white flowers like snow. The "big white golf ball" (the National Weather Service Doppler station) is visible uphill, and the summit gets closer with every step. My son, an expert woodrat nest spotter, pointed out a trailside rodent condo on our winter hike. At 3.5 miles you'll reach a signed junction. The path to the left leads to the trailhead shelter (and parking lot). Turn right for the summit.

After sweeping across a grassy hillside peppered with pines, a flight of steps urges you to the top. And then there it is, the giant old radar building and summit, at 3,486 feet. Views are spectacular—some of the best in the Bay Area, from Monterey Bay north to Mount Saint Helena on a clear day. Take some time to explore the many interpretive panels and exhibits at the summit. When ready, retrace your steps back to the trailhead.

• •

GPS TRAILHEAD COORDINATES N37° 09.570' W121° 52.537'

DIRECTIONS From the CA 1/I-280 junction in San Francisco, drive south about 36 miles on I-280, then take Exit 12 onto CA 85 S. After 10 miles, take the Camden Avenue exit. Turn left (south) onto Camden. Drive 1.7 miles, then turn right onto Hicks Road. Drive 6 miles and, at a stop sign, turn right onto Mount Umunhum Road. Drive uphill 1.7 miles, then turn left into the parking lot.

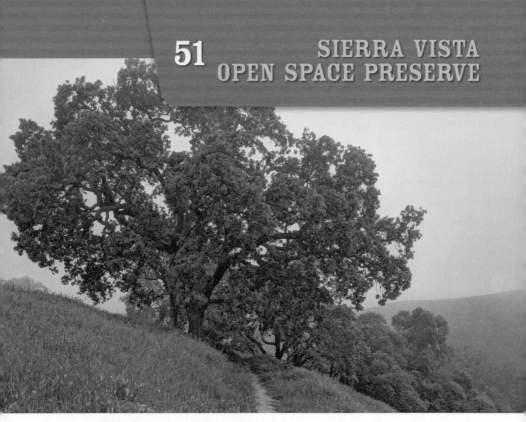

A big oak looms in the fog on Aquila Trail.

THIS PRESERVE STRETCHES across foothills in northeastern San Jose. Miles of trails offer plenty of options, including several loops, all just minutes from very busy and dense city life. This open space abuts Alum Rock Park, permitting hikers to start a journey from the ridge and hike down into the San Jose park, or vice versa.

DESCRIPTION

Sierra Road bisects Sierra Vista Open Space Preserve; one loop is on the north side of the road, and the remaining trails are accessed from the south side. The most popular Sierra Vista option is the Boccardo Loop Trail, just over 4 miles, which drops through grassland from the Sierra Road trailhead down toward Alum Rock City Park. Hikers can also trek east from Sierra Road on Sierra Vista Trail, then loop through chaparral on Calaveras Fault Trail.

I had researched Sierra Vista Open Space Preserve carefully because this Santa Clara County preserve is a long drive from my house and I wanted to make the most of my visit. Late April seemed perfect: wildflowers should be blooming, and if I got there early it wouldn't be too hot. For the first hour and 10 minutes of my drive, everything was great, but as I made the final approach to the trailhead I drove into a wall of fog. I was dismayed. This preserve is famous for its views, and there would be

DISTANCE & CONFIGURATION: 1.1-mile loop

DIFFICULTY: Easy

SCENERY: Grassland, oaks, and views

EXPOSURE: Sun-drenched

TRAIL TRAFFIC: Light

TRAIL SURFACE: Dirt

HIKING TIME: Less than an hour

DRIVING DISTANCE: 59 miles from the CA 1/I-280 junction at the San Francisco–Daly City border

ACCESS: Daily, 8 a.m.–30 minutes after sunset. No fee.

WHEELCHAIR ACCESS: Not recommended for wheelchairs

MAPS: At trailhead and tinyurl.com/sierra vistaospmap

FACILITIES: None

CONTACT: 408-224-7476, openspaceauthority .org/visitors/preserves/sierra

LOCATION: 5341 Sierra Road, San Jose, CA

COMMENTS: No dogs allowed

none for me this day. At home later, I mused on my BAHiker Facebook page about the irony of hiking through the fog at a preserve with "vista" in its name. One of my readers commented, "Foggy hills and trails is also 'vista,' no?" Yes, so right! Some of my favorite hikes happen on foggy days. I love the way the swirling mist creates a hush, pulling my thoughts inward. Fog is an intimate partner, and I was so lucky have it at Sierra Vista, and fortunate to have a wise reader set me straight.

Should you visit on a clear day (of which there are many), you can expect exceptional views before you even set foot on a trail. At the edge of the parking lot, views extend to the southwest, encompassing everything between San Bruno Mountain and Loma Prieta.

Aquila Trail, featured here, is great for beginners. This 1-mile loop has only slight elevation changes and is nicely graded. If you have young kids, consider Aquila for a family hike, but note that the preserve does not have restrooms of any kind or drinking water.

Start across the street from the parking lot at the signed Aquila Trailhead. Once through a cattle gate, the loop splits; either way is an option, but if you want to follow me, turn right. After a short stretch paralleling Sierra Road, the multiuse path bends left. This narrow trail slips between soft rolling hills draped with grassland. Valley oaks punctuate the landscape with their stately posture. In spring look for a variety of wildflowers, including California buttercups, woodland star, mule-ear sunflowers, blue and white lupine, and blue-eyed grass. On clear days, look south for a view to Mount Hamilton and north to Monument Peak. Aquila Trail descends bit by bit, making sweeping turns through the grassland.

At 0.6 mile the path draws near to and then passes a cluster of valley oak. There's a bench on the left that is great for soaking in the lovely vista. Once across a small footbridge, Aquila begins to climb gently. Poison oak hedges slouch across the hillside on the left; on the right look for a lovely, lone buckeye. California poppies add an orange blast of color in May when the grass begins to lose its green glow. Aquila winds uphill through rock-studded grassland, reaching a picnic table on the left at

Sierra Vista Open Space Preserve

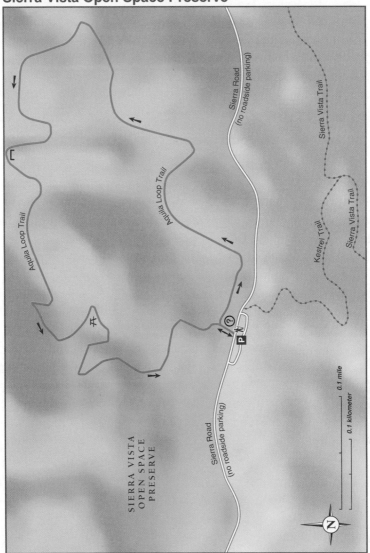

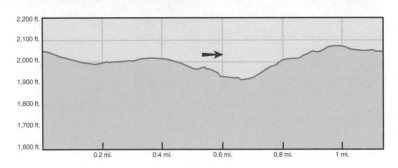

0.9 mile. On the final stretch back to the trailhead, look for Briones Formation rocks along the trail. These rocks originated under the sea, and shells are visible in the sandstone. Geologists call these rocks shell hash. At 1.1 miles the loop closes; bear right to return to the parking lot.

• •

GPS TRAILHEAD COORDINATES N37° 24.541' W121° 48.072'

DIRECTIONS From the CA 1/I-280 junction in San Francisco, drive south on I-280 about 49 miles, then keep left onto I-680 N. Drive about 4 miles, then take the Berryessa Road exit. Turn right and drive east on Berryessa Road about 1 mile, then turn left onto Piedmont Road. Drive about 0.2 mile, then turn right onto Sierra Road. Proceed east on Sierra Road about 3.7 miles, to the signed parking lot on the right.

Shell hash at Sierra Vista Open Space Preserve

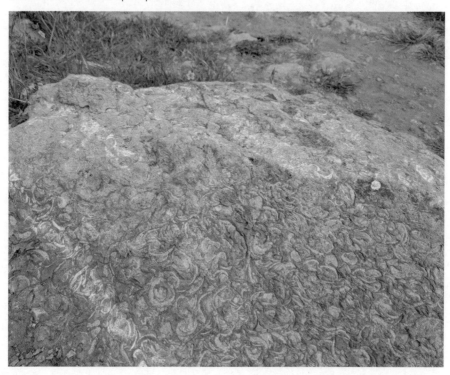

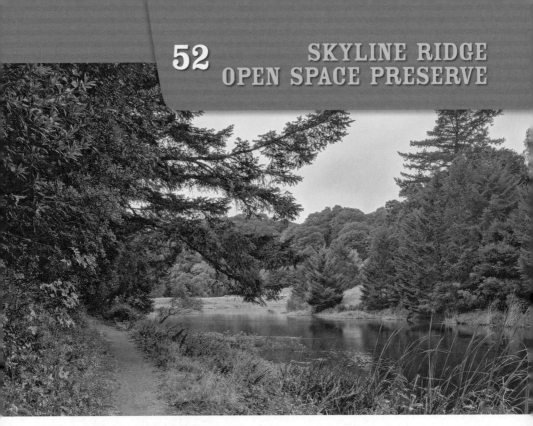

At water's edge on the shore of Horseshoe Lake

IF YOU ENJOY the tranquility of little mountain lakes, I recommend this short but stunning Skyline Ridge hike. This loop skirts Horseshoe Lake, climbs to a chaparral-covered ridge, and then descends through grassland to Alpine Pond. The return route ascends to the ridge, then drops through woods and grassland back to the trailhead.

DESCRIPTION

There are several open-space preserves and parks sprawled on the crest of the Santa Cruz Mountains, but Skyline Ridge is a favorite. The preserve is home to two small man-made lakes that were created to ensure a steady supply of water for former ranches. Horseshoe Lake is partly rimmed with Douglas-fir and Christmas-tree-farm escapees, while Alpine Pond, tucked in the far northern corner of the preserve, hosts Skyline Ridge's nature center. Stretched between the two ponds is a ridge composed of grassland and chaparral, where views extend far to the west, south, and east. This is a good hike for families with kids because it's fairly short and there's good wildlife-viewing at the ponds. You will likely see plenty of waterfowl here, but less-commonly spotted animals visit the ponds as well—on one hike, I came within 10 feet of a bobcat completely engrossed in a shoreline hunt.

DISTANCE & CONFIGURATION: 4.4-mile figure eight

DIFFICULTY: Moderate

SCENERY: Ponds, grassland, chaparral, and views

EXPOSURE: A few pockets of shade; otherwise full sun

TRAIL TRAFFIC: Moderate

TRAIL SURFACE: Dirt fire road and trails

HIKING TIME: 2 hours, plus any additional time spent lollygagging around the ponds

DRIVING DISTANCE: 40 miles from the CA 1/I-280 junction at the San Francisco–Daly City border

ACCESS: Daily, 30 minutes before sunrise–30 minutes after sunset. Good year-round; nice wildflowers in spring. No fee.

WHEELCHAIR ACCESS: There are 2 options for accessing this preserve in a wheelchair: At Skyline Ridge, park in the designated handicapped parking lot (handicapped placard required). There is a 0.2-mile trail segment that is wheelchair accessible. At neighboring Russian Ridge, depart the parking lot, and wheel along Ipiwa Trail to and around Alpine Pond.

MAPS: At trailhead and tinyurl.com /skylineridgemap

FACILITIES: Vault toilets at trailhead and near Alpine Pond; water fountain at Alpine Pond

CONTACT: 650-691-1200, openspace.org /preserves/skyline-ridge

LOCATION: Off CA 35 just south of Page Mill Road, La Honda CA

COMMENTS: No dogs allowed

From the trailhead's information signboard a few feet off the parking lot, bear left, following Sunny Jim Trail toward Horseshoe Lake. This narrow, nearly level path bisects a damp, sloping meadow where coyote brush is mixed through a few yellow bush lupine shrubs. At 0.1 mile the path reaches a parking lot reserved for handicapped visitors. Turn left, walk up the access road a few feet, and then bear right onto a slim path, Horseshoe Lake Trail. The trail ascends slightly, leaving coyote brush for a grassland dotted with Douglas-fir and coast live oak. In spring, look for blue and white lupine, California poppy, blue larkspur, clarkia, and Ithuriel's spear. You'll get a peek at Horseshoe Lake's northern arm, downhill to the right.

The trail crests in the midst of a coast live oak and California bay grove, where two picnic tables on opposite sides of the trail provide secluded spots for lunch. Horseshoe Lake Trail descends to a junction at 0.6 mile, near the equestrian parking lot. Turn right and bisect a damp area where willows huddle on the right. Horseshoe Lake Trail passes through a lush area, with poison oak, blackberry, thimbleberry, and buckeye dominating. The south arm of the lake sits just off to the right.

Once across a tiny footbridge, the trail curves right, leveling in woods where columbine blooms in spring and bigleaf maples toss their orange leaves to the ground in autumn. At 0.95 mile you'll reach a junction. Stay right on Horseshoe Loop Trail, which draws near to the shoreline. From here, you'll have nice lake views; if you want to spend more time on the shoreline, there's a bench on the right. After crossing a sturdy bridge, you'll reach a junction at 1 mile, where Horseshoe Loop Trail bends right. Continue straight and, after a few feet, stay right at a junction with Lambert Creek Trail. The wide trail climbs slightly, through coyote brush, to a junction at 1.1 miles. Turn sharply left onto Sunny Jim Trial, toward Alpine Pond.

Skyline Ridge Open Space Preserve

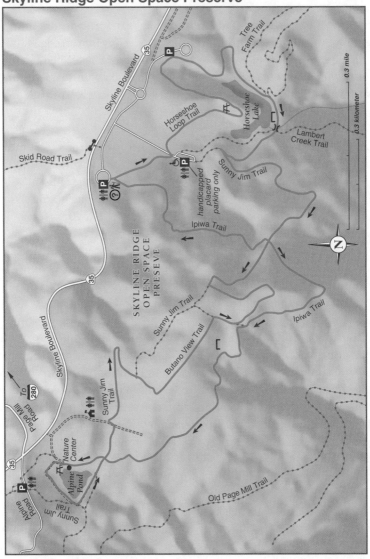

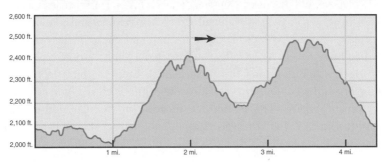

Sunny Jim Trail, here a broad fire road, climbs moderately, passing a few live oaks, buckeyes, California bays, and madrones on the way into grassland. White brodiaea, clarkia, and yarrow bloom along the trail in early June. When the trail bends right, enjoy views of forested ridges to the west, including Portola Redwoods State Park. At 1.6 miles Sunny Jim Trail meets a three-part junction. The path to the right returns to the trailhead—turn left onto Ipiwa Trail.

A sign warns of entry into an area inhabited by rattlesnakes. I've never seen any on this trail, but should you encounter one, here's the protocol: If the snake is stretched out on a trail with plenty of real estate surrounding it, just gingerly walk around it, keeping yourself as far as possible from its head. If the rattlesnake is coiled, that means it's stressed. Back off and wait for it to chill out, uncoil, and slither away. Gopher snakes, also common in this and all parts of the Bay Area, resemble rattlesnakes but are nonvenomous. Both have a cream, tan, and brown pattern, but the easiest way to tell them apart (from a safe distance) is by head shape. Gopher snakes have no distinction from their "necks" to their heads, but rattlers have diamond-shaped heads. Both, by the way, make noises to warn off predators, rattlesnakes by shaking their rattles and gopher snakes by vibrating their tails against the ground. See page 12 for photos of both snakes.

As you climb easily through grassland, the views south and west continue to impress. Spring wildflowers are reliable, with an abundance of owl's clover, clarkia, and California poppy blooming in May. Later, in June, look for yellow mariposa lilies blended through the tall grass with dandelions. As the trail veers right and runs downslope from the ridge, the trailside vegetation shifts to chaparral, with chamise, manzanita, ceanothus, and yerba santa common, along with a few shrubs of silk-tassel and pitcher sage. A pocket of coast live oak provides some unexpected shade. At 1.95 miles, Ipiwa Trail squeezes past a boulder on the right then reaches a junction with a connector trail heading right to the top of the ridge. Continue straight.

The next section is dominated in late spring by orange-blossomed sticky monkey-flower shrubs, overshadowing neighboring sagebrush and lizardtail. Descending easily, Ipiwa Trail offers views to the grassy shoulders of Russian Ridge to the north. The trail leaves grassland and enters woods, where California bays are dwarfed by some positively massive, old live oaks. Now nearly level, Ipiwa Trail reaches a junction at 2.5 miles with a still-somewhat-paved trail. Cross the pavement and continue on Ipiwa Trail, winding through Douglas-fir, California bay, and buckeye. Bear right when a path feeds in from the left. At 2.6 miles you'll reach the south shore of Alpine Pond.

The Daniels Nature Center (open weekends) features exhibits about the preserve's history and wildlife, but even when the center is closed, you can enjoy the pond's shoreline, where I've seen crawfish meandering through mud in the driest months of the year. A wheelchair-accessible pond-viewing station is set up on the side of the building. Shaded picnic tables make this a great spot for lunch.

When you're ready to continue, follow Alpine Pond Loop around the shoreline. At 2.7 miles Sunny Jim Trail departs on the right, toward Alpine Road. Continue straight. After a few steps another trail heads right; stay left on the berm above the pond. Look downhill to the right for a view of American Indian grinding stones. At 2.8 miles Alpine Pond Loop closes. Walk slightly uphill to the junction with Ipiwa Trail, then continue straight, now on Sunny Jim Trail. The sides of wide and paved but crumbling trail host good displays of Chinese houses and fairy lanterns in spring. Ignore a path signed NOT A THROUGH TRAIL, and continue easily uphill to a T-junction with a paved road at 2.9 miles. Turn left and, after a few feet, just before the ranger-station compound, turn right, following the sign toward Horseshoe Lake.

White poplars—non-native trees with silvery leaves—are conspicuous on the right. The broad trail sweeps sharply right and begins to climb, bordering a forest of interior live oak, Douglas-fir, and tanoak on the left. At 3.2 miles Sunny Jim Trail heads left while Butano View Trail continues straight. Both trails converge eventually (consider Sunny Jim if it's hot). Continue straight on Butano View Trail.

The wide trail climbs, passes a water tank, and then bends left. As you ascend along a grassy ridge, savor great views west. At 3.4 miles a connector heads left; turn right, soon reaching a second junction with a path leading to Ipiwa Trail. Proceed left, climbing past tall oaks to a hilltop and the high point of the hike. Butano View Trail begins to descend, then ends at a junction with Sunny Jim Trail at 3.8 miles; turn right. A short, somewhat steep descent reaches the junction with Ipiwa Trail once again. This time, turn left. The trail steps into woods composed of bigleaf maple, live oak, Douglas-fir, California bay, and hazelnut. Descending past a cluster of buckeye, you'll reemerge in grassland, where elegant brodiaea, yellow mariposa lilies, and clarkia bloom in early June. At 4.4 miles the trail ends back at the trailhead.

NEARBY ACTIVITIES

At Skyline Ridge's neighboring preserve, **Long Ridge** (650-691-1200, openspace.org /preserves/long-ridge), you can hike through woods to a grassy hilltop where a stone bench memorializes Wallace Stegner, an author and preservationist who lived the last years of his life in nearby Portola Valley.

• •

GPS TRAILHEAD COORDINATES N37° 18.736' W122° 10.616'

DIRECTIONS From the CA 1/I-280 junction in San Francisco, drive south about 29 miles on I-280, then take Exit 20 onto Page Mill Road. Drive west on Page Mill about 8.6 miles to the junction with CA 35/Skyline Boulevard. Turn left onto Skyline Boulevard and drive south about 0.8 mile; then turn right into the preserve. Stay right and follow the park road to the northern parking lot.

53 SWEENEY RIDGE

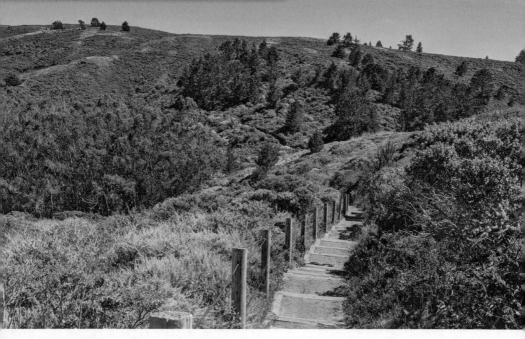

Dropping into "the Notch" at Sweeney Ridge

ALTHOUGH THIS TRAILHEAD is just minutes from San Francisco, a climb through coastal scrub leads to a quiet ridge with sweeping views.

DESCRIPTION

In many ways, Sweeney Ridge exemplifies the past, present, and future of Bay Area open space. In 1769, Spanish explorer Gaspar de Portolà got his first glimpse of San Francisco Bay from the ridge. From 1956 to 1974, Sweeney Ridge was home to a Nike missile site, the remains of which are still visible. Currently, Sweeney Ridge is the gateway to Peninsula Watershed property that stretches from the edge of the ridge across Montara Mountain to CA 92.

Many start from the end of Sneath Lane, at a bare-bones trailhead, climbing to the ridge on Sneath Lane Trail. This route is straightforward and offers excellent views, but it's a paved fire road, not the ideal hiking surface. From the Pacifica side, hikers can begin at Shelldance Nursery or the Baquiano Trailhead at the end of Fassler Lane. Both are fine options, but again, the trails are fire roads (and Mori Ridge Trail is steep). I've finally settled on my favorite trailhead, the one that accesses a lovely little footpath (bracketed by fire roads), the sweetest Sweeney Ridge trail of all.

DISTANCE & CONFIGURATION: 3-mile out-and-back

DIFFICULTY: Easy

SCENERY: Coastal scrub and views

EXPOSURE: Exposed except for a few tiny pockets of shade

TRAIL TRAFFIC: Light

TRAIL SURFACE: Dirt roads and dirt trail

HIKING TIME: 1.5 hours

DRIVING DISTANCE: 7 miles from the CA 1/I-280 junction at the San Francisco–Daly City border

ACCESS: Daily, 8 a.m.–sunset. Good year-round; best late winter–spring.

WHEELCHAIR ACCESS: Not recommended for wheelchairs

MAPS: Available at tinyurl.com/sweeneymap. A good map of the area is Pease Press's *Trails of San Mateo County: Northern Coast, Skyline & Foothills* ($7.95; peasepress.com).

FACILITIES: None

CONTACT: 415-561-4323, nps.gov/goga /sweeney.htm

LOCATION: Between San Bruno and Pacifica, CA, west of CA 35

COMMENTS: No dogs on Notch Trail. Dogs are welcome on Sneath Lane Trail.

Begin at Skyline College from the edge of lot C. Start on a narrow path near an information signboard. The path climbs about 370 feet, then ends at a junction with Notch Trail. Turn right.

This broad fire road ascends through coastal scrub, mostly sagebrush, coffee-berry, sticky monkeyflower, and coyote brush, with some Monterey pines. Fennel is common. In summer, pink clarkia blooms in grassy patches. At about 0.5 mile Notch Trail crests near an old shack. Here the trail narrows to a path and drops off to the right. The San Francisco County Jail is downhill on the left. Fog provides moisture for late-summer wildflowers here, including orchids, buckwheat, wild carrot, and coyote mint. Steps route the trail down into a saddle, then after a brief, mostly level interlude, the path snakes uphill, and then steps take over again. Look for snow-berry and twinberry. When the steps end, the trail keeps climbing, and coastal scrub gives way to grassland punctuated with shrubs. At about 1 mile Notch Trail ends at a signed junction. Turn left onto Sweeney Ridge Trail.

This is a quiet part of Sweeney Ridge. The wide dirt fire road climbs steadily, offering good 360-degree views when the day is clear. Trailside vegetation thickens and includes osoberry, ceanothus, coffeeberry, thimbleberry, poison oak, coyote brush, and twinberry.

At 1.5 miles Sweeney Ridge Trail sweeps left, then right, and ends at the old Nike Missile Control Site. These ruins are all that remains from the Cold War era, and we have them to thank for accidentally preserving Sweeney Ridge as open space. From here you could continue south, on paved Sweeney Ridge Trail, following the ridgeline to the Portola Discovery Site (about another mile), or go even farther to the Portola Gate (nearly 2 miles from the Nike Missile Site). For me, this is the turn-around spot. Retrace your steps back to the trailhead.

Sweeney Ridge

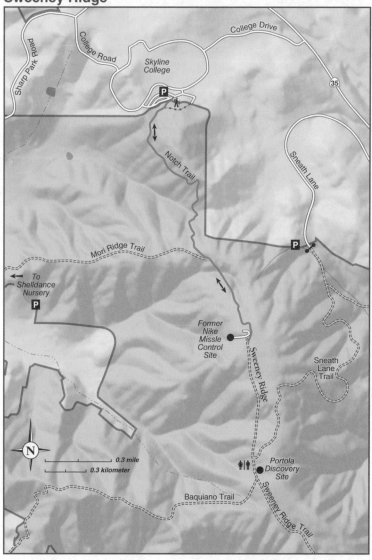

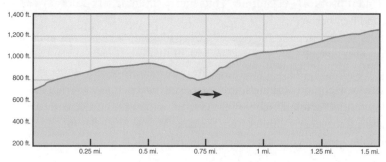

NEARBY ACTIVITIES

The main trailhead for Sweeney Ridge is at the end of Sneath Lane: from the junction of College Drive and Skyline Boulevard, drive south 0.7 mile, then turn right onto Sneath Lane and follow the road to the trailhead.

• •

GPS TRAILHEAD COORDINATES N37° 37.701' W122° 27.901'

DIRECTIONS From the CA 1/I-280 junction in San Francisco, drive about 5.5 miles south on I-280, then take Exit 45 onto Westborough Boulevard. Drive west 1 mile to the junction with CA 35/Skyline Boulevard. Turn left and drive south on Skyline 0.7 mile. Turn right onto College Drive. After 0.7 mile turn left onto College Road. Follow the road past the baseball field on the right, and turn left at the Lot C sign. Immediately turn right and drive 300 feet to the small trailhead, on the left side of the parking lot. There is free parking for four cars (use the spots reserved for Golden Gate National Recreation Area only). If those spots are full, pay to park at one of the Skyline College parking kiosks.

A foggy summer day on Notch Trail

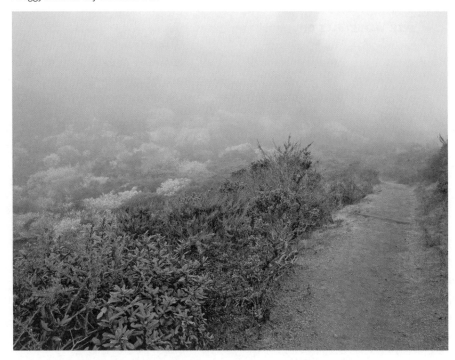

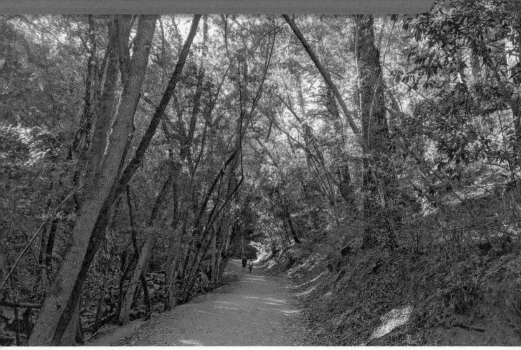

Hikers in the shade at Uvas Canyon County Park

WITH WATERFALLS ON four different creeks, Uvas Canyon Park has a premium waterfall-to-mileage quotient. Most Bay Area waterfalls require substantial hikes, but that's not the case at Uvas, where three of the falls can be reached with very little effort; the fourth requires a bit more grunt. You can visit all of the falls on this tour through the canyon's woods and chaparral.

DESCRIPTION

Uvas' hikes are all about waterfalls. It's no wonder, given the park's location, tucked back in a canyon. Steep hillsides channel runoff to a series of creeks that flow with the greatest intensity after sequential winter rainstorms. However, if you enjoy autumn foliage (such as it is in the Bay Area), you might make a special trip to Uvas in October or November, when the leaves on the park's many bigleaf maple trees flush orange and drift slowly down onto the creekbeds and trails.

Part of Uvas' charm is that the journey to the park is such a pleasant prelude to a day hike. Once you get off the highway, back roads travel through bucolic countryside, a landscape of rolling hills studded with oaks. This part of Santa Clara County has largely escaped the era of the tech boom, when developers dug up orchards and installed acres of tilt-up buildings. There are a few megamansions but still lots of old horse ranches and lonely stretches where you might see wildlife. On one visit to

DISTANCE & CONFIGURATION: 4.4-mile balloon with 2 very short spurs and 1 out-and-back stretch

DIFFICULTY: Moderate

SCENERY: Woods, waterfalls, and chaparral

EXPOSURE: Mostly shaded

TRAIL TRAFFIC: Light–heavy, depending on season

TRAIL SURFACE: Dirt trails and fire roads, with some rocky stretches along Swanson Creek

HIKING TIME: 2 hours

DRIVING DISTANCE: 70 miles from the CA 1/I-280 junction at the San Francisco–Daly City border

ACCESS: Daily, 8 a.m.–sunset; best in winter for waterfalls. Pay $6 fee at entrance station (credit card only when unattended). Reservations are required seasonally; reserve at gooutsideandplay.org.

WHEELCHAIR ACCESS: Not recommended for wheelchairs

MAPS: Available at entrance station, the start of Waterfall Loop, and tinyurl.com/uvascanyon parkmap

FACILITIES: Restrooms and water at trailhead

CONTACT: 408-779-9232, sccgov.org

LOCATION: 8515 Croy Road, Morgan Hill, CA

COMMENTS: Dogs welcome

Uvas, I spotted a huge bobcat along the side of McKean Road, ambling through the far reaches of a golf course.

Park in the day-use lot just uphill and around the corner from the park entrance and the ranger station. From the lot, ascend a flight of steps toward the restrooms, then walk up the park road; where it forks, bear right. After a short stretch downhill, turn left onto the signed Waterfall Loop Trail.

Begin following the self-guided tour if you have the pamphlet. The trail ascends on some steps and reaches a junction and bridge. Turn left, remaining on the Waterfall Loop Trail. On the right, savor Granuja Falls—the first of the waterfalls on this hike. Waterfall Loop Trail, here wide and nearly flat, runs above Swanson Creek beneath California bays and tanoaks. At about 0.15 mile you'll reach a signed two-part junction (like a triangle). Stay right on Waterfall Loop Trail.

A sturdy bridge crosses the creek, and a few yards later the footpath section of the waterfall loop breaks off on the left, heading to the far side of the creek. Check the water level for a possible return leg of the loop; it requires a ford here, but if the water is high, crossing is not recommended (you can connect to the fire road farther up the creek, if necessary). Continue straight uphill on the fire road.

Waterfall Loop Trail stiffens a bit, ascending through a forest of California bay, Douglas-fir, bigleaf maple, oak, and some young redwoods. On the right side of the trail, a sunny stretch fosters a grassy hillside peppered with buckeyes. Look for snoozing ladybugs on trailside vegetation in winter. At about 0.6 mile a spur to Black Rock Falls departs on the right from a signed junction. (Skip this if you're hiking in the drier months.) Turn right and head uphill to the falls. When I visited one February, maples and boulders surrounding the falls were swathed in green moss, and a few milkmaids bloomed along the trail. Return to the fire road and continue uphill.

Uvas Canyon County Park

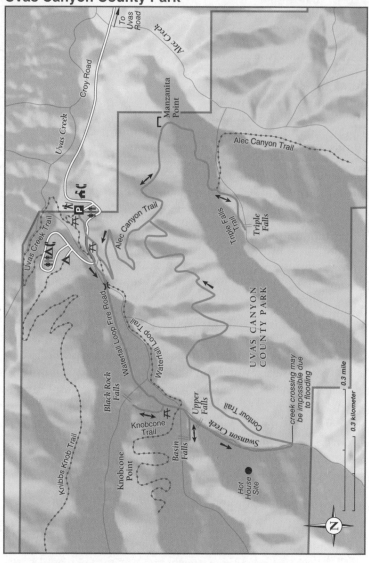

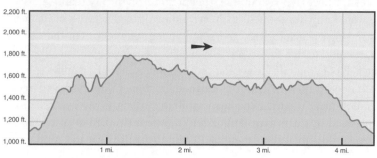

The trail ascends to signed Myrtle Flat and a junction at 0.8 mile. Knobcone Point Trail starts on the right. This is the turnaround spot for the waterfall loop, and a picnic table makes a good rest spot. A cabin used to stand here—look for the foundation, surrounded by invasive vinca (otherwise known as myrtle). The trail steepens considerably from here, so if you want to return to the trailhead, do so by descending on the narrow path that starts near the picnic table. Otherwise, cross the bridge and continue uphill, now on Contour Trail.

Lean a bit to the left for a lovely view of Upper Falls. Then, on the right, a short side spur sets off to Basin Falls. Check it out, then return to Contour Trail. A sign warns that when the creek (0.4 mile ahead) is high, fording is unsafe. The path climbs steeply along a narrow canyon. Starflower blooms here in spring; ferns add a lush feel. Big boulders litter the creekbed. Other than the sounds of water rushing downhill, it's very quiet. Some steps stabilize a steep stretch. Contour Trail dips once and climbs some more. The trail passes the Hot House Site (plumbing remnants jut out on the side of the path) then reaches the creek crossing at about 1.2 miles. If the water is rushing (or if you just want to return via the Waterfall Loop), turn back here. Otherwise, cross through the creek.

Contour Trail is a bit chaotic for a few feet, but then tall stone steps turn the trail away from the creek and head into the forest. The vegetation cover is heavy, with few views of the surrounding hillsides. Contour Trail is very narrow through-out, and the drop-off on the left side is steep. Woods consisting of madrone, tanoak, Douglas-fir, and California bay, with ferns and moss-covered rock formations in the understory, shade the path as it heads gradually downhill. Look for manzanitas in a small patch of chaparral. At 2.3 miles Contour Trail ends at a signed junction with Alec Canyon Trail. To head back to the trailhead, turn left. If you want to visit Triple Falls (as described below), turn right on Alec Canyon Trail.

Alec Canyon Trail descends a bit, cutting through chaparral with good views to the east. At 2.9 miles turn right toward Triple Falls.

The narrow path quickly ascends into a canyon and reaches the falls, perhaps the loveliest in the park. Retrace your steps back to the junction with Contour Trail, and continue straight (north).

Alec Canyon Trail descends at a moderate grade. At a viewpoint, there's a bench right next to a pink-flowering currant bush. In winter the bush's blossoms attract hummingbirds and butterflies. Later in the year, the berries are edible (although cur-rants are not the most delicious wild berry). The view from the bench fans out of the canyon to the east. The trail returns to a forest of California bay, Douglas-fir, tanoak, and madrone. After a sharp turn near a water tank, the trail drops to a signed junc-tion at 4.25 miles. Turn right.

At a nearly level grade, the wide fire road returns to the main park area. You'll reach a gate and the end of the trail at 4.3 miles. Pass through the picnic area on the paved road, and retrace your steps back to the parking lot.

● ●

GPS TRAILHEAD COORDINATES N37° 05.049' W121° 47.566'

DIRECTIONS From the CA 1/I-280 junction in San Francisco, drive south about 37 miles on I-280, then take Exit 12 onto CA 85 S. After about 12 miles, take Exit 6 for Almaden Expressway. Turn south onto Almaden, drive about 5 miles to the end of the expressway, and turn right onto Harry Road. Almost immediately, turn left onto McKean Road. Drive south on McKean, which turns into Uvas Road after about 6.5 miles. Continue on Uvas another 3.7 miles, then turn right onto Croy Road (look for a brown county-park sign before the turnoff). Drive about 4.4 miles to the park entrance, at the end of the road. *Note:* The last stretch of Croy passes through the Swedish American private community of Sveadal; drive slowly.

Bigleaf maple leaves floating in the creek along Waterfall Loop Trail

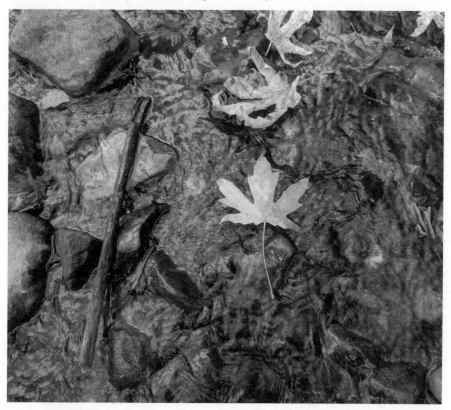

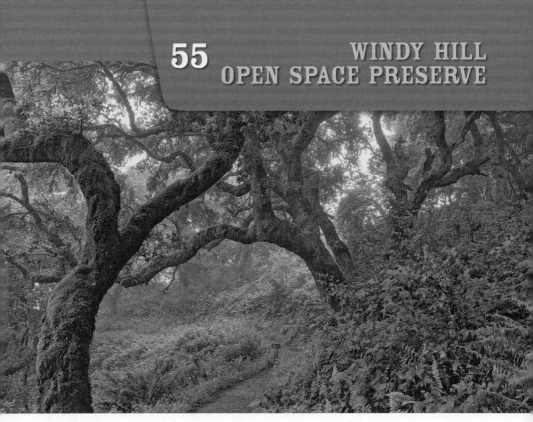

There's green everywhere you look on Windy Hill's Lost Trail.

WINDY HILL SHOWCASES the micro and macro sides of nature. From the highest reaches of this preserve, there are excellent views from ocean to East Bay; on narrow, winding paths that climb through quiet woods, there are spectacular displays of wildflowers and autumn foliage. At Windy Hill, you can see the woods for the trees, and then some. This loop begins at the edge of Portola Valley, then ascends through woods to the top of Windy Hill. The return leg is a fast descent on a fire road with a quick detour around Sausal Pond.

DESCRIPTION

I've enjoyed many magical hikes at Windy Hill over the years, in every season. In summer the woods are cool; spring brings tons of flowers; in autumn, maple leaves blaze with color; and winter is lonely with starkly naked oaks and quiet trails. The preserve has two major trailheads at the top and bottom of the mountain. I like to start in Portola Valley, get the climbing out of the way first, and cruise downhill back to the trailhead. If, however, you prefer to face the ascent on the return, begin at the CA 35 trailhead, but note that Spring Ridge Trail is significantly steeper than Hamms Gulch Trail.

The lower trailhead, just off Portola Road, is a parking lot next to the Sequoias retirement community. Begin on a connector trail that winds through oak, buckeye,

DISTANCE & CONFIGURATION: 7.1-mile loop

DIFFICULTY: Moderate

SCENERY: Grassland, woods, views, and pond

EXPOSURE: Nearly equal parts shaded and exposed

TRAIL TRAFFIC: Moderate

TRAIL SURFACE: Dirt fire roads and trails

HIKING TIME: 3.5 hours

DRIVING DISTANCE: 31.6 miles from the CA 1/I-280 junction at the San Francisco–Daly City border

ACCESS: Daily, 30 minutes before sunrise–30 minutes after sunset. Good year-round, although Spring Ridge Trail is very hot in summer. No fee.

WHEELCHAIR ACCESS: No designated handi-capped parking at this trailhead, but trail access is unobstructed, and folks in wheelchairs should be able to travel at least 0.3 mile along Sausal Pond.

MAPS: At trailhead's information signboard and openspace.org/sites/default/files/map_WH.pdf

FACILITIES: Vault toilets and water at trailhead

CONTACT: 650-691-1200, openspace.org /preserves/windy-hill

LOCATION: 555 Portola Road, Portola Valley, CA

COMMENTS: Leashed dogs are permitted on this hike but not on all Windy Hill trails.

poison oak, and coyote brush. After about 300 feet, you'll reach a junction near Sausal Pond. Turn left onto Spring Ridge Trail.

At a level grade, the broad trail creeps along the preserve boundary. Native shrubs, including currant and toyon, help to block the noise from the Sequoias complex, visible on the left. Sausal Pond sits off to the right behind tangles of blackberry, poison oak, and young coast live oak. Spring Ridge Trail begins to ascend a bit, passing huge old valley oaks. You may see or hear red-winged blackbirds and quail in this area. At 0.6 mile Spring Ridge Trail curves right and heads uphill, and a path leaves the preserve on the left. Continue straight, following the sign toward Alpine Road.

Madrone; California bay; bigleaf maple; and coast live, black, and valley oaks shade the level trail, where hound's tongue and buttercups bloom in late spring. In autumn, you might notice shrubs with marble-size white berries—the aptly named snowberry plant. Quite a few hawthorn shrubs blend into the vegetation on the right. Hawthorn is not a plant commonly spotted in natural areas in these parts, and it's easy to pick out in autumn, when its red berries dangle from tooth-leaved branches.

You'll reach an important series of junctions at about 0.8 mile: First the trail crosses a paved private road; then a trail leads left to Alpine Road. Continue straight onto Hamms Gulch Trail. A few steps later Meadow Trail, the connector to Spring Ridge Trail, departs to the right. Continue straight.

In the grassy understory beneath gorgeous black and valley oaks, blue dicks and blue-eyed grass bloom in early spring. Watch out for poison oak, which is common along this slim path. Hamms Gulch Trail enters the woods. A creek runs slightly downslope to the left, and this riparian microclimate hosts plants that prefer a damp environment, including currant, California bay, and buckeye, plus trilliums and milkmaids in late winter.

The trail dips to cross a creek, then reaches a junction with Eagle Trail at 1.1 miles. Stay right on Hamms Gulch Trail, which abandons the waterway and begins to climb.

Windy Hill Open Space Preserve

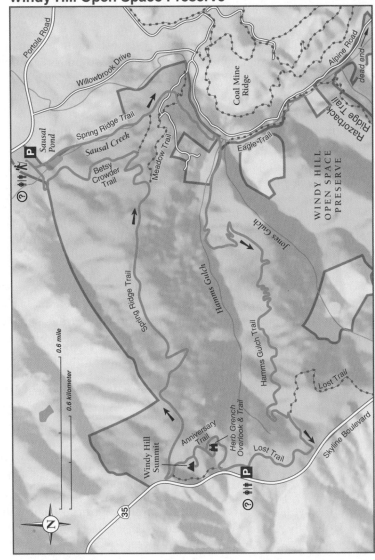

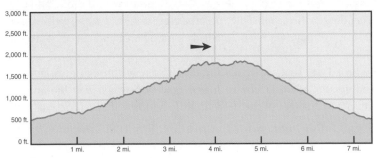

In early March, hound's tongue is usually prolific, blooming in giant colonies along the length of the trail, but you'll also likely see many other wildflowers, including shooting stars, trilliums, and milkmaids. The forest is a pretty mix of madrone; oaks; California bay; and some maple, redwood, and Douglas-fir. Hazelnut, creambush, poison oak, currant, and gooseberry compose the bulk of the understory.

Hamms Gulch Trail is well graded with many switchbacks and, except for a few short steeper sections, makes for an easy climb. Occasional breaks in the forest reveal views across the gulch to Spring Ridge Trail. In a sunny patch of chaparral, nearly hidden in thick stands of coyote brush, look for western leatherwood, an extremely rare shrub that is easiest to spot when yellow blossoms appear in late winter.

After another foray through the woods, Hamms Gulch Trail skirts the edge of a sloping, grassy meadow—the only significant grassland on the trail. Benches here and there along the trail are a welcome sight for weary hikers. The trail just keeps climbing, and you may begin to notice some incredibly large Douglas-firs mixed through tanoak, bigleaf maple, oaks, and madrone. At 3.3 miles, Hamms Gulch Trail ends at a T-junction. Turn right onto Lost Trail.

Lost Trail makes its way out of the forest, then runs along the edge of the woods, allowing good close-up views of those giant Douglas-firs. On the left side of the trail, coyote brush dominates, with some currant mixed in. This level stretch is a nice intermission between the ascent of Hamms Gulch and the descent of Spring Ridge.

Within audible range of CA 35 on the left, Lost Trail cuts across grassland on the high flanks of Windy Hill. Blue-eyed grass, mule-ear sunflowers, fiddlenecks, and California poppies are common in early spring. Views east extend to Mount Diablo. At 4 miles you'll reach a picnic area on the left, near the CA 35 trailhead. More than once I've seen hikers sprawled on top of the picnic tables, resting at either the midpoint or end of their journey. Continue straight past the trailhead, now on Anniversary Trail, built and named to commemorate the 10th anniversary of Windy Hill's preservation.

The trail parallels CA 35 then veers right and makes the brief ascent to the hilltop. If you want the bragging rights for bagging the peak, turn left at a bench onto a 0.1 mile spur. If you've been wondering why the preserve is named Windy Hill, visit on a breezy day and the mystery will be revealed—air rushes unimpeded east from the ocean to this prominent Santa Cruz Mountains hilltop. A 360-degree panorama encompasses the Santa Clara Valley, Mounts Hamilton and Diablo, and soft grassy hills descending to the ocean. Once past the crest at 4.6 miles, the trail drops through coyote brush to a junction near a roadside parking area and CA 35. Turn right onto Spring Ridge Trail.

The broad fire road descends somewhat steeply through grassland. Look for blue-eyed grass, California poppy, lupine, and popcorn flower blooming in early spring. In the first stages of the descent, little huddles of coast live oak provide the only shade, but as Spring Ridge Trail heads downhill, woods begin a gradual squeeze toward the trail. Meadow Trail, the connector to Hamms Gulch Trail, sets off on the right at 6 miles. In April, blue and white lupines put on a good show in the grass on both sides of the trail at this junction. Continue left on Spring Ridge Trail. The grade thankfully eases to moderate as the trail winds through madrone, coast live oak, California bay, toyon, buckeye, and poison oak. California coffeeberry dangles red and black berries in late autumn to the delight of Windy Hill's bird and coyote population. Spring Ridge Trail emerges in an area dominated by coyote brush and offers views east. The quad-aching descent finally ends at 6.4 miles at a junction with Betsy Crowder Trail. Turn left.

This gentle grade is welcome after Spring Ridge's descent. The trail is named in honor of a guidebook author and Midpeninsula Regional Open Space District board member who died in 2000. Her namesake trail drifts through a grassy meadow favored by deer, then drops into a forest of California bay, madrone, buckeye, hazelnut, coffeeberry, and coast live oak. Sausal Pond is barely visible. In early spring, look for the dregs of blooming hound's tongue, plus trilliums and blue dicks. The path curves right, around a few massive eucalyptus, and draws near a road outside the park boundary. Vinca, a non-native ground cover, sprawls through the understory. If you peer through the trees on the right, you may notice a tall, level berm that contains the north side of Sausal Pond.

At 7 miles, Betsy Crowder Trail ends. Turn left and return to the trailhead on the connector trail.

• •

GPS TRAILHEAD COORDINATES N37° 22.517' W122° 13.408'

DIRECTIONS From the CA 1/I-280 junction in San Francisco, drive south about 27 miles on I-280, then take Exit 22 for Alpine Road. Head west on Alpine about 3 miles, then turn right onto Portola Road. Drive about 1 mile and turn left into the preserve parking lot.

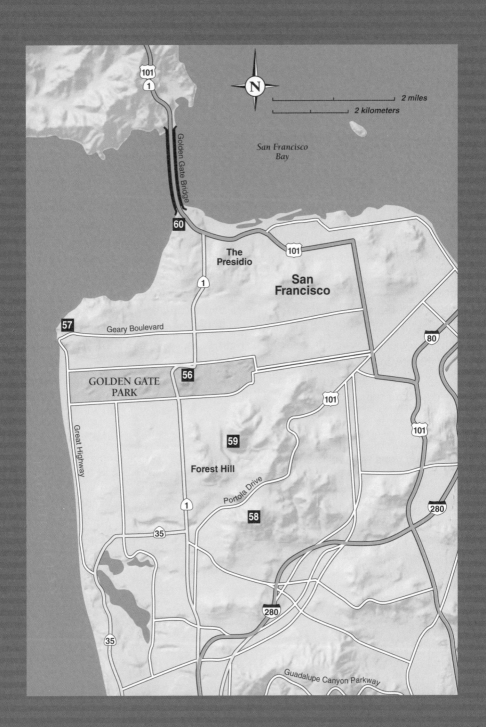

101
1

Golden Gate Bridge

60

San Francisco
Bay

2 miles
2 kilometers

The
Presidio

101

San
Francisco

1

57

Geary Boulevard

56

80

GOLDEN GATE
PARK

101

101

59

Great Highway

Forest Hill

1

Portola Drive

58

280

35

35

280

Guadalupe Canyon Parkway

CITY OF SAN FRANCISCO

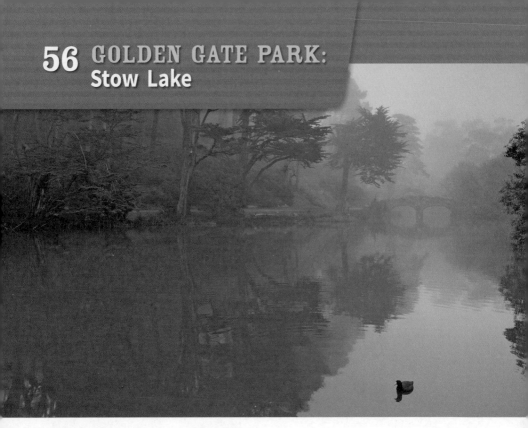

A foggy morning at Stow Lake

SOMEWHERE BETWEEN a walk and a hike (a wike? a halk?), this little jaunt spirals around Stow Lake and up to the top of Strawberry Hill.

DESCRIPTION

Beautiful Golden Gate Park (GGP) is a manufactured masterpiece, transformed in the late 1800s from a sand-blown landscape of dunes. Over time, the land has been planted, shaped, and tweaked a million ways, and today GGP's more than 1,000 acres host an incredible assortment of activities: There are museums, sports fields, ponds, playgrounds, and grassy meadows for picnics.

The park's paths range from wide and paved to narrow and dirt, but there is little actual hiking to be found. Many areas of the park offer lovely strolls, and if that's what you're after, consider the Botanical Garden, the Japanese Tea Garden, or North Lake.

My favorite GGP destination for a hybrid walk/hike is Strawberry Hill, which is perhaps better known for its surrounding artificial moat, Stow Lake. A flat, paved trail rings the lake, and dirt paths and stairs wind up and down the hill, allowing walkers to create a variety of exercise routes. The hill and lake offer excellent city bird-watching with frequent surprises, like glimpses of great horned owls, red-tailed hawks, and great blue herons.

DISTANCE & CONFIGURATION: 2.1-mile spiral

DIFFICULTY: Easy

SCENERY: Pond and woods

EXPOSURE: Mixture of shade and sun

TRAIL TRAFFIC: Heavy

TRAIL SURFACE: Paved path and dirt trails

HIKING TIME: 1 hour

DRIVING DISTANCE: 4 miles from the San Francisco Civic Center

ACCESS: Daily, 5 a.m.–midnight. Good year-round. No fee.

WHEELCHAIR ACCESS: To explore in a wheelchair, park at designated spots near the

boathouse. The outer ring around Stow Lake is paved and wheelchair accessible.

MAPS: Available at tinyurl.com/ggparkmap. *The Walker's Map of San Francisco,* published by Pease Press, is a good option ($7.95, peasepress.com).

FACILITIES: Restrooms, water, and food at boathouse

CONTACT: 415-831-2700, sfrecpark.org/parks -open-spaces/golden-gate-park-guide

LOCATION: Golden Gate Park, San Francisco

COMMENTS: Dogs welcome if leashed or under voice control

Start at the yellow-gated bridge on the lake's north side. For a quicker walk, you can head right over the bridge, but to get the most out of your excursion, begin walking east on the paved trail, in the same direction as the one-way park road. The trail is a popular route for walkers and stroller pushers. Look to the right for a view to one of the lake's small tree-dotted islands. Common waterfowl, including American coots and mallards, are year-round natives around the lake. You'll also likely see (and hear) Canada geese, Brewer's blackbirds, pigeons, and crows. I was surprised once to come across a softshell turtle along the trail—it must have been dumped here, as is the fate of some Muscovy ducks who have been "retired" at the lake.

The paved trail curves around the east edge of the lake, offering great views across the water to man-made Huntington Falls and the Chinese Pavilion. On the south shore, at 0.6 mile, you'll pass one of GGP's treasures, Rustic Bridge, constructed in 1893. This pretty little bridge crosses the lake and connects to Strawberry Hill, but our route continues straight around the lake on the paved path.

Traffic noise from Transverse Drive (out of sight to the west) is heavy here as the path bends north and heads toward the boathouse area. Look right to the lake's largest island, where great blue herons commonly nest in spring. Pass the boathouse (or stop here for a bathroom break, food and drink, or a boat rental), and now follow the path east. At 1 mile you'll reach the walk's starting point, at the yellow gate. Turn right across the bridge.

At the end of the bridge, turn left onto the dirt trail. For now ignore the stairs and paths that head uphill to the right, continuing on the flat trail as it crosses the bottom of Huntington Falls, a popular destination for wedding photos, then passes through a tiny grove of planted redwoods. Once past the Chinese Pavilion, the path bends right. You'll typically encounter tons of squirrel beggars along the trail here. At 1.3 miles pass the other side of the stone bridge and continue on the dirt

Golden Gate Park: Stow Lake

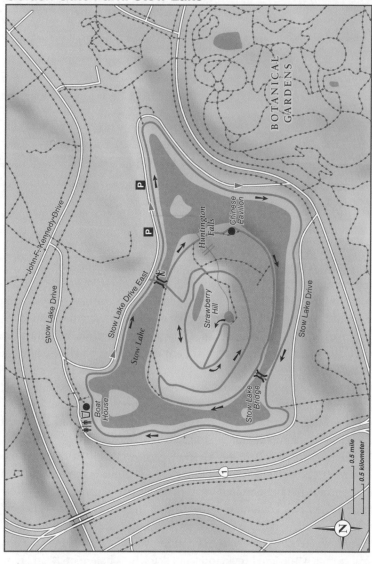

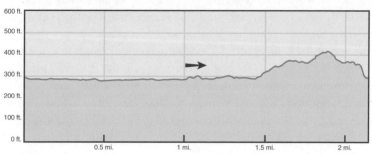

path, which sweeps slightly uphill to the right and reaches an unsigned junction at 1.4 miles. Turn right and then, after a few steps uphill, right again.

The wide dirt trail climbs gently through some Monterey pines, which block most of the views south. At 1.7 miles the trail flattens at a junction. Steps head back downhill to the right. A wide trail doubles back toward the left, heading to the hilltop, but continue straight on the trail that runs along a small fenced reservoir.

Lucky, sharp-eyed hikers might get a glimpse of great horned owls, which often nest in the trees in this part of Golden Gate Park. I seem to be blind to them, but many more-skilled birders spot them during nesting season and sometimes after the birds have fledged. The trail is level along the reservoir but then climbs again, passing a grove of toyon and coast live oak on the left. At 1.8 miles pass a set of steps on the left and continue straight.

As you make the final push to the hilltop, notice surprisingly tall and sturdy pines and cypress trees along the trail. At 1.9 miles the trail reaches the flattened top of Strawberry Hill. An interpretive panel prompts visitors to look for butterflies here, and sure enough, there are commonly swallowtails, admirals, and ladies fluttering about in warm, sunny weather. Turn left to admire a partial view north to the Golden Gate Bridge and Marin Headlands. The rocky rubble on the east side of the hilltop is the remains of an observatory that was destroyed by the 1906 earthquake.

When ready, follow a sandy path west along the crest of the hill. The path descends through a cluster of native shrubs, including lizardtail, coyote brush, lupine, and native blackberry. Buckwheat blooms here in summer. Old stone steps drop to a junction with the fire road. Turn right.

Retrace your steps past the reservoir back to the junction at 2.1 miles. Turn left onto a trail (with a green handrail) that quickly descends and forks. Bear left and descend more steps to a junction, at lake level, at 2.1 miles. Retrace your steps back across the bridge to the trailhead.

• •

GPS TRAILHEAD COORDINATES N37° 46.175' W122° 28.476'

DIRECTIONS From northbound 19th Avenue in San Francisco, just as you enter Golden Gate Park, turn right onto Martin Luther King Jr. Drive. After 0.2 mile turn left onto Stow Lake Drive. Follow the road around the lake and past the boathouse, and where the road splits, stay right. Park near the yellow gate on the right.

From southbound Park Presidio Boulevard in San Francisco, in Golden Gate Park, turn right onto Crossover Drive. After 0.1 mile turn left onto Transverse Drive, then left again onto John F. Kennedy Drive. After 0.4 mile turn right onto Stow Lake Drive; where the road splits, stay left. Park near the yellow gate on the right.

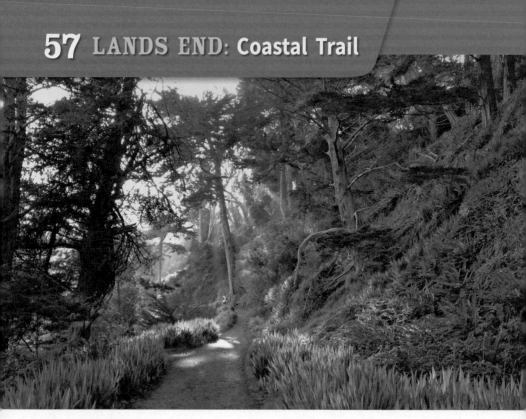

Coastal Trail at Lands End

LANDS END IS a rugged bit of coastline in the northwestern corner of San Francisco, around the bend from the historic Cliff House and the flat expanse of Ocean Beach. Locals come here to jog or walk the trails, while tourists enjoy the views of the Golden Gate Bridge.

DESCRIPTION

Coastal Trail is the "Main Street" at Lands End, popular with local runners, dog walkers, stroller-pushing parents, and folks from out of town. In addition to trekking out and back on Coastal Trail, hikers can explore spur paths leading to the Sutro Bath ruins and Lands End proper. Veteran hikers will likely find Coastal Trail lovely but tame. The round trip to Eagle's Point is less than 3 miles, and the elevation change (albeit for two sets of steps) is slight. It's a good choice for beginners because it's an out-and-back hike—simply head back to the trailhead when you've had enough.

If you're new to San Francisco, or to hiking, do use caution at Lands End: stay back from the steep, unprotected drop-offs along some stretches of the trail; stay on the trails; and learn to recognize and avoid poison oak. I would not normally issue these cautions, but it's not uncommon for folks to get lost or stranded at Lands End, particularly on the rocks at the coastline. Don't wreck your day with a helicopter rescue!

DISTANCE & CONFIGURATION: 2.8-mile out-and-back

DIFFICULTY: Easy

SCENERY: Coastline, with views of the Golden Gate Bridge

EXPOSURE: Mixture of shade and sun

TRAIL TRAFFIC: Heavy

TRAIL SURFACE: Dirt fire road and trail with many steps

HIKING TIME: 2 hours

DRIVING DISTANCE: 5.5 miles from the San Francisco Civic Center

ACCESS: Daily, sunrise–1 a.m. Good year-round. No fee.

WHEELCHAIR ACCESS: There is designated handicapped parking, and this hike is wheelchair friendly for about the first 0.3 mile.

MAPS: Under glass at trailhead's information signboard and available at tinyurl.com/lands endcoastaltrail. *The Walker's Map of San Francisco,* published by Pease Press, shows all trails in the area ($7.95, peasepress.com).

FACILITIES: Restrooms, water, and food at Lands End Lookout

CONTACT: 415-426-5240, nps.gov/goga /planyourvisit/landsend.htm

LOCATION: (Lands End Lookout) Point Lobos Avenue, 0.1 mile south of its intersection with El Camino del Mar (just east of the Cliff House), San Francisco, CA

COMMENTS: Dogs welcome if leashed or under voice control. Be mindful of the additional dog regulations posted along the trails.

Begin from the parking lot at Merrie Way. A big, pleasant parking lot and an information display greet you. The Lands End Lookout contains interpretive displays, restrooms, and a café. Ascend a few stairs to a kiosk with a map under glass and information about Lands End; then begin hiking north on Coastal Trail. Tall Monterey pines tower over a restored area with a lovely assortment of native plants, including buckwheat, bush lupines, coyote brush, monkeyflower, lizardtail, and yarrow. Just before the wide paved trail sweeps back to the right, a signed trail descends left to the Sutro Bath area. Continue straight on Coastal Trail.

A second gentle curve swings the trail north again, climbing slightly (a shortcut trail to the left is an option here). Where a second paved trail enters from the right at 0.2 mile, bear left. Soon you'll reach the first interpretive panel—although Lands End appears relatively untouched by civilization, a railroad ran along the coast here in the 1880s, and in the 1900s ships wrecked on the rocks (some sharp-eyed hikers can spot the wrecks during low tide). Visit on a foggy day and get an earful of the foghorns described on one panel—each horn has a different tone to assist ships navigating through our local pea soup.

At 0.3 mile Coastal Trail reaches a signed junction and overlook. On a clear day, views sweep north across the water to the Marin Headlands and the Golden Gate Bridge. A set of steps leads up the War Memorial area, but our route continues straight on Coastal Trail.

A retaining wall on the right holds up a hillside dotted with Monterey pines. At a second overlook, the trail shifts to dirt but remains nearly flat—if you're visiting with a stroller or in a wheelchair, you'll most likely want to turn around here. Beware of a massive hedge of poison oak on the left shortly before Coastal Trail passes an

Lands End: Coastal Trail

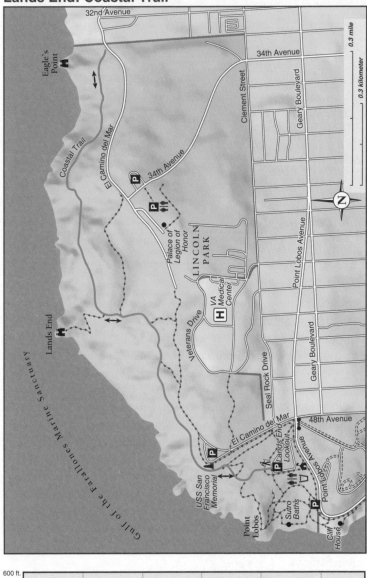

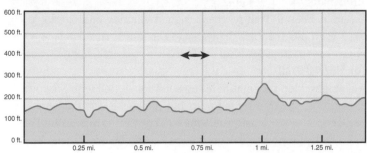

unmarked path heading uphill on the right. Continue straight. The trail rolls up and down a bit over loose, sandy soil. Another trail, this one signed, breaks off to the right. Again, continue straight on Coastal Trail.

Thickets of willow and cypress crowd the trail. Cheerful orange nasturtiums drape over the trailside shrubs; you might also see poison hemlock, with white, lacy flowers and purple-blotched stems. At 0.7 mile a paved trail enters from the right, leading up through the Lincoln Park golf course to the Palace of the Legion of Honor. Continue left on Coastal Trail.

Shortly past the junction, a signed trail near the emergency call box heads downhill to the left, leading to the actual Lands End—this is a nice side trip to a rocky beach (not described here), but note that the climb back up is rough.

On Coastal Trail, a set of ascending steps brings the easy section of this hike to an end. Look for native strawberry and yerba buena plants on the grassy hill to the right. The trail crests and almost immediately begins to drop, again on steps. Eucalyptus and Monterey cypress trees shade the trail and screen most of the view, but as the trail sweeps downhill, a dramatic vista north across the Golden Gate opens up.

The trail hugs the coast, then turns slightly inland near Deadman's Point, passing through more eucalyptus before emerging to coastal views that now include the posh Sea Cliff neighborhood slightly northeast. You may see or hear some common Bay Area birds here, including chickadees and a variety of sparrows. At 1.4 miles the golf course is visible on the right and Coastal Trail reaches Eagle's Point on the left.

The trail ends here, at 32nd Avenue and El Camino del Mar. After soaking in the views, retrace your steps back to the trailhead.

• •

GPS TRAILHEAD COORDINATES N37° 46.841' W122° 30.703'

DIRECTIONS Lands End is in northwest San Francisco. Drive west on Geary Boulevard, which becomes Point Lobos Avenue at 39th Avenue. Continue west on Point Lobos, cross 48th Avenue/El Camino del Mar, and turn right into the parking lot, on the right—if you reach the Cliff House, you've gone too far.

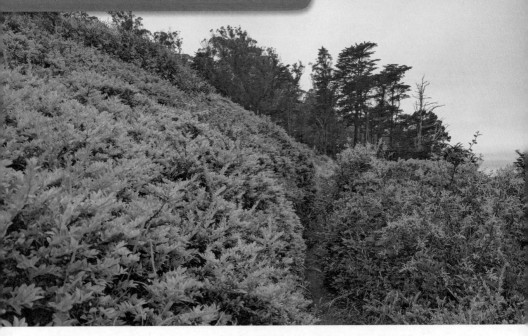

A dense thicket of coastal scrub on the north slope of Mount Davidson

AT 938 FEET, Mount Davidson is the highest natural point in San Francisco but is often overlooked as a hiking destination. Most locals recognize it as the hill with the cross on top; film buffs remember it from *Dirty Harry*. But there's more! The 40-acre Mount Davidson Park is laced with trails that offer expansive views. This easy hike winding through woods and grassland is also enjoyable in the fog, when the swirling mist muffles noise from the surrounding city and sporadic birdsong drifts through the woods.

DESCRIPTION

Although Mount Davidson is a small park completely surrounded by development, the trails are unsigned and it's surprisingly easy to get lost in the woods. Be sure to follow my directions closely and check to make sure you're on the right track, especially at the junction in the woods at the end of the Native Garden segment.

Starting from the bus stop at the junction of Dalewood Way and Lansdale Avenue, head up the unsigned but obvious trail. Within a few feet, a forest of eucalyptus and Monterey pine shades the broad dirt path. The understory consists mostly of blackberry and non-native plants, including some showy fuchsias. After a brief climb, you'll reach an unsigned junction at 0.1 mile. Bear right.

The trail moves away from the woods into grassland, initially hugging a tall fence on the right. The rocky cut on the left is a good place to spot blue dicks

DISTANCE & CONFIGURATION: 0.9-mile
balloon loop

DIFFICULTY: Easy

SCENERY: Grassland, woods, coastal scrub,
and city views

EXPOSURE: Mix of shade and sun

TRAIL TRAFFIC: Moderate

TRAIL SURFACE: Dirt

HIKING TIME: 1 hour or less

DRIVING DISTANCE: 4.6 miles from the San
Francisco Civic Center

ACCESS: Daily (no hours posted). Good year-
round. No fee.

WHEELCHAIR ACCESS: Not recommended
for wheelchairs

MAPS: Available at tinyurl.com/mtdavidsontrail
map. *The Walker's Map of San Francisco,* published by Pease Press, is a good option ($7.95,
peasepress.com).

FACILITIES: None

CONTACT: 415-831-6326, sfrecpark.org
/destination/mt-davidson-park

LOCATION: Off Portola Drive, 1.5 miles east of
CA 1/19th Avenue, San Francisco, CA

COMMENTS: Dogs welcome if leashed or under
voice control

blooming in spring. Red-tailed hawks are often seen hunting on this part of the hill, and crowned sparrows and phoebes are common. Descending gently, the trail sweeps through grassland dotted with ferns and coyote brush, just upslope from the park boundary on the right. It then rises a bit and crosses a rocky outcrop. Views to downtown San Francisco unfold. The trail squeezes past a second fence. At 0.3 mile, paths head uphill (left) and out of the park (right). Continue straight.

As the trail curves around to the north slope of the mountain, trailside vegetation shifts from grassland to coastal scrub. Some hikers call this next stretch the Native Garden Trail. There are lots of lovely plant treasures to enjoy here, including huckleberry, creambush, monkeyflower, coyote brush, currant, and snowberry. A few feet before the trail heads back into the woods, at about 0.35 mile, a rough path ascends on the left. Continue straight.

A large serviceberry shrub stands off to the left—to my knowledge, Mount Davidson is the sole San Francisco home for this native shrub. Eucalyptus and Monterey pine shade the trail as it keeps to an easy grade. This is a good stretch of woods for bird-watching—look (and listen) for chickadees, northern flickers, and wrens. Scrub jays are common, but I've seen Steller's jays too, as well as many hummingbirds. Mixed through red elderberry and ferns, the understory blackberry bushes produce tasty fruit during warm summers, but in cold years they fail to thrive. At 0.4 mile you'll reach an important but unsigned junction; bear left. The trail ascends through Monterey pine and eucalyptus (invasive ivy blocks out nearly every understory plant save blackberry), passes a rock outcrop, and bends left. At 0.5 mile the trail ends at a fire road. Cross the road and continue straight.

Ascend a set of pretty stone steps. Look for yerba buena, a tiny-leaved trailing native plant, growing on the right. Crush a leaf to release its powerful, sweet mint scent. As the stone steps end, continue a few feet, then turn left and ascend again.

Mount Davidson

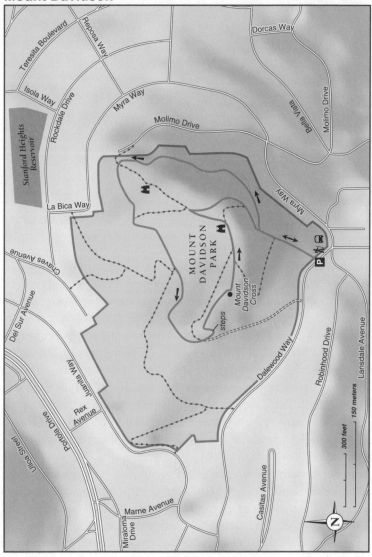

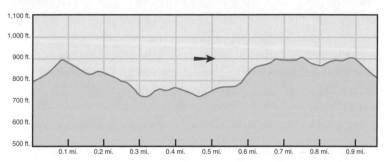

The steps, constructed from wood planks and logs, are steep. Notice that the bunchgrasses crowding the trail remain green year-round. The first time I ascended to the top of Mount Davidson, it was socked in, and as I walked, the soft, pale, billowing fog wrapped around me like a fleece blanket. It's so damp on this part of the mountain that ferns grow in the crooks and stumps of some of the eucalyptus, Monterey pine, and Monterey cypress trees. The steps end at a clearing, to the left. Bear right and ascend the final steps to the mountaintop and the cross.

This flat summit is a broad clearing dominated by the Mount Davidson cross. Constructed in 1934, the cross and lands immediately surrounding it were sold by the city in 1997 to the Council of Armenian American Organizations of Northern California to commemorate the Armenian genocide of 1915–1923. Throngs of people visit on Easter, but the rest of the year is quite peaceful. After inspecting the cross, walk east along the wide, flat trail toward the viewpoint.

Butterflies love hilltops, and butterfly lovers will be delighted by their colorful fluttering at the mountaintop in summer and autumn. Sometimes I see common red admirals and painted ladies, but often there are dozens of swallowtails here too.

From the viewpoint, enjoy wonderful scenery east and north. Unfortunately, the city's geography permits no glimpses of the Golden Gate Bridge. When you're ready, descend the set of steps to the left of the large metal water-department box. This hillside has been seeded with lupine, yarrow, and sagebrush. Look for more serviceberry shrubs here, with conspicuous white flowers in April and May. At 0.7 mile the trail continues straight to a lower viewpoint (explore it if you like), but our route continues right.

The trail passes over rocky ground where I've seen garter snakes (the only snakes I've ever encountered within San Francisco's city limits). In spring, California poppies and buckwheat bloom along the path. After a brief descent—watch for poison oak mixed through blackberry on the right—you'll return to the hike's first junction. Continue straight downhill to the bus stop and trailhead.

• •

GPS TRAILHEAD COORDINATES N37° 44.211' W122° 27.234'

DIRECTIONS From northbound CA 1/19th Avenue in San Francisco, bear right onto Junipero Serra Boulevard. Junipero Serra ends at Sloat Boulevard; continue straight/ right, now on Portola Drive. After about 0.7 mile turn right at a traffic light onto Marne Avenue (same junction as Miraloma Drive). Drive one block on Marne and turn right onto Juanita Way. Drive one short block and continue straight onto Lansdale Avenue. Drive one short block and turn left onto Dalewood Way. Drive one block uphill on steep Dalewood to the park entrance, at the junction of Lansdale and Dalewood.

Note: Feel free to consult a map and create your own directions. Many other streets reach the park, but you'll need a map unless you're familiar with the neighborhood.

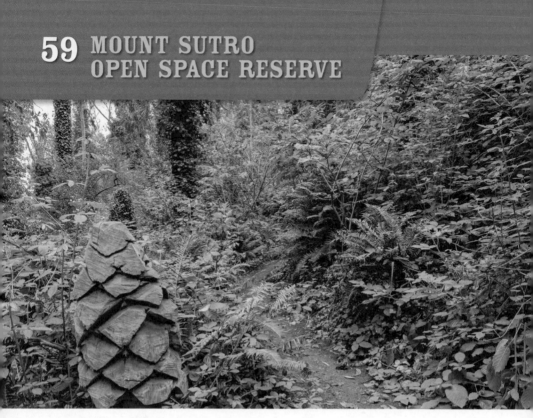

A touch of whimsy on Mystery Trail at Mount Sutro

WITH SO MANY PARKS, large and small, in San Francisco, Mount Sutro is often overlooked. This 61-acre parcel in the middle of the city has an awesome trail network winding through woods and a surprise at the top.

DESCRIPTION

The trails here are not well known, perhaps because the forest blocks views and the land is quietly managed by the University of California San Francisco (UCSF). The hill (which doesn't feel much like a mount) was part of a massive land grant owned by Adolph Sutro, who planted acres of Monterey cypress, Monterey pine, and eucalyptus, transforming grassland and coastal scrub into dense forest. The property eventually became part of UCSF, and in the early 2000s volunteers restored some old trails and built new ones, creating a compact trail network great for quick jogs and short hikes.

Start at the side of Clarendon Avenue near the intersection with Christopher Drive, from the signed trailhead. Narrow Clarendon Connector Trail begins to climb through eucalyptus woods at the edge of UCSF's Aldea San Miguel housing community. The path passes the Sutro Nursery (plants, not babies), makes a sharp right, and reaches a junction at 0.25 mile. Turn left onto Quarry Road.

The grade slackens but the eucalyptus remains. At 0.4 mile you'll reach a multiple junction. Turn right onto South Ridge Trail. After a few steps, a small path breaks off to

DISTANCE & CONFIGURATION: 2.1-mile balloon loop

DIFFICULTY: Easy

SCENERY: Woods and hilltop meadow

EXPOSURE: All shade except for hilltop

TRAIL TRAFFIC: Moderate

TRAIL SURFACE: Dirt

HIKING TIME: 1 hour

DRIVING DISTANCE: 3.3 miles from San Francisco City Hall

ACCESS: Open daily. Good year-round. No fee.

WHEELCHAIR ACCESS: Not recommended for wheelchairs

MAPS: Available at peasepress.com/sutro map.pdf

FACILITIES: None

CONTACT: ucsf.edu/about/locations/mount-sutro-open-space-reserve

LOCATION: Neighboring UCSF's Parnassus Heights campus, San Francisco, CA

COMMENTS: Leashed dogs welcome

the left. Continue straight. On foggy days, this part of the hill is bathed in quiet. South Ridge climbs easily through woods to a junction at 0.45 mile. Turn left onto Nike Road.

The wide paved trail climbs a bit sharply. Look for vibrant pink-flowering currant in bloom on the left in winter. A large sign announces the entrance to Rotary Meadow. This summit area was the location of a Nike radar base in the 1950s. When the military cleared out, the hilltop returned to UCSF control. Volunteers have planted many native trees and shrubs here, and you are likely to see many birds and butterflies enjoying the plants.

At about 0.5 mile you'll reach a junction and information signboard. Continue right. The path ascends easily, through sagebrush, coyote brush, manzanita, silk-tassel, and many other natives. At 0.6 mile take a moment (perhaps on a bench along the meadow) to savor the peace at the actual summit. The surrounding forest blocks views. When ready, continue, now on East Ridge Trail.

Three switchbacks route the path through eucalyptus to a junction at 0.7 mile. East Ridge drops to the right, then ends at a paved road in Aldea. Turn left onto Mystery Trail.

Although Mystery is only 0.1 mile long, it's a sweet path. At a nearly level grade, the trail edges across a lush hillside with a good assortment of native plants, including snowberry and ferns (watch for poison oak). You'll discover some whimsical natural decorations along Mystery Trail, sure to delight your hiking partners, especially children. Mystery Trail ends at 0.8 mile. Turn right onto North Ridge Trail.

North Ridge Trail descends easily through a thin eucalyptus forest with native shrubs in the understory. At 1.1 miles it ends at Medical Center Way. Carefully cross the pavement and resume hiking on Fairy Gates Trail (you can shave a bit off the hike by walking downhill along the road to Historic Trail, but be cautious of traffic).

After a few steps, Fairy Gates continues straight at a signed junction; turn left. The path weaves downhill through woods where wild plum trees bloom in February. This is excellent bird habitat—on one hike I watched a brown creeper twirl up

Mount Sutro Open Space Reserve

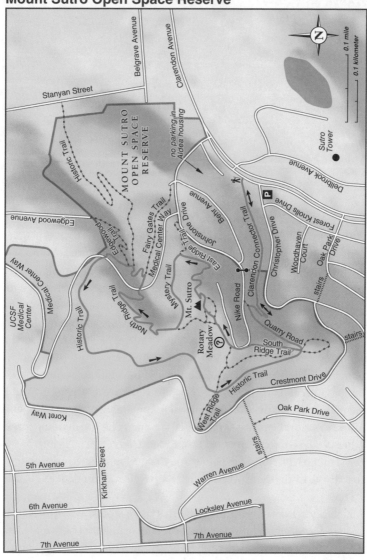

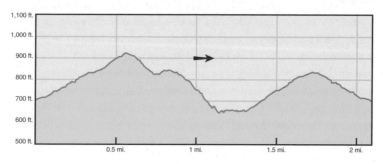

a tree trunk. At 1.1 miles Edgewood Trail heads out of the forest straight ahead, and Historic Trail does the same (on a longer route) to the right. Turn left.

Historic Trail climbs through eucalyptus and crosses Medical Center Way at 1.2 miles. Watch for traffic. On the other side of the road, the path begins to easily ascend through woods. Noise from UCSF Medical Center is strong but fades as the trail bends left. On this west slope of the hill, ferns are common, including some growing in the crooks of eucalyptus trees. At a few spots where the tree cover permits, there are partial views of the Golden Gate Bridge. The grade remains easy—be alert for cyclists. At 1.6 miles steep West Ridge Trail crosses the trail. Continue straight on Historic Trail.

Huge boulders perch along the trail. Look for iris, fairy bells (a rare find in the city), and hummingbird sage blooming here in spring. At 1.7 miles Historic Trail ends. Even though you will have been at this four-way junction earlier in the hike, it's still confusing. Continue straight onto Quarry Road (look for a small BART symbol on a tree), and retrace your steps back to the trailhead.

• •

GPS TRAILHEAD COORDINATES N37° 45.438' W122° 27.247'

DIRECTIONS From the CA 1/I-280 junction in San Francisco, drive north on CA 1/19th Avenue 2.5 miles, and turn right onto Taraval Street. Head east on Taraval about 0.6 mile to a traffic circle. Take the third exit, onto Dewey Boulevard. Drive 0.3 mile to a traffic light. Continue straight, now on Laguna Honda Boulevard. Drive north on Laguna Honda Boulevard 0.5 mile, then turn right onto Clarendon Avenue. Drive uphill about 0.6 mile, then turn left onto Oak Park Drive. After one very short block, turn right onto Forest Knolls Drive. Drive 2 blocks, then turn left at the T-junction onto Christopher Drive. Park on the side of the road, then walk east on Christopher to the intersection with Clarendon. Turn left, and after about 40 feet, turn left again onto the signed trail.

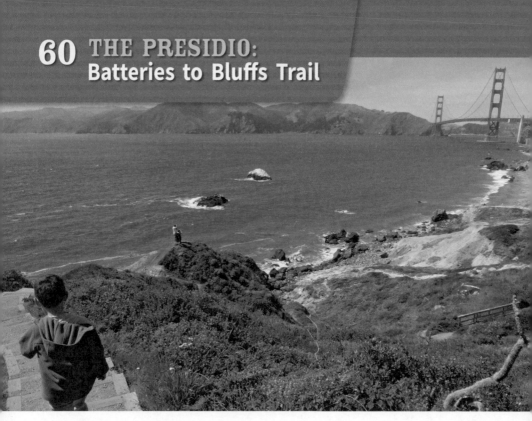

Golden Gate Bridge view from Batteries to Bluffs Trail

THINK OF A dream San Francisco hike: a path overlooking the ocean, with gorgeous views of the Golden Gate Bridge; a peaceful place where you could sit and watch the waves crash or get your morning exercise running through a scenic landscape while birds sing and flowers bloom. You don't have to imagine this trail because it already exists—it's the Batteries to Bluffs Trail in The Presidio.

DESCRIPTION

Batteries to Bluffs Trail runs parallel to and downslope from Lincoln Boulevard and consists mostly of sets of steps and some flat sections of trail. You can hike in either direction, starting from the parking lot at the Golden Gate Overlook, as described here, or from the street-side parking on Lincoln Boulevard (the latter is my preferred trailhead, but there isn't much parking).

Begin at the parking area near Golden Gate Overlook. If you want to take in the view of the Golden Gate, follow the paved path to the north, then return to the parking lot when ready. Three paths depart to the south: one edging along Lincoln, the second where a driveway connects two segments of parking lots, and a third on the western edge of the second parking lot. All three join, but for this hike, take the middle path.

The wide dirt trail weaves through a thin forest of Monterey cypress and Monterey pine. The understory is mostly invasive ivy. At 0.1 mile bear right (the path left

DISTANCE & CONFIGURATION: 1.6-mile out-and-back

DIFFICULTY: Easy

SCENERY: Coastline, beach, and Golden Gate Bridge views

EXPOSURE: Almost completely exposed

TRAIL TRAFFIC: Moderate

TRAIL SURFACE: Dirt fire roads and trail with many steps

HIKING TIME: 1 hour

DRIVING DISTANCE: 5 miles from the San Francisco Civic Center

ACCESS: Open 24/7. No fee.

WHEELCHAIR ACCESS: There is designated handicapped parking. Batteries to Bluffs Trail is not wheelchair accessible, but folks in wheelchairs can visit the Golden Gate Overlook.

MAPS: At trailhead's information signboard and tinyurl.com/presidiotrailmap. *The Walker's Map of San Francisco,* published by Pease Press, is another good option ($7.95, peasepress.com).

FACILITIES: None

CONTACT: 415-561-5300, presidio.gov/trails/batteries-to-bluffs-trail

LOCATION: Golden Gate Overlook, San Francisco, CA

COMMENTS: No dogs allowed

leads to the Pacific Overlook on Lincoln). A sign at the top of wooden steps marks the start of Batteries to Bluffs Trail.

Here you begin the descent, with the trail already showing off fantastic views south to Lands End. In autumn you may see white-crowned sparrows flitting from ceanothus to coyote brush shrubs. Poison oak is a near-constant companion along the path. In spring look for purple irises in bloom. The steps keep dropping, and the trail passes a bare, rocky hillside. At 0.2 mile note an overlook with a bench on the right—this is an excellent rest stop on the way back uphill. The trail descends again, passing through a clump of willows. At 0.4 mile turn right at the junction with Marshall Beach Trail.

The narrow path descends, then ends at one last set of stairs leading to the beach, at 0.5 mile. Here you can gaze north to the Golden Gate Bridge and the Marin Headlands. I often see brown pelicans flying in formation overhead, and on one September visit, I was delighted to watch a pod of porpoises cavorting offshore. Explore the beach, if you like; when ready, retrace your steps back to the junction with Batteries to Bluffs Trail, then turn right.

The trail crosses a year-round trickling stream. Toyon, coyote brush, and coffeeberry thrive here. Soon Batteries to Bluffs Trail begins to climb—yes, more steps! At the top, the trail heads over the top of Battery Crosby; use caution here so you don't fall down to the left. As you enjoy views south to Baker Beach, watch for lizards scampering about. A few more steps head down to join a wide dirt track that leads up to Lincoln Boulevard. You could start back toward the Golden Gate Overlook now, at 0.8 mile, but consider walking up to Lincoln and the official end of the trail. If you do, you'll likely see purple bush lupine as well as San Francisco wallflower, buckwheat, and other lovely wildflowers blooming here in spring. This is also the section of trail where I commonly spot coyote scat.

When you're ready, retrace your steps back to the trailhead.

The Presidio: Batteries to Bluffs Trail

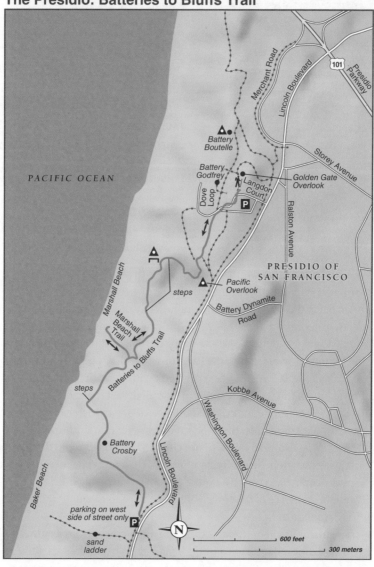

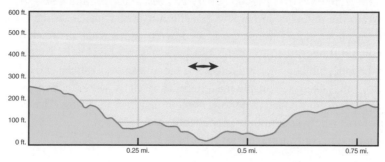

• •

GPS TRAILHEAD COORDINATES
N37° 48.207' W122° 28.609' (north parking lot)
N37° 47.805' W122° 28.766' (street-side parking on Lincoln Boulevard)

DIRECTIONS From southbound US 101 in San Francisco, just past the Golden Gate Bridge toll plaza, turn right onto Merchant Road. After about 500 feet, turn right onto Lincoln Boulevard, then almost immediately right again into the parking lot at Golden Gate Overlook, or continue to street-side parking on Lincoln near Kobbe Avenue.

From northbound 19th Avenue in San Francisco, bear left onto Crossover Drive in Golden Gate Park. Continue, now on 25th Avenue, to the junction with El Camino del Mar. Turn right. Continue, now on Lincoln, into The Presidio, to street-side parking near the junction with Kobbe Avenue, or to the parking lot on the left at Golden Gate Overlook.

An iris blooming in spring

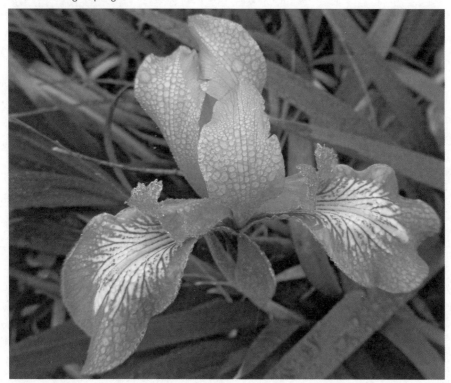

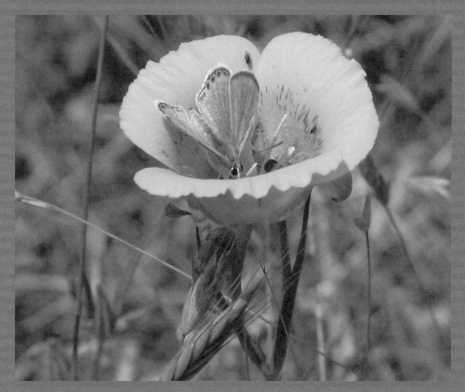

Blue butterfly on mariposa lily in Mount Burdell Open Space Preserve (Hike 5, page 35)

APPENDIXES AND INDEX

APPENDIX A:
Hiking Clubs and Information

BAY AREA HIKER bahiker.com
I created this website in 1999 to explore the diverse and wonderful spectrum of hikes in the San Francisco Bay Area. Here you'll find detailed descriptions and photos of more than 200 hikes, along with discussion forums. Bay Area Hiker is also an exceptional resource (if I do say so myself) for identifying local flora and fauna. For the companion Facebook page, go to tinyurl .com/bahiker. —J. H.

BAY AREA RIDGE TRAIL COUNCIL
ridgetrail.org
1007 General Kennedy Ave., Ste. 3
San Francisco, CA 94129; 415-561-2595

CALIFORNIA ALPINE CLUB
calalpineclub.org
P.O. Box 2180
Mill Valley, CA 94942

CALIFORNIA DEPARTMENT OF PARKS AND RECREATION parks.ca.gov
1416 Ninth St.
Sacramento, CA 95814
800-777-0369; info@parks.ca.gov

CHAOS (California Hiking and Outdoor Society) chaosberkeley.org
University of California
432 Eshleman Hall, MC 4500
Berkeley, CA 94720

CONFUSED (Commonwealth of Nature Fanatics Unofficial SF/South Bay Excursion Division) OUTDOOR CLUB
confused.org

EAST BAY REGIONAL PARK DISTRICT
ebparks.org
2950 Peralta Oaks Court
Oakland, CA 94605; 888-327-2757

FRIENDS OF MT TAM
friendsofmttam.org
P.O. Box 7064
Corte Madera, CA 94976

GREENBELT ALLIANCE greenbelt.org
312 Sutter St., Ste. 510
San Francisco, CA 94108; 415-543-6771

INTREPID NORTHERN CALIFORNIA HIKERS (INCH) rawbw.com/~svw/inch

MARIN COUNTY PARKS
marincountyparks.org
3501 Civic Center Dr., Ste. 260
San Rafael, CA 94903; 415-473-6387

MIDPENINSULA REGIONAL OPEN SPACE DISTRICT openspace.org
330 Distel Cir.
Los Altos, CA 94022; 650-691-1200

MOUNT DIABLO INTERPRETIVE ASSOCIATION mdia.org
P.O. Box 346
Walnut Creek, CA 94597; 925-927-7222

SAN MATEO COUNTY PARKS
parks.smcgov.org
455 County Center, Fourth Floor
Redwood City, CA 94063; 650-363-4020

SANTA CLARA COUNTY PARKS
sccgov.org/sites/parks
298 Garden Hill Dr.
Los Gatos, CA 95032; 408-355-2200

THE SANTA CRUZ MOUNTAINS TRAIL ASSOCIATION scmta-trails.org

SIERRA CLUB, Loma Prieta Chapter
sierraclub.org/loma-prieta
3921 E. Bayshore Road, Ste. 204
Palo Alto, CA 94303; 650-390-8411

SIERRA CLUB, San Francisco Bay Chapter
sierraclub.org/san-francisco-bay
2530 San Pablo Ave., Ste. I
Berkeley, CA 94702; 510-848-0800

TRAIL CENTER
trailcenter.org
3921 E. Bayshore Road
Palo Alto, CA 94303; 650-968-7065

ANY MOUNTAIN anymountain.net

- **Corte Madera**
  71 Tamal Vista Blvd.
  Corte Madera, CA 9492; 415-927-0170

- **Redwood City**
  928 Whipple Ave.
  Redwood City, CA 94063; 650-361-1213

PEASE PRESS

peasepress.com
1717 Cabrillo St.
San Francisco, CA 94121; 415-387-1437

REI rei.com

- **Berkeley**
  1338 San Pablo Ave.
  Berkeley, CA 94702; 510-527-4140

- **Concord**
  The Willows Shopping Center
  1975 Diamond Blvd., Ste. B-100
  Concord, CA 94520; 925-825-9400

- **Corte Madera**
  213 Corte Madera Town Center
  Corte Madera, CA 94925; 415-927-1938

- **Dublin**
  7099 Amador Plaza Road
  Dublin, CA 94568; 925-828-9826

- **Fremont**
  43962 Fremont Blvd.
  Fremont, CA 94538; 510-651-0305

- **Mountain View**
  2450 Charleston Road
  Mountain View, CA 94043; 650-969-1938

- **San Carlos**
  1119 Industrial Road, Ste. A
  San Carlos, CA 94070; 650-508-2330

- **San Francisco**
  840 Brannan St.
  San Francisco, CA 94103; 415-934-1938

- **Saratoga**
  400 El Paseo de Saratoga
  San Jose, CA 95130; 408-871-8765

- **Santa Rosa**
  2715 Santa Rosa Ave.
  Santa Rosa, CA 95407; 707-540-9025

REDWOOD HIKES

redwoodhikes.com

SONOMA OUTFITTERS

sonomaoutfitters.com
2412 Magowan Drive
Santa Rosa, CA 95405; 800-290-1920

TOM HARRISON MAPS

tomharrisonmaps.com

ANY MOUNTAIN anymountain.net
See page 289 for locations.

REI rei.com
See page 289 for locations.

SONOMA OUTFITTERS
sonomaoutfitters.com
2412 Magowan Drive
Santa Rosa, CA 95405
800-290-1920

SPORTS BASEMENT
sportsbasement.com

- **Berkeley**
  2727 Milvia St.
  Berkeley, CA 94703; 510-984-3907

- **Campbell**
  The Pruneyard Shopping Center
  1875 S. Bascom Ave., Ste. 240
  Campbell, CA 95008
  408-899-5783

- **Novato**
  100 Vintage Way
  Novato, CA, 94945; 415-493-2623

- **Redwood City**
  202 Walnut St.
  Redwood City, CA 94063; 650-421-7440

- **San Francisco–Bryant Street**
  1590 Bryant St.
  San Francisco, CA 94103
  415-575-3001

- **San Francisco–Presidio**
  610 Old Mason St.
  San Francisco, CA 94129
  415-934-2900

- **San Ramon**
  1041 Market Place
  San Ramon, CA 94583; 925-498-6130

- **Santa Rosa**
  1970 Santa Rosa Ave.
  Santa Rosa, CA, 95407; 707-921-3147

- **Sunnyvale**
  1177 Kern Ave.
  Sunnyvale, CA 94085; 408-598-4240

- **Walnut Creek**
  1881 Ygnacio Valley Road
  Walnut Creek, CA 94598; 925-941-6100

OPPOSITE: Big Basin Redwoods State Park (Hike 38, page 187)

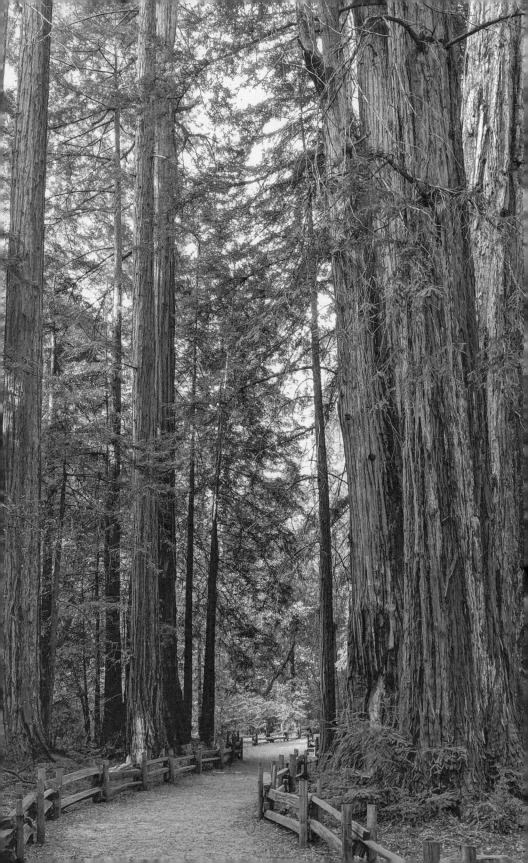

INDEX

FOLLOWING SPREAD: A bird's-eye view from San Bruno Mountain
State & County Park (Hike 48, page 231)

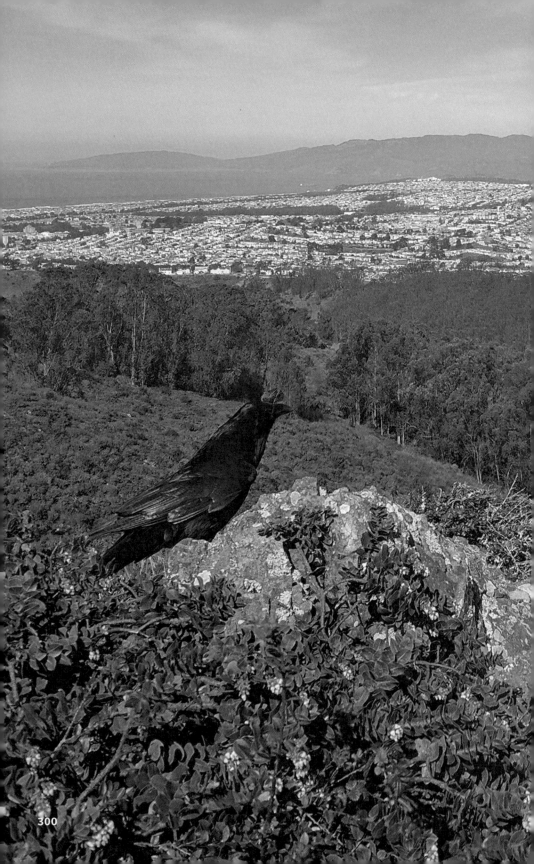

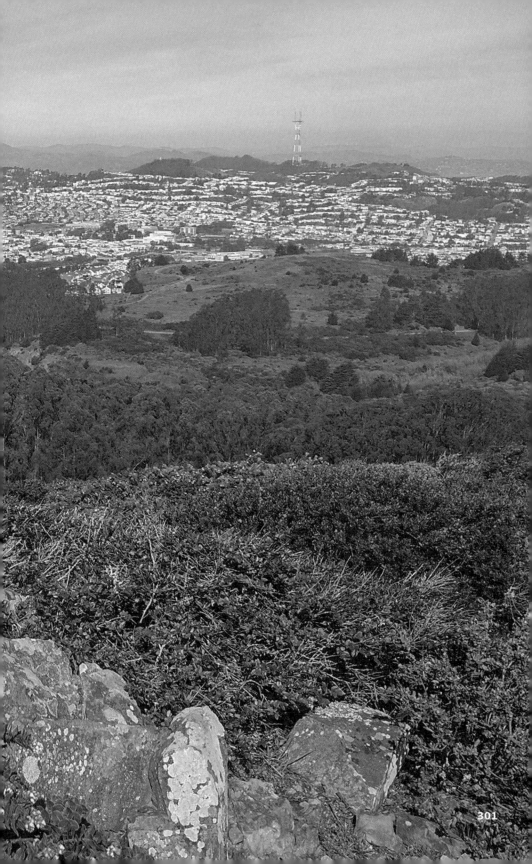

DEAR CUSTOMERS AND FRIENDS,

SUPPORTING YOUR INTEREST IN OUTDOOR ADVENTURE, travel, and an active lifestyle is central to our operations, from the authors we choose to the locations we detail to the way we design our books. Menasha Ridge Press was incorporated in 1982 by a group of veteran outdoorsmen and professional outfitters. For many years now, we've specialized in creating books that benefit the outdoors enthusiast.

Almost immediately, Menasha Ridge Press earned a reputation for revolutionizing outdoors- and travel-guidebook publishing. For such activities as canoeing, kayaking, hiking, backpacking, and mountain biking, we established new standards of quality that transformed the whole genre, resulting in outdoor-recreation guides of great sophistication and solid content. Menasha Ridge Press continues to be outdoor publishing's greatest innovator.

The folks at Menasha Ridge Press are as at home on a whitewater river or mountain trail as they are editing a manuscript. The books we build for you are the best they can be, because we're responding to your needs. Plus, we use and depend on them ourselves.

We look forward to seeing you on the river or the trail. If you'd like to contact us directly, visit us at menasharidge.com. We thank you for your interest in our books and the natural world around us all.

SAFE TRAVELS,

Bob Sehlinger

BOB SEHLINGER
PUBLISHER